Ultrasound Review of the

Abdomen, Male Pelvis, & Small Parts

Ultrasound Review of the
Abdomen, Male Pelvis, & Small Parts

Janice Hickey, RT(R), RDMS
St. Luke's Hospital
Bethlehem, Pennsylvania
Lehigh Valley Hospital
Allentown, Pennsylvania

Franklin Goldberg, MD
Assistant Professor of Radiology
Hotel Dieu Hospital
Kingston General Hospital
Queens University
Kingston, Ontario
Canada

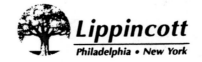
Lippincott
Philadelphia • New York

Acquisitions Editor: Lawrence McGrew
Assistant Editor: Holly Chapman
Project Editor: Sandra Cherrey Scheinin
Senior Production Manager: Helen Ewan
Production Coordinator: Patricia McCloskey
Design Coordinator: Doug Smock

Library of Congress Cataloging-in-Publication Data

Hickey, Janice.
    Ultrasound review of the abdomen, male pelvis, and small parts /
Janice Hickey, Franklin Goldberg.
        p.   cm.
    Includes bibliographical references and index.
    ISBN 0-397-51691-6 (alk. paper)
        1. Abdomen—Ultrasonic imaging—Outlines, syllabi, etc.
    2. Pelvis—Ultrasonic imaging—Outlines, syllabi, etc.
    3. Generative organs, Male—Ultrasonic imaging—Outlines, syllabi,
    etc.   I. Goldberg, Franklin.   II. Title.
        [DNLM: 1. Abdomen—ultrasonography outlines.   2. Genitalia,
    Male—ultrasonography outlines.   3. Pelvis—ultrasonography outlines.
    WI 18.2 H628u 1999]
    QM543.H53   1999
    611'.95—dc21
    DNLM/DLC
    for Library of Congress
                                                    98-15839
                                                    CIP

Care has been taken to confirm the accuracy of the information presented and to describe generally accepted
practices. However, the authors, editors, and publisher are not responsible for errors or omissions or for any
consequences from application of the information in this book and make no warranty, express or implied, with
respect to the contents of the publication.

The authors, editors, and publisher have exerted every effort to ensure that drug selection and dosage set forth
in this text are in accordance with current recommendations and practice at the time of publication. However, in
view of ongoing research, changes in government regulations, and the constant flow of information relating to drug
therapy and drug reactions, the reader is urged to check the package insert for each drug for any change in
indications and dosage and for added warnings and precautions. This is particularly important when the
recommended agent is a new or infrequently employed drug.

Some drugs and medical devices presented in this publication have Food and Drug Administration (FDA)
clearance for limited use in restricted research settings. It is the responsibility of the health care provider to
ascertain the FDA status of each drug or device planned for use in their clinical practice.

I would like to thank my husband Jim and daughters Julie and Jessica for their constant love and encouragement that gave me the motivation to complete this book. I am also blessed with a family of enthusiastic supporters for which I am forever grateful: my parents Elizabeth and William Bygrave and my siblings and their spouses William and Lorie Bygrave, Robert and Laura Bygrave, and Jennifer and Glenn Schmelzle.

JDH

For the next generation . . . Hailey, Stephanie-Rose, Justin, Hartley, and Helene.

FG

PREFACE

As we did with our first book, *Ultrasound Review of Obstetrics and Gynecology,* we have presented a vast amount of information in a format that is unique. The information in *Ultrasound Review of the Abdomen, Male Pelvis, and Small Parts* is organized in a succinct, orderly fashion, and is arranged alphabetically, in point form, with lots of images and diagrams.

The amount of "stuff" that we are required to know is daunting. With research and the constant improvement and advancement in technology, our ability to discriminate subtle and small findings increases. It almost seems that the more we see the less we know! But, common findings being common, this book is a resource for the clinical practice—offering the type of "stuff" you will see day after day at the other end of the transducer. We hope this book helps the sonographer as a student and as a professional, as well as residents and radiologists in their practice of ultrasound.

Janice Hickey, RDMS
Frank Goldberg, MD

ACKNOWLEDGMENTS

This book has been enhanced by the help and contributions of the following talented people:

- Sonographers and radiologists at Lehigh Valley Hospital, Allentown, Pennsylvania—especially Michael DeSantis, RDMS, RVT; Sherie Mohn, RDMS, RVT; Kim Goff, RDMS; Nancy Wagner, RDMS; Kristin Winterson, RDMS; Cathy-Jo Sitko, RDMS; Alan Wolson, MD; and Thomas Fitzsimons, MD
- Sonographers and radiologists at Kingston General Hospital and Hotel Dieu Hospital, Kingston, Ontario—especially Donald Soboleski, MD; Eric Sauerbrei, MD; Angie Henson, RDMS; Jan Veenstra, RDMS; Anne Joslin, RDMS; and Tina Cadieux, RDMS
- Sonographers at McMaster University Medical Center, Chedoke-McMaster Hospitals, Hamilton, Ontario—especially Ray Lappalainen, RDMS
- Kathleen Foran, RDMS, RVT, Ottawa Civic Hospital, Ottawa, Ontario
- Carol Anderson, RDMS, Hamilton, Ontario
- Janet Markotich, MD, Calgary, Alberta
- Diane Kawamura, PhD, RT(R), RDMS, Weber State University, Ogden, Utah
- JoAnn Meiers, BS, RT, RDMS and Rhonda Knighton, RDMS, RDCS, RVT, RT, Clinical Specialists at Siemens Medical Systems, Inc., Issaquah, Washington

CONTENTS

Abbreviations and Key Terms .... *xiv*

1 Adrenal Glands...1
  A Normal Anatomy and Sonographic Appearance 1
  B Vasculature 3
  C Physiology...3
  D Lab Tests 4
  E Anomalies..4
  F Technical Factors 10

2 Bile Ducts...11
  A Normal Anatomy and Sonographic Appearance 11
  B Physiology...14
  C Lab Test 14
  D Anomalies..15
  E Technical Factors 22

3 Breasts (Mammary Glands)..23
  A Normal Anatomy and Sonographic Appearance 23
  B Vasculature 26
  C Physiology...26
  D Anomalies..27
  E Technical Factors 32

4 Gallbladder 36
  A Normal Anatomy and Sonographic Appearance 36
  B Physiology...41
  C Lab Tests 41
  D Anomalies..42
  E Technical Factors 55

5 Gastrointestinal Tract 56
  A Normal Anatomy and Sonographic Appearance 56
  B Physiology...60
  C Lab Tests 61
  D Anomalies..62
  E Technical Factors 74

6 Kidneys...75
  A Normal Anatomy and Sonographic Appearance 75
  B Vasculature 79
  C Physiology...81
  D Lab Tests 82
  E Anomalies..83

7 Liver..116
  A Normal Anatomy and Sonographic Appearance 116
  B Vasculature 123
  C Physiology...127

    D Lab Tests *128*
    E Anomalies *130*
    F Technical Factors *150*

8 **Neck and Head**
    Salivary, Thyroid, and Parathyroid Glands *151*
    A Normal Anatomy and Sonographic Appearance of
        Salivary Glands *151*
    B Vasculature of Salivary Glands *152*
    C Physiology of Salivary Glands *152*
    D Anomalies of Salivary Glands *153*
    E Technical Factors for Salivary Glands *154*

    A Normal Anatomy and Sonographic Appearance of Thyroid and
        Parathyroid Glands *155*
    B Vasculature of Thyroid and Parathyroid Glands *158*
    C Physiology of Thyroid and Parathyroid Glands *159*
    D Lab Tests for Parathyroid and Thyroid Glands *160*
    E Anomalies of Parathyroid and Thyroid Glands *161*
    F Technical Factors for Thyroid and Parathyroid Glands *168*

9 **Pancreas** *169*
    A Normal Anatomy and Sonographic Appearance *169*
    B Vasculature *175*
    C Physiology *175*
    D Lab Tests *177*
    E Anomalies *178*
    F Technical Factors *184*

10 **Peritoneum and Cavity, Mesenteries, Retroperitoneum,**
    Diaphragm, and Abdominal Wall *185*
    A Normal Anatomy and Sonographic Appearance *185*
    B Anomalies *194*
    C Technical Factors *206*

11 **Prostate and Seminal Vesicles** *207*
    A Anatomy and Sonographic Appearance of Prostate Gland and
        Seminal Vesicles *207*
    B Physiology of Prostate Gland *212*
    C Lab tests *213*
    D Anomalies *214*
    E Technical Factors *218*

12 **Scrotum and Testes** *219*
    A Normal Anatomy and Sonographic Appearance *219*
    B Vasculature *223*
    C Physiology *224*
    D Lab Tests *224*
    E Anomalies *225*
    F Technical Factors *238*

13 **Spleen and Lymphatic System** *239*
    A Normal Anatomy and Sonographic Appearance *239*
    B Vasculature *242*
    C Physiology *242*
    D Lab and Other Tests *243*
    E Anomalies *245*
    F Technical Factors *252*

14   Urinary Bladder and Ureters..*253*
    A Normal Anatomy and Sonographic Appearance *253*
    B Physiology..*256*
    C Anomalies...*257*
    D Technical Factors...*265*

15   Vasculature System *267*
    A Normal Anatomy and Sonographic Appearance *267*
    B Physiology..*276*
    C Anomalies...*282*
    D Technical Factors...*297*

Bibliography *310*

Index...*311*

AA	abdominal aorta; aortic arch
AAA	abdominal aortic aneurysm
AAo	ascending aorta
ABC	acalculous biliary colic
ABE	acute bacterial endocarditis
AC	acute cholecystitis
Acid phos	acid phosphatase
ACKD	acquired cystic kidney disease
ACP	acid phosphatase
ACT	acute tubular necrosis; anticoagulant therapy
ACTH	adrenocorticotrophic hormone
AD	autosomal dominant
ADCH	adrenocorticotrophic hormone
Adeno Ca	adenocarcinoma
ADH	antidiuretic hormone
ADPD	adult dominant polycystic disease
AFP	α-fetoprotein
AFS	anterior fibromuscular stroma
AIDS	acquired immunodeficiency syndrome
AKA	also known as
Alk Phos	alkaline phosphatase
ALL	acute lymphocytic leukemia
ALT	alanine aminotransferase; alanine transaminase (SGPT)
ALP	alkaline phosphatase
ALS	amyotrophic lateral sclerosis
ant.	anterior
Ao	aorta
AP	anterioposterior
APKD	adult polycystic kidney disease
ARF	acute renal failure
ARPD	autosomal recessive polycystic disease
AST	aspartate aminotransferase; aspartate transaminase (SGOT)
ATN	acute tubular necrosis
AV	arteriovenous
b-HCG	β-human chorionic gonadotrophin
BCS	Budd-Chiari syndrome
BPH	benign prostatic hypertrophy
BR	bilirubin
BSO	bilateral salpingo-oophorectomy
BTx	blood transfusion
BUN	blood urea nitrogen
Bx	biopsy
Ca	cancer; carcinoma
CA	celiac axis
CAB(G)	coronary artery bypass (graft)
CAD	coronary artery disease
CAH	chronic active hepatitis; congenital adrenal hyperplasia
CAPD	continuous ambulatory peritoneal dialysis
CAT	computer assisted (axial) tomography
CAVG	coronary artery vein graft
CBC	complete blood count
CBD	common bile duct
CC	Crohn's colitis
CCA	common carotid artery
CC(H)F	congestive cardiac (heart) failure
CCK	cholecystokinin
CD	Crohn's disease
CD	color Doppler; common duct; Crohn's disease
CDE	color Doppler energy imaging
CDH	congenital dislocation of the hip
CDI	color Doppler imaging
CF	cystic fibrosis

CFI	color flow imaging
CHA	common hepatic artery
CHD	common hepatic duct; congenital heart disease; coronary heart disease
CHF	congestive heart failure
chemo.	chemotherapy
CIS	carcinoma in situ
CIV	common iliac vein
CMJ	corticomedullary differentiation
CML	chronic myelocytic leukemia
CMV	cytomegalovirus
CNS	central nervous system
cor.	coronal
CP	chest pain
CPH	chronic persistent hepatitis
CR	creatinine
CRF	chronic renal failure; corticotropin-releasing factor
CSF	cerebrospinal fluid
CT	computed tomography
CW	continuous wave
CXR	chest x-ray
CZ	central zone
DCI	Doppler color imaging
DD(x.)	differential diagnosis
DIC	disseminated intravascular coagulation
DM	diabetes mellitus
DRE	direct rectal exam
DST	dexamethasone suppression test
DVT	deep vein thrombosis
ECA	external carotid artery
EC(K)G	electrocardiogram
EJV	external jugular vein
ERCP	endoscopic retrograde cholangiopancreatography
ESR	erythrocyte sedimentation rate
ETOH	ethanol-ethyl alcohol
EVS	endovaginal sonography
FAS	fetal alcohol syndrome
FBS(G)	fasting blood sugar (glucose)
FMD	fibromuscular dysplasia
FN	false negative
FNA	fine needle aspiration
FNAB	fine needle aspiration biopsy
FNH	focal nodular hyperplasia
FP	false positive
FYI	for your information
GB	gallbladder
GDA	gastroduodenal artery
GE	gastroenteritis; gastroesophageal
GET	gastric emptying time
GFR	glomerular filtration rate
GH	growth hormone
GHRH	growth hormone-releasing hormone
GI	gastrointestinal
Glu.	glucose
Gn-RH	gonadotropin-releasing factor
GPT	glutamate pyruvate transaminase
GTT	glucose tolerance test
GU	genitourinary; gastric ulcer
HBsAg	hepatitis B surface antigen
HBV	hepatitis B virus
HCC	hepatocellular disease
Hct	hematocrit
HD	hemodialysis; Huntingdon's disease; Hodgkin's disease
HDL	high-density lipoprotein

Hep A/B/C	hepatitis A,B,C,	PCKD	polycystic kidney disease
Hgb; Hb.	hemoglobin	PD	peritoneal dialysis; pancreatic duct
HGH	human growth hormone	PDS	penile Doppler studies
HIDA	hepatoiminodiacetic acid (lidofenin)	PE	pulmonary embolism; pulmonary effusion
HIV	human immunodeficiency virus	PHA	proper hepatic artery
HLTx	heart-lung transplant	PI	pulsitivity index
H/O; Ho	history of	PID	pelvic inflammatory disease
HPD	home peritoneal dialysis	Plts	platelets
HPS	hypertrophic pyloric stenosis	PMN	polymorphonuclear
HPV	hepatic portal vein	post.	posterior
HRT	hormone replacement therapy	PP	postprandial
HVT	hepatic vein thrombosis	PRF	pulse repetition frequency
IBD	inflammatory bowel disease	PSA	prostate specific antigen
IBS	irritable bowel syndrome	PSAD	prostate specific antigen density
ICA	internal carotid artery	PT	prothrombin time; parathyroids
IDS	insulin-dependent diabetes mellitus	PTA	percutaneous transluminal angioplasty
IgA	immunoglobulin A	PTBD	percutaneous transhepatic biliary drainage
IJV	internal jugular vein	PTH	parathyroid hormone
IMA	inferior mesenteric artery	PTT	partial prothrombin time
IMV	internal mesenteric vein	PTV	posterior tibial vein
inf.	inferior	PUD	peptic ulcer disease
IOUS	intraoperative ultrasound	PUJ(O)	pelvic-ureteric junction (obstruction)
IPKD	infantile polycystic kidney disease	PUO	pyrexia (fever) of unknown origin
IUD	intrauterine device	PUV	posterior urethral valves
IV	intravenous	PV	portal vein
IVC	inferior vena cava	PVD	peripheral vascular disease
IVP	intravenous pyelography	PZ	peripheral zone
JV	jugular vein	RAIU	radioactive iodine uptake
KTx	kidney transplant	RAO	right anterior oblique
KUB	kidney ureter bladder	RAR	renal artery-to-aortic ratio
Lap.	laparoscopic	RAS	renal artery stenosis
LCCA	left common carotid artery	RBC	red blood cell (count)
LDH	lactic acid dehydrogenase	RCCA	right common carotid artery
LFT	liver function test	RF	renal failure
LHD	left hepatic duct	RHD	right hepatic duct
LHV	left hepatic vein	RHL	right hepatic lobe
LLL	left lobe liver	RHV	right hepatic vein
LLQ	left lower quadrant	RI	resistive index
long.	longitudinal section	RLL	right lobe of liver
LP	lumbar puncture	RLQ	right lower quadrant
LPO	left posterior oblique	RPV	right portal vein
LPV	left portal vein	RUQ	right upper quadrant
LUQ	left upper quadrant	RVT	renal vein thrombosis
LV	ligamentum venosum	SALP; SAP	serum alkaline phosphatase
MCDK	multicystic dysplastic kidney	SBE	subacute bacterial endocarditis
MCK	multicystic kidney	SBO	small bowel obstruction
MCL	midclavicular line	SCM	sternocleidomastoid (muscle)
Mets	metastases	SFA (V)	superficial femoral artery (vein)
MHV	middle hepatic vein	SGOT	serum glutamic oxaloacetic transaminase
mHz	megahertz	SGPT	serum glutamic pyruvic transaminase
MM	malignant melanoma	SLE	systemic lupus erythematosus
MPV	main portal vein	SLR	splenorenal ligament
MRA	magnetic resonance angiography	SMA	superior mesenteric artery
MRI	magnetic resonance imaging	SMV	superior mesenteric vein
MRM	magnetic resonance mammography	SOB	shortness of breath
MTC	medullary thyroid carcinoma	SS	signs and symptoms
NAD	no active disease; no abnormalities demonstrated; nothing abnormal detected	sup.	superior
		SVBG	saphenous vein bypass graft
NIDDM	non–insulin-dependent diabetic	SVC	superior vena cava
NMR	nuclear magnetic resonance	TB	tuberculosis
NPO	nil per oram (nothing by mouth)	TBG	thyroid-binding globulin
NVB	neurovascular bundles	TCC	transitional cell carcinoma
OD	overdose	TCD	transcranial Doppler sonography
PBS	peripheral blood smear	TE	tracheoesophageal (fistula)
PC	portalcaval; presenting complaint	TGC	time-gain compensation (curve)

ABBREVIATIONS AND KEY TERMS (*Continued*)

TIA	transient ischemic attack	TZ	transitional zone
TIPS	transjugular intrahepatic portosystemic shunts	UC	ulcerative colitis
TNM	tumor-nodes-metastases	UGI	upper gastrointestinal
TPN	total parenteral nutrition	ULQ	upper left quadrant
TR	transverse; transrectal	UPJ	ureteropelvic junction
TRH	thyroid-releasing hormone	US	ultrasound
TRS	transvaginal sonography	UT (I)	urinary tract (infection)
TRUS	transrectal ultrasound	UVJ	ureterovesical junction
TRUSP	transrectal ultrasound of the prostate	VMA	vanillylmandelic acid
TSC	technetium sulfur colloid	WBC	white blood count
TSH	thyroid-stimulating hormone	WC	white count
TURP	transurethral resection of the prostate	WES sign	wall-echo-shadow sign
Tx.	transplant; treatment; therapy		

TERMS

A) POSITION

TERM	DEFINITION	EXAMPLE
INFRA	something is <u>below</u> the thing that is identified by "infra"	subclavian artery can be palpated infraclavicular
SUPRA	something is <u>above</u>	adrenal glands are suprarenal
INTRA	within	cerebrum is intracranial
INTER	between	interventricular septum lies between the cardiac ventricles
ANTE	comes <u>before</u> something else	fetal testing is antepartum
POST	comes <u>after</u> something else	postpartum is after the delivery
SUB	below something	subclavian artery is below clavicle
PERI	surrounding, adjacent	perigastric is adjacent to or surrounding the stomach

B) POSITION

TERM	DEFINITION	EXAMPLE
CRANIAL or CRANIAD, SUPERIOR, CEPHALAD	toward head	thorax is superior to abdomen neck is cranial to thorax blood flow in IVC moves cephalad
CAUDAL or CAUDAD, INFERIOR	toward feet	calf is inferior to thigh blood flow in descending aorta moves caudad
MEDIAL	toward midline	IVC is medial to kidney
LATERAL	away from midline	right lobe of liver is lateral to left lobe of liver
ANTERIOR VENTRAL	front half of body	pancreas is anterior to splenic vein
POSTERIOR DORSAL	back half of body or opposite of anterior	psoas muscle is posterior to kidneys
IPSILATERAL	same side as	right arm is ipsilateral to right leg
CONTRALATERAL	opposite side as	left arm is contralateral to right arm

CHAPTER 1 - ADRENAL GLANDS
A) NORMAL ANATOMY AND SONOGRAPHIC APPEARANCE

DEFINITION	• paired structures also known as suprarenal glands

STRUCTURE	
• covered by a fibrous capsule • each adrenal is comprised of two distinct structural and functional glands: **1. CORTEX** • outer aspect of gland • secretes steroids **2. MEDULLA** • central 20% of gland • functionally related to sympathetic nervous system • secretes catecholamines	

SHAPE	• both are basically triangular in shape Right: pyramidal shaped Left: semilunar or crescent shaped and usually larger and more superior than right

SIZE	INFANTS	ADULTS
	• proportionately larger at birth • 1/13 size of kidney	• 1/13 size of kidney Length: 0.8–1 cm Width: 2–4 cm Thickness: 3–6 mm

LOCATION	• superior and anteromedial aspects of each kidney • retroperitoneal • within renal fascia connected to Gerota's fascia	

REGIONAL ANATOMY		
	RIGHT ADRENAL • more superior to kidney	**LEFT ADRENAL** • more superomedial to kidney
ANTERIOR	• IVC • right lobe of liver	• cardia of stomach • lesser sac peritoneum • tail of pancreas • splenic vein
POSTERIOR	• right crus of diaphragm • superior pole of right kidney	• upper pole of left kidney
MEDIAL	• right crus of diaphragm	• aorta • left crus of diaphragm
SUPERIOR	• liver	• spleen
INFERIOR	• upper pole of right kidney	• upper pole of left kidney

SONOGRAPHIC APPEARANCE

- mainly hypoechoic structures surrounded by echogenic retroperitoneal fat
- crescent-shaped structure anterior to diaphragmatic crus

1. Medulla
- echogenic central linear structure within adrenal gland

2. Cortex
- hypoechoic outer region surrounding echogenic medulla
- isoechoic to normal liver/spleen

VISUALIZATION DEPENDS ON:
- age of patient
- size of patient
- amount of perirenal fat surrounding gland
- presence of bowel gas
- ability to change patient's position

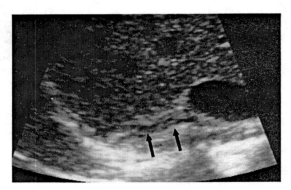

Adult

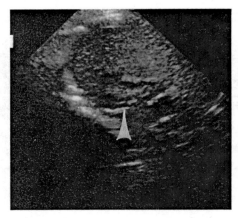

Neonate

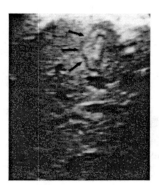

Fetal

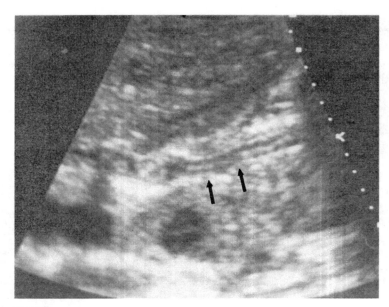

Neonate

B) VASCULATURE

ARTERIAL SUPPLY	VENOUS RETURN
• supplied by many small arteries	• drained usually by one vein
phrenic artery →→ superior suprarenal arteries (1) aorta →→ mid suprarenal arteries (3) (2) renal artery →→ inferior suprarenal arteries (4)	(5) right suprarenal vein →→ IVC (7) (6) left suprarenal vein →→ left renal vein (8)

C) PHYSIOLOGY

PHYSIOLOGY
• stimulated by anterior pituitary
• each gland consists of 2 layers that function as separate endocrine glands

	CORTEX—outer layer "Salt, Sugar and Sex"	MEDULLA—inner layer "Fight or Flight" Reaction
STRUCTURE AND FUNCTION	• derived from mesoderm • differentiated into 3 zones that each secrete a specific hormone • these hormones are essential for life	• derived from ectoderm • functionally related to sympathetic nervous system • consists of cords of secretory and nerve cells, and its secretions are involved in the regulation of acute responses of the body to environmental stimuli and help body resist stress • medullary hormones are <u>not</u> essential for life
OPERATION	• Divided into 3 layers or zones that each secrete a different steroid 1. Zona glomerulosa—outermost zone "salt" secretes: • **mineralocorticoids** primarily aldosterone and deoxycorticosterone affects fluid/electrolyte balance, particularly sodium and potassium 2. Zona fasciculata—middle zone "Sugar" secretes: • **glucocorticoids** primarily cortisol and corticosterone promotes normal protein, fat, and carbohydrate metabolism secretion stimulated by ACTH (adrenocorticotropic hormones) from the anterior pituitary 3. <u>Zona reticularis</u>—inner zone "Sex" secretes: • **gonadocorticoids and small amounts of sex hormones** promote normal development of the bones and reproductive organs	• two principal hormones synthesized are: • **epinephrine (adrenaline)** dilates coronary vessels, constricts skin and kidney vessels • **norepinephrine (noradrenaline)** constricts all arterial vessels except coronary arteries, which dilate essential regulator of blood pressure • stimulate the metabolic rate and the breakdown of starch (glycogen) and lipids (fatty acids) resulting in more available energy • causes increased nervous system activity: dilated pupils increased blood supply to critical areas increased pulse increased respiration rate

D) LAB TESTS

TESTS	ELEVATED	DECREASED
ADRENOCORTICOTROPIC HORMONE (ACTH) • hormone released by anterior pituitary • stimulates adrenal cortex to secrete cortisol, androgens, and aldosterone	primary adrenal hypofunction (Addison's disease) Cushing's disease	
ALDOSTERONE • mineralocorticoid secreted by adrenal cortex • helps to maintain blood pressure and volume • higher levels will increase serum sodium and decrease serum potassium • lower levels will lead to higher serum potassium and lower serum sodium	adrenocortical hyperplasia adenoma adrenal carcinoma	Addison's disease
CORTISOL • could be measured by blood samples or urine • glucocorticoid secreted by the adrenal cortex • helps metabolize nutrients, mediate stress, and regulate the immune system	adrenal hyperfunction (Cushing's disease) hyperthyroidism stress some types of obesity	adrenal hypofunction (Addison's disease) hypothyroidism liver disease
DEXAMETHASONE SUPPRESSION TEST (DST) AKA ADRENOCORTICOTROPIC HORMONE (ACTH) • ACTH is produced by anterior pituitary gland and stimulates the secretion of cortisol and other glucocorticoids • dexamethasone suppresses normal pituitary release of ACTH and therefore will decrease the production of cortisol • test performed when there is evidence of glucocorticoid excess • test used to distinguish the etiology and origin of the excess steroid production (adrenal cortex pathology versus hypopituitarism)		
CATECHOLAMINES • catecholamines are hormones (epinephrine and norepinephrine) secreted by the adrenal medulla • urine catecholamine test is considered more reliable than a serum test • vanillylmandelic acid (VMA) is a product of catecholamine breakdown and a VMA test for screening can be ordered because it is easy to perform	strenuous exercise malignant neuroblastoma $100 \times$ normal = pheochromocytoma	

E) ANOMALIES

ADRENAL MASSES—where they arise from:	
CORTEX	**MEDULLA**
adenomas carcinomas hyperplasia	ganglioneuroma neuroblastoma pheochromocytoma
CONNECTIVE TISSUE	**METASTASES (Most Commonly Arise From)**
lipoma fibroma cysts	breast lung ovary melanoma GI and urinary tracts

DISPLACEMENT OF REGIONAL ANATOMY BY ADRENAL MASSES		
DISPLACED DIRECTION	**RIGHT ADRENAL**	**LEFT ADRENAL**
ANTERIOR	retroperitoneal fat line IVC right renal vein	splenic vein
POSTERIOR	right kidney	left kidney

ANOMALY SS = signs and symptoms	US DESCRIPTION US = ultrasound
ADENOMA • primary nonfunctioning tumor arising from cortex • can result in endocrine abnormalities as small percentage are hyperfunctioning (Cushing's) • usually an incidental finding SS • usually asymptomatic	• variable size, but usually <3 cm • nodular in appearance • solid, hypoechoic lesion • may be bilateral and multiple • can have calcifications
CARCINOMA • rare, aggressive, and highly malignant primary tumor of cortex • 50% may function and produce steroids and simulated any hyperfunction adrenal syndrome such as Cushing's • may extend through the adrenal veins into the IVC • metastases to lymph glands SS • in women with functioning tumor may produce virilism symptoms • clinical symptoms as seen in Cushing's disease	• thrombus may be seen in the adrenal vein and IVC • enlarged lymph nodes • size can range from 3 cm to larger than 20 cm • well defined homogenous mass when tumor is 2–6 cm • calcifications and a more heterogeneous appearance due to necrosis and hemorrhage when larger
CYST • rarely seen sonographically • usually asymptomatic, unilateral • include pseudocysts, hemorrhagic, epithelial, cystic degeneration of adenoma, parasitic, lymphangiomatous • occur more frequently in women SS • asymptomatic • patient may be hypertensive	• anechoic with increased through transmission and posterior enhancement • well defined walls • can be small to large, uni- or multiloculated • can have scattered internal echos (secondary to hemorrhage) • posterior displacement of superior pole of kidney
HEMORRHAGE • more common in children and neonates due to very vascular adrenals, which are highly susceptible to trauma • difficult delivery can cause hemorrhage • hemorrhage can also occur with infection most commonly with a meningococcemia infection (known as Waterhouse-Friderichsen syndrome) • this can induce acute adrenal cortical insufficiency SS <u>Neonates:</u> • long labor, <32 week gestation, ↓ hematocrit, palpable flank mass, jaundice, ↑ bilirubin <u>Adult:</u> • signs of acute adrenal insufficiency, which can be life threatening	• cystic to complex mass anterosuperior to kidney • neonatal hemorrhage is usually bilateral • initially echogenic region in adrenal that becomes over time more hypoechoic to anechoic and smaller

ANOMALY	US DESCRIPTION

HYPERFUNCTION OF CORTEX (HYPERADRENALISM)
• oversecretion of adrenal cortex
• caused by:
  anterior pituitary tumor secreting excess ACTH, which causes hyperplasia
  cortisol-secreting adrenal tumor (adenoma, carcinoma, or a pituitary adenoma)
  nonendocrine neoplasm, which secretes ACTH (usually a lung cancer)
  iatrogenic cause from prolonged administration of steroids
3 types:
 	
1. ADRENOGENITAL SYNDROMES
• excess of androgens causes disorders of sexual differentiation
 	
SS
• variety of forms including, hermaphroditism, virilization in female, precocity in male
 	
2. CUSHING'S SYNDROME/HYPERCORTISOLISM
• symptom complex produced by an excess of adrenal corticosteroids
• usually caused by:
  pituitary overproduction of ACTH leading to bilateral hyperplasia
  adrenal adenoma or carcinoma
  excess production of ACTH from a nonpituitary source
  iatrogenic ingestion of excess corticosteroids
 	
SS
• redistribution of fat resulting in truncal obesity, "moon face," and fat deposit on upper back area (buffalo hump)
• flushed facial skin, muscle wasting, diabetes, hirsutism, hypertension, osteoporosis neuropsychiatric abnormalities
 	
3. HYPERALDOSTERONISM (CONN'S SYNDROME)
• aldosterone promotes potassium secretion and sodium retention
• increased levels cause hypokalemia (low potassium levels in blood), hypernatremia (high sodium levels in blood), and hypertension
• in 90% of cases the excess aldosterone is from an adrenal adenoma
• remaining cases are due to primary bilateral adrenal hyperplasia or rarely adrenal carcinoma
 	
SS
• hypokalemia (from renal potassium wasting), which causes weakness, paresthesias, visual problems
• ↑ serum sodium level
	• depending on the etiology there could be an adrenal adenoma, bilateral adrenal enlargement, or adrenal mass

HYPOFUNCTION OF CORTEX (HYPOADRENALISM)
• atrophy of cortex leads to diminished secretion of mineralocorticoids, glucocorticoids, androgens
 	
1. PRIMARY ADRENAL INSUFFICIENCY
• impairs output of cortical steroids
• due to anatomic or metabolic lesion of the cortex
i) Acute: adrenal crisis
  caused by too rapid withdrawal of steroids, massive destruction of adrenals (e.g., hemorrhage), stress that causes the gland to not respond correctly
 	
ii) Chronic: Addison's disease
  failure of adrenals to produce sufficient amounts of adrenal corticosteroids caused by:
    autoimmune destruction (80% of cases)
    adrenal destruction by tuberculosis (20% of cases)
    other more rare causes include: hemorrhage, infarction, tumor, other infections, radiation, drugs, amyloidosis, sarcoidosis, congenital abnormalities, removal of adrenal gland
 	
SS
• can be asymptomatic until most of gland is destroyed
• weakness, fatigue, nausea, vomiting, anorexia, weight loss, hypotension, hyperpigmentation of the skin
 	
2. SECONDARY ADRENAL INSUFFICIENCY
• any disorder of the hypothalamus or pituitary that reduces the amount of ACTH leading to underproduction of glucocorticoids
• causes include, carcinoma, infection, infarction
	• due to the small size of the adrenal glands in Addison's disease it is usually not detected by ultrasound
	• if the Addison's is secondary to infection or tumor mass, those lesions may be detected

ANOMALY	US APPEARANCE
MEDULLA TUMORS 1. GANGLIONEUROMA • rare benign tumor • most commonly occurs in patients younger than 20 SS • asymptomatic, hypertension 2. NEUROBLASTOMA • highly malignant pediatric tumor of adrenal medulla with poor prognosis • almost always found in children under age 8 • >1 year of age has greater chance of malignancy and often present with metastatic spread • 30% survive 5 years when discovered in 1st year of life, although spontaneous regression does occur, especially in very young infants • metastatic sites usually found in liver and bone although nearly every organ can be affected SS • asymptomatic or • anemia, failure to thrive, fever 3. PHEOCROMOCYTOMA • originates from adrenal medulla • causes hypersecretion of medullary hormones • increases production of catecholamines usually norepinephrine and epinephrine • known as the "10% tumor": 10% are malignant, 10% bilateral, and 10% occur outside adrenal glands • can be familial SS • asymptomatic or • related to secretion of the hormones adrenaline and norepinephrine • palpitations, pounding headaches, sweating, nausea • causes hypertension	1. GANGLIONEUROMA • discrete mass with partial capsule • may contain calcifications 2. NEUROBLASTOMA • bizarre presentations • heterogeneous, irregular solid mass mixed with hypoechoic areas • echogenic mass that may be quite large • calcifications are common • displaces kidney rather than distorting it • displaces aorta, IVC • retroperitoneal metastatic involvement • spread to liver Diff. Dx.: • Wilms' tumor 3. PHEOCHROMOCYTOMA • >2 cm, usually large (5–6 cm) • primarily solid hypoechoic lesions with low-level echos • can have a variety of appearances including cystic, solid, and calcified components • well encapsulated, sharply marginated • can occur extra-adrenally • can be bilateral, usually unilateral
METASTASES • can be found incidentally • 4th most common metastatic site • lung, breast, stomach, melanoma, and renal cell carcinomas are common primaries • 25% of non-Hodgkin's lymphoma has adrenal involvement	• usually bilateral • variable size and echogenicity • hypoechoic to hyperechoic solid mass in adrenal area • nonspecific sonographic appearance

ULTRASOUND SCANS

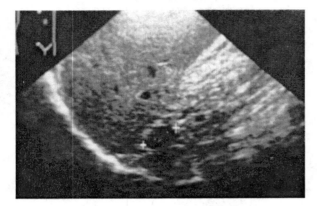

Adenoma: between calipers on sagittal scan plane

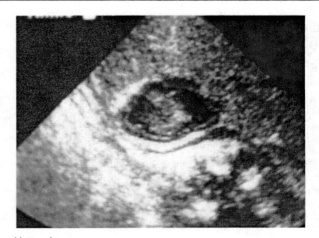

Hemorrhage

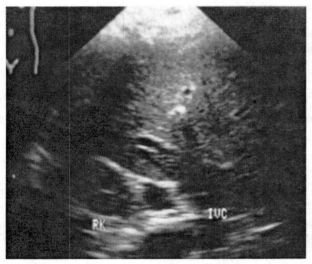

Adrenal enlargement: between right kidney (RK) and IVC in transverse scan plane

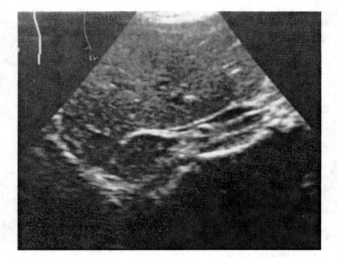

Metastasis from a lung primary: sagittal scan plane, displacing IVC

ULTRASOUND SCANS

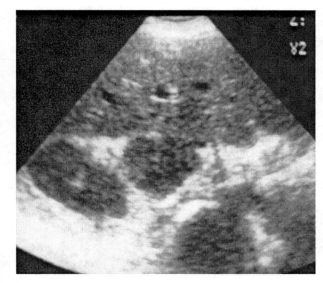

Carcinoma: transverse scan plane

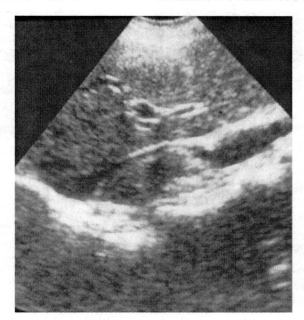

Carcinoma: sagittal scan plane displacing IVC anteriorly

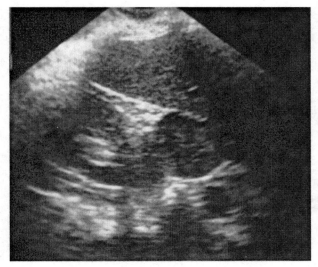

Neuroblastoma

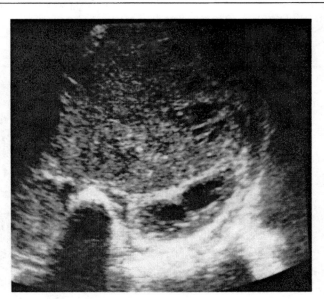

Neuroblastoma

9

F) TECHNICAL FACTORS

- transverse and longitudinal planes in both supine and decubitus positions can be used
- success of visualization of normal adrenal depends on examiner skill, persistence, and knowledge of surrounding anatomy and landmarks, patient size, amount of perirenal fat and bowel gas
- sometimes even with optimum conditions the adrenal gland cannot be visualized

	RIGHT ADRENAL GLAND	LEFT ADRENAL GLAND
PATIENT POSITION	• supine, left posterior oblique, left lateral	• right posterior oblique, right lateral
SCAN PLANE	• coronal scan plane using liver as acoustic window	• coronal scan plane using spleen as acoustic window
TECHNIQUE	• localize superior aspect of right kidney and IVC • angle posterior from IVC should be localized medial and anterior to the upper pole of the right kidney • concentrate on the lateral posterior border of the IVC • the resulting longitudinal section should show the right adrenal behind the IVC, anterior to right crus	• localize superior aspect of the left kidney and aorta • search area between left diaphragmatic crus, aorta, and left kidney • adrenal lies medial to the upper pole and lateral to the aorta, posterior to the tail of the pancreas between • the resulting longitudinal section should show the left adrenal between the spleen and upper pole of left kidney anterior to the aorta
VASCULAR LANDMARKS	IVC	aorta

LOCATING THE ADRENAL GLAND—common approaches

1. Right Lateral Approach	2. Right Anterior Approach	3. Left Posterior Approach
LIVER ↓ UPPER POLE RIGHT KIDNEY ↓ RIGHT ADRENAL	LIVER ↓ IVC (Right renal artery can also be seen) ↓ RIGHT ADRENAL ↓ RIGHT CRUS	SPLEEN ↓ LEFT KIDNEY ↓ RIGHT ADRENAL ↓ AORTA

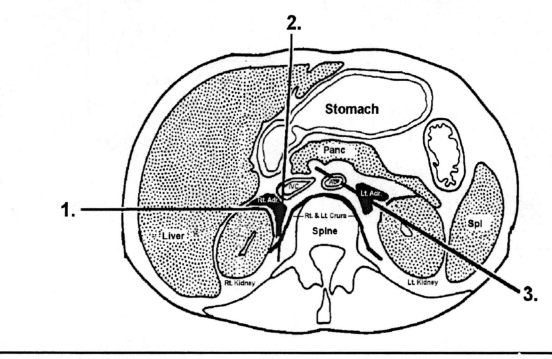

CHAPTER 2 - BILE DUCTS

A) NORMAL ANATOMY AND SONOGRAPHIC APPEARANCE

DEFINITION	• system of tubules or ducts that carry bile from the liver to the gallbladder (GB) and the duodenum

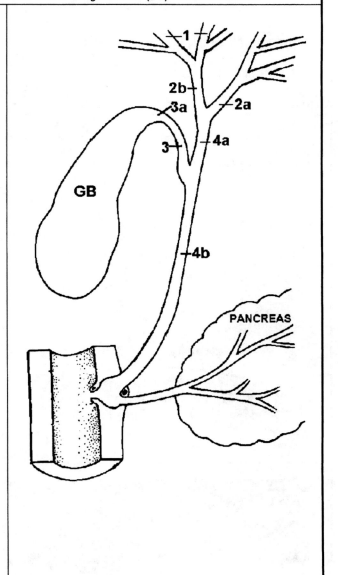

STRUCTURE

1. INTRAHEPATIC BILE DUCTS
• in liver they follow the same course as portal veins and hepatic arteries
• encased in common sheath to form portal triad, which consists of a:
  1. portal vein branch
  2. hepatic artery branch
  3. intrahepatic bile duct

2. HEPATIC DUCTS
a) Left hepatic duct (LHD)
b) Right hepatic duct (RHD)
  • emerge from liver in porta hepatis where they meet to form the hepatic duct
  • travel anterior to left and right portal veins

3. CYSTIC DUCT
• connects GB with hepatic duct to form the common bile duct (CBD)
• not normally seen sonographically
a) Spiral valve
  • tortuous portion of cystic duct

4. COMMON DUCT
• in ultrasound there is no differentiation between common hepatic and common bile ducts and both are referred to as the CBD sonographically
a) Common hepatic duct (CHD)
  • superior (proximal) portion of common duct
  • travels caudad and medial in porta hepatis
  • from the junction of the right and left hepatic duct to the point of insertion of the cystic duct
b) Common bile duct (CBD)
  • mainly composed of elastic and fibrous tissue that is capable of expanding and retracting
Path:
1st part of CBD
  • runs downward in the right free margin of the lesser omentum (hepatoduodenal ligament)
  • hepatic artery is left of CBD
  • portal vein is posterior to CBD
2nd part of CBD
  • passes behind 1st part duodenum to enter the posterior pancreatic head
3rd part of CBD
  • lies in a groove on the posterior surface of the pancreas or through the pancreatic head
  • exits pancreas when it enters the posteromedial wall of the 2nd part of the duodenum where it usually joins the main pancreatic duct at the hepatopancreatic ampulla (ampulla of Vater)

COMMON BILE DUCT SIZE

ADULT FASTING	4–6 mm • there is a normal taper in the distal portion of the CBD Helpful Hint: • If you can visualize the indentation of the right hepatic artery into the CBD, this is a good indicator that the CBD is not obstructed and is of normal size
GERIATRIC PATIENT	• Add 1 mm to normal size for every decade after 50 years • becomes increasingly ectatic
POSTCHOLECYSTECTOMY	7–10 mm • dimensions are slightly greater than before surgery
AFTER FATTY MEAL	• normally contracts and decreases in diameter

WHERE TO MEASURE?
• proper measurement of all ducts is from the inner wall to the inner wall
• measure in its long axis in a plane perpendicular to its course
• ideally measure at the point where it crosses the right hepatic artery, parallel to the right portal vein

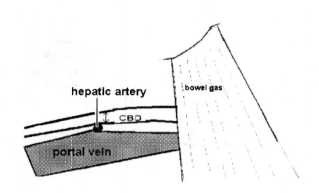

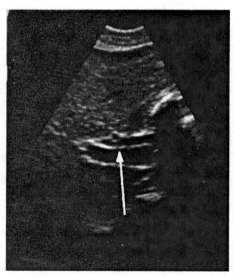

CBD (arrow)

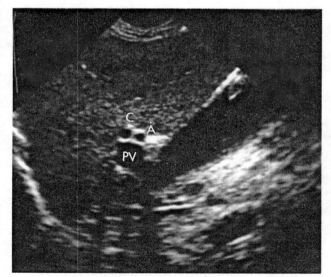

"Mickey Mouse" appearance: cross-section scan of 3 anechoic structures: CBD (C), hepatic artery (A), and portal vein (PV)

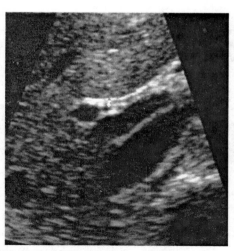

Nonfasting CBD: measures at just over 1 mm

VARIATIONS IN LOCATION OF HEPATIC ARTERY

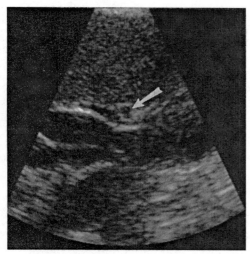

Right hepatic artery (arrow), can cross above CBD in about 1/3 of the population

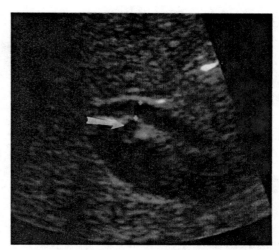

Right hepatic artery (arrow) is more commonly located between CBD and portal vein (2/3 of people)

NORMAL SONOGRAPHIC APPEARANCES: IS IT A VEIN OR A DUCT?

Helpful Hint:
Color and pulsed Doppler are the best way to distinguish veins from ducts. If these features are not available, the following can be useful to help determine the difference:
• to help differentiate veins and enlarged ducts, follow biliary ducts into CBD and track main portal vein into its intrahepatic branches

Ducts do....	Ducts do not....
• acoustically enhance • run anterior to portal veins • branch repeatedly	• dilate with Valsalva maneuver (as will venous structures)
NORMAL BILIARY TREE	**DILATED BILIARY TREE**
• smooth, symmetrical walls • intrahepatic biliary ducts not visualized normally • right and left hepatic ducts may be demonstrated as tubular structures running parallel to the left and right portal veins, respectively	• appear as several tributaries converging centrally giving a characteristic stellate pattern of tubes near porta hepatis • double barrel or parallel channel appearance, which gives the appearance of too many tubes • the minor intrahepatic ducts that are deep within the liver are not normally seen, even with dilatation

SONOGRAPHIC APPEARANCE OF DILATED BILIARY SYSTEM

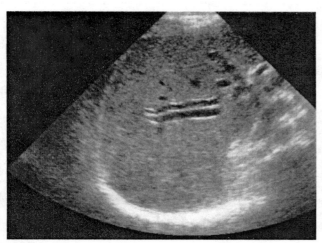

Right lobe liver

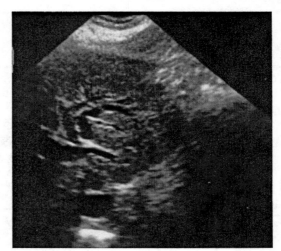

Left lobe liver

(*continued*)

SONOGRAPHIC APPEARANCE OF DILATED BILIARY SYSTEM (*Continued*)

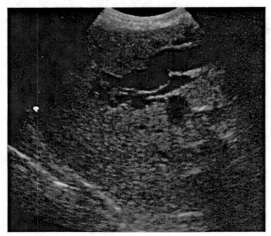

Right lobe liver

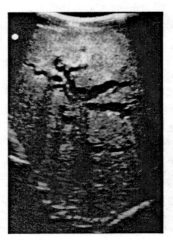

Left of liver

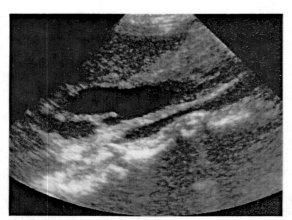

Enlarged CBD due to obstruction in the head of the pancreas, which shows the insertion of the cystic duct in the CBD

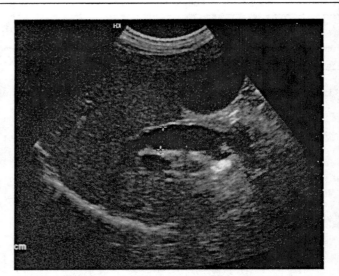

Enlarged CBD measuring almost 1.6 cm: level of obstruction should be documented

B) PHYSIOLOGY

PURPOSE	• transport bile from the liver cells to the duodenal lumen • bile ducts have no motor role in bile flow

OPERATION	• bile flow can be:
	  1. increased by contraction of GB
	  2. decreased by contraction of the sphincter of Oddi in the distal end of the CBD
	
	• bile flows secondary to pressure differences, which depend on:
	  1. rate of bile flow from liver into bile ducts
	  2. GB function (filling and resorption)
	  3. contractility of the distal sphincter of Oddi, which has a regular cycle of contractions and relaxations

C) LAB TEST

SEE GALLBLADDER AND LIVER SECTIONS

14

D) ANOMALIES

ANOMALY	US APPEARANCE
ASCARIASIS • a type of roundworm that inhabits the intestines usually the jejunum • can be 15–50 cm long and about 3–6 mm thick • once a relatively rare occurrence, but now more frequently encountered with increasing travel to heavy endemic countries and is the most common parasitic infection worldwide • can migrate through the biliary system causing cholecystitis, cholangitis, biliary obstruction, and hepatic abscess SS • passage of works via rectum or vomiting US • echogenic, nonshadowing linear intraductal filling defects (tube within a tube) • can have coiled or spaghetti-like appearance • can be seen to move on real-time imaging • do not shadow unless dead and calcified	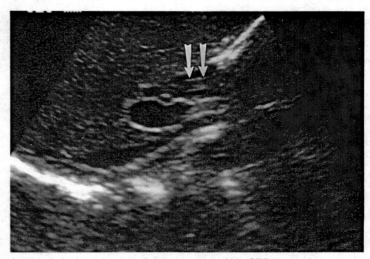 Ascariasis is the echogenic linear structure within CBD (arrows) 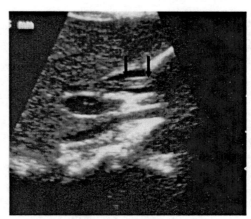 Echogenic tube within a dilated CBD (arrows)
BILIARY ATRESIA • congenital anomaly whereby part or all of the bile duct is not formed 1. INTRAHEPATIC ATRESIA • may be due to intrauterine infection • fatal disorder • no evidence of biliary radicals • hepatomegaly 2. EXTRAHEPATIC ATRESIA (commonest form) • anastomosis of biliary tree to jejunum • probably due to chronic cholangitis in utero • dilated intrahepatic radicals 3. FOCAL ATRESIA • probably due to intrauterine vascular accident Diff. Dx.: • neonatal hepatitis (normal GB supports diagnosis of hepatitis) • neonatal jaundice Helpful Hint: • presence of GB reduces the likelihood but does not exclude diagnosis	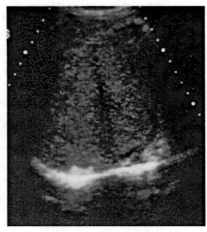 Transverse scan of neonatal liver showing no evidence of a biliary tree

ANOMALY	US APPEARANCE

BILIARY NEOPLASMS

1. CHOLANGIOCARCINOMA
- rare primary carcinoma of bile ducts
- location:
  intrahepatic
  junction of cystic duct and CBD
  common hepatic duct and bifurcation (see Klatskin tumor below)

i) Klatskin tumor
- 10%–25% of bile duct carcinomas arise at the hepatic duct bifurcation (porta hepatis) and are then called Klatskin tumors
- gives rise to enlarged intrahepatic but normal extrahepatic ducts, solid mass at hilum in region of junction of right and left hepatic ducts

SS
- anorexia, weight loss, RUQ pain, jaundice
- ↑ direct bilirubin, ALP, SGOT/SGPT

US
- abrupt stop of duct seen on long axis view
- marked obstruction of biliary ducts with normal pancreas
- mass in duct with coarse shadow
- evaluate both RHD and LHD because cholangiocarcinoma may obstruct one branch and not the other

2. CYSTADENOCARCINOMA AND CYSTADENOMA
- rare hepatic neoplasms
- intrahepatic cysts of bile duct origin
- primary seen in right lobe of liver

SS
- painful epigastric mass
- intermittent jaundice

US
- cystic, multiloculated intrahepatic mass (3–10 cm) with thick echogenic internal septations and papillary projections

Diff. Dx.:
- hydatid echinococcal disease
- abscess
- hematoma
- complicated cyst
- cystic metastases

3. METASTATIC DISEASE TO BILIARY SYSTEM
- pancreatic carcinoma is the most common cause of malignant obstruction to bile ducts
- others include gallbladder carcinoma, hepatocellular carcinoma

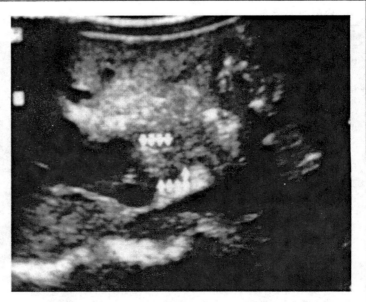

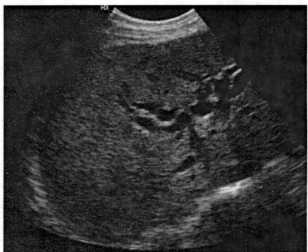

Klatskin tumor

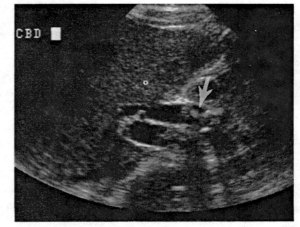

Mass within distal CBD (arrow)

ANOMALY	US APPEARANCE
CAROLI'S DISEASE • segmental saccular dilatation of intrahepatic ducts (congenital duct ectasia) with sparing of the extrahepatic ducts • unknown etiology • biliary stasis causes infection and stones US • normal CBD • beaded appearance of intrahepatic ducts, which appear as multiple cystic structures in liver • sludge and calculi can appear in dilated ducts • "central dot sign": dilated bile duct surrounds the adjacent hepatic artery and portal vein, which appears sonographically as a central echogenic focus in the middle of the dilated duct <u>Helpful Hint:</u> • make sure these dilated ducts communicate with biliary tree for diagnosis	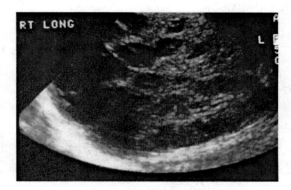 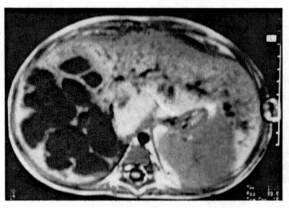

ANOMALY	US APPEARANCE

CHOLANGITIS

- inflammation of the bile ducts caused by bacterial infection
- usually associated with obstruction (choledocholithiasis, neoplasms)

1. AIDS CHOLANGITIS

- dilated ducts, ↑ liver function tests (LFTs), jaundice
- caused by cytomegalovirus, cryptosporidium, mycobacterium avium intracellulare
- sclerosing cholangitis pattern may develop

US
- very thick GB wall
- gallstones are typically absent
- dilatation of cystic duct can be seen

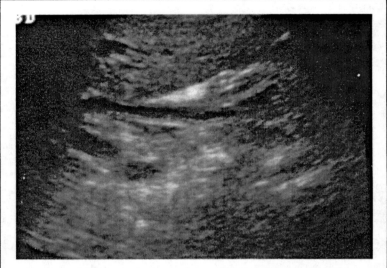

2. ORIENTAL (RECURRENT PYOGENIC CHOLANGITIS)

- etiologies include acquired or congenital stricture, coliform bacterial infection of bile, parasitic infestation
- if untreated leads to intrahepatic bile stasis and liver failure

SS
- repetitive attacks of cholangitis, fever, chills, epigastric or RUQ pain, jaundice

US
- distended intrahepatic ducts
- huge CBD (3–4 cm)
- GB large and palpable
- ductal stones and cholelithiasis may be seen

<u>Diff. Dx.:</u>
- biliary obstruction
- Caroli's disease

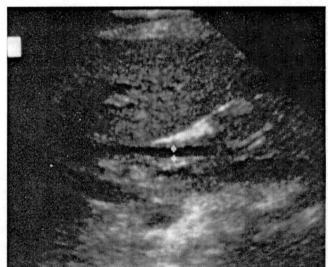

3. SCLEROSING CHOLANGITIS

- chronic inflammatory process of bile ducts
  intrahepatic ducts—20%
  extrahepatic ducts—80%
- increased incidence in patients with ulcerative colitis
- unknown etiology but may be secondary to either bacterial or metabolic alteration of bile acids

SS
- chronic intermittent obstructive jaundice
- pain (biliary colic), chills, and fever
- leukocystosis, ↑ serum bilirubin, ↑ ALP

US
- periportal fibrosis of bile ducts, which causes them to become thickened and irregular
- biliary obstruction associated with thickening of intra- and extrahepatic biliary tree

ANOMALY

CHOLEDOCHAL CYST

- rare form of cystic dilatation of the biliary system
- most accepted etiology is that an anomalous insertion of CBD into pancreatic duct causes reflux of pancreatic juice leading to cholangitis and dilatation
- commonly presents in infants, 1st decade of life, or in utero
- 4 types:
  1. cystic dilatation of CBD (most common)
  2. diverticulum of CBD
  3. choledochocele
  4. multiple intrahepatic and extrahepatic cysts

SS
- jaundice
- RUQ pain
- RUQ palpable mass
- fever

US
- large cystic mass in porta hepatis
- enlarged CBD or CHD entering cystic mass, although the communication with biliary tree may not be apparent
- must demonstrate GB separate from cyst
- calculi may be present within cyst

Diff. Dx.:
- hepatic cyst
- pancreatic pseudocyst
- hepatic artery aneurysm
- duplication cyst
- perforation of extrahepatic bile ducts

US APPEARANCE

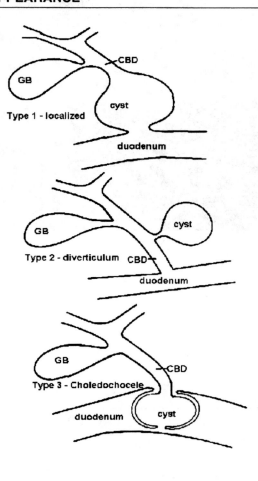

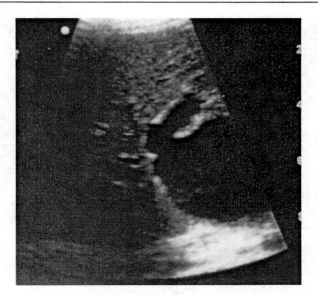

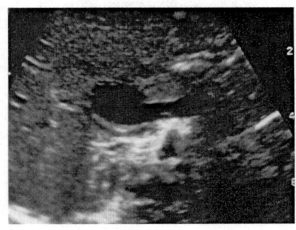

ANOMALY	US APPEARANCE

CHOLEDOCHOLITHIASIS

- stone(s) in bile ducts
- usually stones form in GB and pass through into bile ducts
- small stones may spontaneously pass through to duodenum
- obstruction can be complete or intermittent

SS
- biliary colic, jaundice, GB stones
- ↑ serum ALP, ↑ serum bilirubin

US
- hyperechoic structure (stone) in duct with or without shadowing
- careful scanning required as this is often difficult to image as not much (if any) bile surrounding stone, to create good acoustic contrast

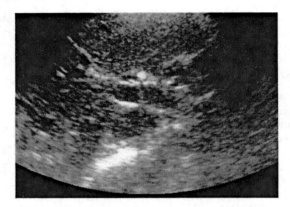

1. MIRIZZI SYNDROME
- rare condition
- CBD obstruction resulting from a stone in the cystic duct or GB neck
- the mass effect of the impacted stone and/or the associated inflammation pushes on CBD
- this causes partial mechanical obstruction and dilatation of CBD
- uncommon, surgically correctable cause of extrahepatic obstruction

SS
- jaundice, recurrent cholangitis, formation of bilobilary fistula, cholangitic cirrhosis

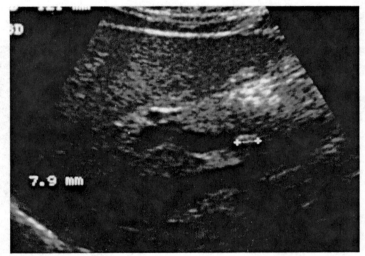

US
- impacted stone in cystic duct, cystic duct remnant, or GB neck
- partial mechanical obstruction of CHD by compression or inflammatory reaction around stone
- CHD increased in size with normal diameter CBD below site of obstruction
- hepatobiliary nuclear medicine often suggested

Pitfalls:
- shadowing from adjacent bowel
- right hepatic artery crossing CBD and indenting it
- postoperative cholecystectomy clips
- pneumobilia

ANOMALY	US APPEARANCE
PNEUMOBILIA • presence of air/gas in biliary tree • caused by fistula (e.g., caused by cholecystitis or tumor), more commonly seen due to recent surgery or endoscopic retrograde cholangiopancreatography (ERCP) US • multiple echogenic foci causing acoustic shadow in the region of bile ducts Diff. Dx.: • gallstones • surgical clips	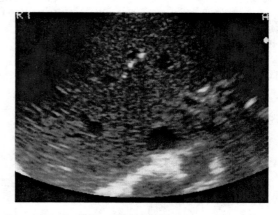 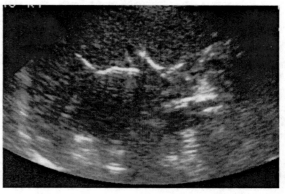

BILE DUCT PATHOLOGY DIFFERENTIAL

INTRALUMINAL FOCUS	• biliary calculus • ascaris • tumor • sludge, blood clot, debris, pus
INTRINSIC DUCT WALL DISEASE	• postinflammatory or operative fibrous stricture • malignant stricture (cholangiocarcinoma) • congenital atresia of CBD • sclerosing cholangitis
EXTRINSIC COMPRESSION	• pancreatic head tumor • acute pancreatitis • choledochal cyst • enlarged portal lymphadenopathy • liver masses
UNOBSTRUCTED DILATED BILE DUCTS	• age related • Caroli's disease • choledochal cyst • immediately following removal of obstruction • postcholecystectomy
BILE DUCT WALL THICKENING	• AIDS cholangiopathy • ascending cholangitis • cholangiocarcinoma • CBD stones • oriental cholangiohepatitis • pancreatitis • sclerosing cholangitis

ABNORMAL BILIARY TREE IN RELATION TO GALLBLADDER

	GALLBLADDER	DUCTS
COUVASIER'S SIGN/ PANCREATIC HEAD MASS	palpable thin wall ↑ size	all enlarged
ORIENTAL CHOLANGITIS	palpable thin wall ↑ size	huge CBD (3–4 cm)
MERRIZZI SYNDROME	enlarged	↑ common hepatic duct ↑ intrahepatics normal CBD
KLATSKIN TUMOR	normal	normal extrahepatics ↑ intrahepatics
CYSTADENOMA, CYSTADENOCARCINOMA	normal	↑ focal/peripheral intrahepatics
CAROLI'S DISEASE	normal	normal CBD intrahepatic ectasia of bile ducts
CHOLEDOCHAL CYST	GB appears small compared to huge CBD	huge CBD

E) TECHNICAL FACTORS

PATIENT PREP	• fasting for 8–12 hours guarantees maximum biliary tract dilatation • it is important to verify with patients when they last ate
TRANSDUCER	3.0–5.0 MHz
TECHNIQUE	• usually CBD is best seen by placing patient in left lateral decubitus or left posterior oblique position and scan from a right anterior oblique approach • deep held respiration is used • scanning from the right lateral even intercostal approach with patient on the left side can be helpful to visualize a difficult to obtain duct
MINIMUM PROTOCOL	• measure CHD anterior to the right hepatic artery and the right portal vein • document any intrahepatic biliary dilation • CBD into head of pancreas • if biliary dilation is present, try to demonstrate cause
HELPFUL HINTS	BEST SCAN PLANES • due to small size of CBD it is best visualized in the longitudinal scan plane • transverse imaging of the CHD is best seen at GB neck and CBD best seen at head of pancreas DISPLACING DUODENAL GAS • use transducer pressure to push gas out of way • have patient drink water to displace gas out of stomach and duodenum • change the patient's position to upright, or decubitus ENLARGED DUCT • measure duct 45 minutes after patient has eaten or 5–10 minutes after injection of cholecystokinin to see if contracts normally • if you can visualize the indentation of the right hepatic artery as it crosses the CBD, this is a good indicator that the CBD is not obstructed and is of normal size

CHAPTER 3 - BREASTS (MAMMARY GLANDS)
A) NORMAL ANATOMY AND SONOGRAPHIC APPEARANCE

DEFINITION	• paired subcutaneous organs that are accessory organs of female reproduction • modified (differentiated apocrine) sweat glands

STRUCTURE

Breast = fibrous + glandular + adipose tissue

1. SUSPENSORY LIGAMENTS (COOPER'S LIGAMENTS)
• strands of connective tissue that divide gland into lobes and lobules
• run from the deep fascia, between the lobes of the breast tissue to attach to the skin and areola
• support the weight of the breast

2. LOBES
• 15–20 compartments separated by adipose tissue made up of several small lobules
• epithelial cells embedded in connective tissue of lobules secrete milk via secondary tubules
• tail of Spence is an axillary tail of breast glandular tissue that reaches the axilla

3. LACTIFEROUS DUCTS
• one in each lobe opens individually into the nipple
• convey milk from one of the lobes to the exterior

4. MAMMARY DUCTS
• milk passes from secondary tubules through mammary ducts to nipple

5. AMPULLAE/LACTIFEROUS SINUSES
• formed by expanded mammary ducts
• store milk

6. AREOLA
• circular pigmented area of skin surrounding nipple
• contain sebaceous glands
• the male breast consists primarily of nipple and areola

7. DEEP FASCIA
• retromammary space is the fat-filled space between the breast and deep fascia

8. PECTORALIS MAJOR MUSCLE
• lies posterior to the deep fascia

9. FAT

10. RIB

11. INTERCOSTAL MUSCLE

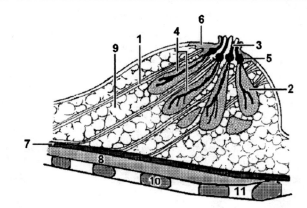

NORMAL ANATOMY

SIZE & SHAPE	• size and shape of breast depends and varies with amount of adipose tissue, which is highly dependent on body weight
LOCATION	• located on the anterior thorax • within the superficial and deep layers of the superficial pectoral fascia
RELATIONSHIPS	Muscles: • lie over pectoralis major and serratus anterior muscles • connected to muscle by layer of connective tissue • sometimes breast tissue can be found within the chest posterior to breast

US APPEARANCE		
ANATOMY	**MAMMO APPEARANCE**	**US APPEARANCE**
SKIN		• most superior linear structure
SUBCUTANEOUS FAT	black	• quality varies with age, parity, and hormonal status • hypoechoic
FAT LOBULES	black areas	• hypoechoic as fat does not have many vessels • oval in one plane, elongated in opposite plane
COOPER'S LIGAMENTS		• tentlike structures that arise from surface of breast and create a saw-tooth pattern • can cause shadowing due to intersection of apices • shadow should disappear with a change in the angle of the transducer

PARENCHYMA/ FIBROGLANDULAR TISSUE	white areas	• fibroglandular is echogenic
		• separated by fascial planes
		  1. Juvenile—hyperechoic breasts with very little fat
		  2. Premenopausal—partly involuted with increasing amount of hypoechoic fat
		  3. Postmenopausal—mostly involuted with increasing amount of fat
		  4. Pregnancy and lactating—increased amount of glandular tissue that leads to fine granular pattern

DUCTS	white	• echopoor tubular structures • progressive luminal enlargement as they converge at nipple
RETROMAMMARY FAT		• narrow hypoechoic layer deep to the base • may be completely absent • defines posterior boundaries of glandular tissue
PECTORALIS MUSCLE	white	• low-level echo areas posterior to retromammary layer • parallel to skin • sheathed in echogenic fascial plane
NIPPLE REGION		• dense connective tissue at areolar region and around the converging ducts • this attenuates sound, which results in posterior acoustic shadowing • position transducer tangentially to nipple to visualize subareolar region
RIBS	white	• oval, hypoechoic structures with few internal echos posterior to pectoralis muscle • can be mistaken as lesions • attention must be paid to location and other structures deep in breast to avoid misidentifying these structures • attenuate sound, which results in posterior acoustic shadowing
AXILLARY VESSELS	white	• tubular structures in axilla that show flow with Doppler ultrasound
LYMPH NODES	white and black areas	• normal nodes contain a peripheral hypoechoic rim containing an echogenic fatty hilus

CHANGES WITH AGE		• in the older patient:
		  • the amount of fatty tissue increases and the fibroglandular tissue decreases (increase of fat/parenchyma ratio)
		  • this process is reversed with patients receiving hormonal therapy

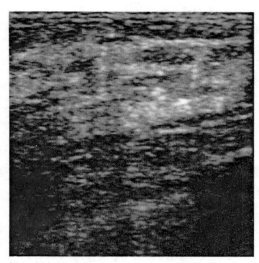

Normal breast tissue

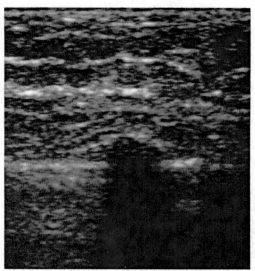

Pitfall: Do not mistake shadowing from a rib as a lesion. This is a sagittal scan plane through a normal breast, showing shadowing from a rib. Image all suspicious areas in two planes to avoid this pitfall.

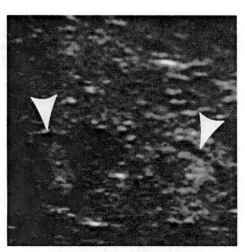

Lymph nodes within breast tissue (arrows)

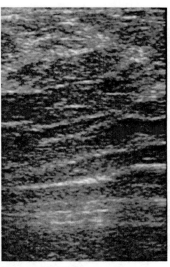

Normal breast tissue

B) VASCULATURE

ARTERIAL AND VENOUS

thoracic aorta ↓ posterior intercostal arteries ↓ TO lateral aspect of breast	subclavian artery ↓ internal thoracic artery ↓ TO medial aspect of breast	branch of axillary artery ↓ lateral thoracic artery ↓ TO posterior aspect of breast

- veins follow course of arteries

LYMPHATICS

- lymphatics of each breast communicate with each other
- continuous with the superficial lymphatics of the skin of the abdomen and neck
- drain 3 major routes
  1. Axillary—receive most of the lymph stream
  2. Inter- or transpectoral
  3. Internal mammary

- drain fat molecules in milk as they are generally too big for the veins
- transfer infection or malignancy from breast to more distant areas

SUPERFICIAL (SUBAREOLAR)	DEEP	
central gland, skin, nipple, areolar ↓ pectoral nodes ↓ axillary nodes ↓ subclavian nodes	lateral aspect of breast ↓ axillary nodes ↓ subclavian nodes	medial aspect of breast ↓ parasternal and mediastinal nodes (along internal thoracic artery)

C) PHYSIOLOGY

PURPOSE		• lactation; milk secretion and ejection
OPERATION		Milk secretion: • largely due to hormone prolactin from anterior pituitary • under influence of progesterone and estrogen Milk ejection: • occurs in presence of oxytocin from posterior pituitary released by stimulation of infant sucking
DEVELOPMENT	PUBERTY	• estrogen from ovary stimulates development
	MATURITY (AFTER OVULATION)	• progesterone influences formation of lobules • enlarge slightly during menstrual cycle due to water retention • during reproductive years breasts are composed mainly of fibroglandular tissue • increase in fat deposits
	PREGNANCY	• proliferation of ductal system and lobules
	MENOPAUSE	• glandular tissue atrophies and breasts become mainly composed of fatty tissue • ducts become ectatic

D) ANOMALIES

ANOMALY	US APPEARANCE
AUGMENTATION/PROSTHESIS	

AUGMENTATION/PROSTHESIS

- placement of silicone gel or saline implants in the retromammary space for enlargement of small breast OR used for postmastectomy purposes since the early 1960s
- after implantation a fibrous capsule develops around the implant that may cause hardening and breast pain
- Many varieties:
  single double lumen
  saline (newer implants have a thicker outer shell and appear smaller in the AP plane due to the speed of sound in saline, which is closer to tissue than is silicone
  silicone; older implants

US
Pitfalls:
- difficulty in imaging due to fibrous changes that occasionally occur in tissue adjacent to silicone gel implant and scar tissue along incision site
- sound travels faster in silicone gel; therefore, implants appear deeper than truly are
- reverberation artifacts in anterior part of implant must not be misinterpreted as abnormal echos

1. RUPTURE
- complications related to breast implants include rupture
- best detected with magnetic resonance imaging (MRI)
- caused by vigorous manipulation of the implant through the skin, compression mammography, trauma

SS
- change in appearance and consistency of breast
- breast tenderness
- breast lump

US
Intracapsular rupture
- rupture of the prosthesis but the fibrous capsule around it remains intact
- "stepladder sign": multiple linear and curvilinear echogenic lines within implant from extravasation of silicone gel surrounding collapsed implant shell. This is the ultrasound finding that correlates with the "linguini" sign of MRI
- irregular globules of silicone between implant surface and fibrous capsule

Extracapsular rupture
- rupture of both the prosthesis and the fibrous capsule
- diffusely echogenic echo pattern resembling bowel gas within an implant
- caused by globules of silicone smaller than the ultrasound beam

Intracapsular implant rupture
a) stepladder sign from overlapping layers of ruptured implant
b) globules of silicone (arrows) outside implant

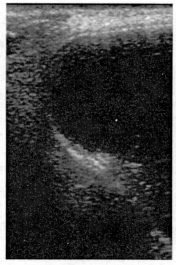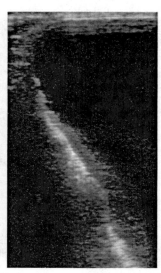

Saline implant in postmastectomy patient

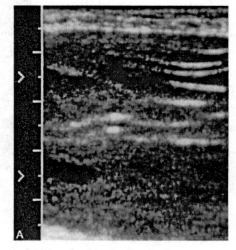

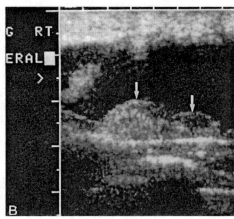

ANOMALY	US APPEARANCE

CARCINOMA

- risks: female, age, family history, reproductive history, but most commonly arises in patients with no known risk factors
- genetic testing for breast cancer can determine if a gene mutation that increases the risk is present
- early diagnosis is key to effective treatment
- on physical exam are usually relatively fixed, nontender, solitary hard masses with irregular, ill-defined margins
- 1% occur in males, in whom lymphatic spread is early and extensive
- although all distant visceral sites are potential sites, the major metastatic sites include:
  bone
  lung
  brain
  liver

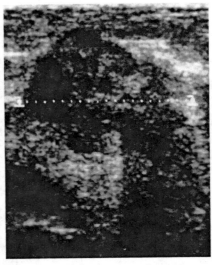

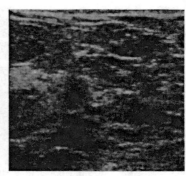

Calipers measuring breast malignant neoplasm

1. INFILTRATING LOBULAR CARCINOMA

- second in frequency of occurrence after ductal carcinoma
- frequently found in upper outer quadrants
- poorly circumscribed
- arises from the extralobular terminal ducts the same as ductal carcinoma
- identical gross appearance on pathology to ductal carcinoma
- diagnosis is histologic
- can be difficult to detect on mammography

2. INVASIVE DUCTAL CARCINOMA (SQUAMOUS CELL CARCINOMA)

- most common malignancy (80%)
- arise from extralobular terminal ducts
- subgroups include:

a) Medullary carcinoma
- rare, but occur with greater frequency in women under 50 years of age
- sonographically similar to adenoma, which can appear homogeneous and hypoechoic
- well circumscribed mass that may have posterior acoustic enhancement

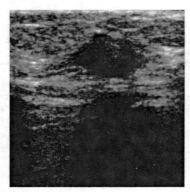

Infiltrating lobular carcinoma   Invasive carcinoma

b) Mucinous (colloid) carcinoma
- rare form
- better prognosis than infiltrating ductal carcinoma
- mass full of mucin with malignant cells
- low echogenicity, lack of posterior attenuation

c) Papillary carcinoma
- occurs most commonly in postmenopausal women
- initially arises as an intraductal mass
- first clinical symptom is bloody nipple discharge
- rare
- intracystic papilloma grows from a stalk into the lumen of a serous or hemorrhagic cyst

d) Tubular carcinoma
- rare form
- well differentiated ductal carcinoma with an excellent prognosis if small
- ultrasound findings are nonspecific

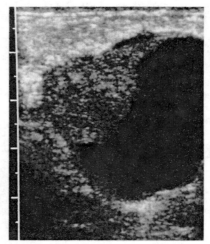

Intracystic papilloma

ANOMALY	US APPEARANCE
US FOR CARCINOMA • ULTRASOUND IS NOT A SCREENING TEST! • solid, hypoechoic mass with irregular margins • echogenic band around periphery due to fibrous reaction • posterior acoustic shadowing (may only visualize a shadow with no mass) • displace suspensory ligaments and disrupts normal breast architecture if large enough Diff. Dx.: • abscess, hematoma, hamartoma Doppler: • Doppler assessment of tumor vascularity is still being researched • current studies are showing an increase in detection of Doppler signals in malignant lesions versus nonmalignant lesions • a frequency shift > 1 kHz indicates a high probability for malignancy • negative findings with pulsed Doppler US cannot be used to exclude malignancy Pitfall: • if lesion isoechoic to fat, it can be missed	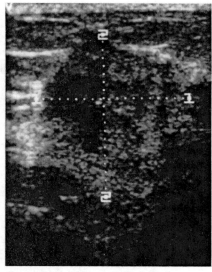 Carcinoma: solid mass with irregular borders

CYSTS AND CYSTIC STRUCTURES
1. ABSCESS
• caused by surgery, iatrogenic causes, breast feeding
• single or multiple
 	
SS
• tenderness, redness, and swelling of breast
 	
US
• mass with irregular borders, low-level echos and posterior enhancement
  acute abscess—poorly defined border
  mature abscess—well encapsulated with sharp borders
 	
2. DILATED DUCTS
• ducts in pregnancy and lactation fill with colostrum then milk
• become enlarged and have a linear tubular hypoechoic appearance
 	
3. GALACTOCELES
• localized accumulation of milk behind obstructed duct during lactation
 	
US
• variable appearance
• low-level echo mass with poorly defined margin
 	
4. HEMATOMA
• caused by trauma, surgery anticoagulants
• appears as a hematoma as in anywhere in body
 	
US
• variable appearance depending on age of injury
 	
5. HEMORRHAGIC CYSTS
• can be caused by tumor in wall (mural nodule)/intracystic cancer
• any cyst that contains blood must be investigated for a tumor
• needle aspiration can assist in diagnosis
 	
US
• should distinguish between simple hemorrhagic cyst or hemorrhagic cyst within a neoplasm
• neoplastic cyst would have irregular wall thickening or papillary projections from wall
• can both have enhanced through transmission and internal echos
	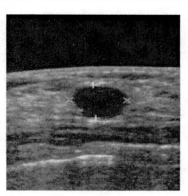
	Simple cyst
	
	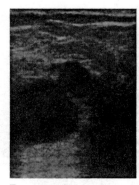 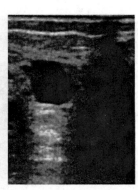
	Two cysts that appear connected Simple cyst with irregular shape

ANOMALY	US APPEARANCE

6. MASTITIS
- results from infection, trauma, or mechanical obstruction of ducts
- most frequently occur in lactating patient
- often is confined to one area of the breast

US
- diffuse decrease in echogenicity secondary to edema with scattered small fluid collections

7. SIMPLE CYSTS
- fluid imbalance of how much fluid is made and how much is absorbed
- terminal ductal lobular unit expands
- often cyclic appearing in last half of menstrual cycle and associated with pain and tenderness
- common in women aged 35–50 years

US
- anechoic
- sharply defined back wall with well defined margins
- posterior acoustic enhancement
- not fixed
- lateral edge shadowing
- if echos within, differential includes hemorrhagic cyst (simple or neoplastic), infection

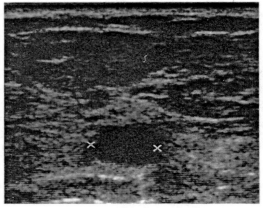

Simple cyst

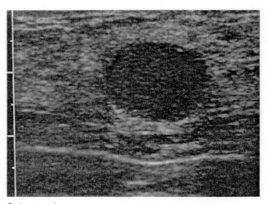

Galactocele

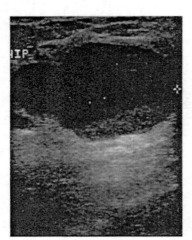

Hemorrhagic cyst: particulate material (blood) is seen within posterior portion of cyst

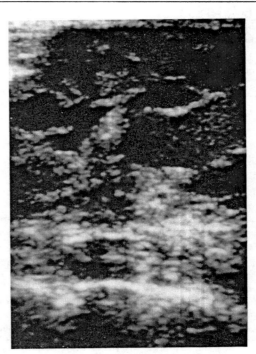

Mastitis: collection with dilated ducts

ANOMALY	US APPEARANCE
FIBROADENOMAS/PAPILLOMA • common solid benign breast mass • encountered at all ages, but most commonly in a young woman • primarily unilateral (multiple in 10%–20% of cases) • growth is stimulated by estrogen • may be partially calcified US • variable appearances • hypoechoic to fibroglandular parenchyma and isoechoic to fat lobules • well defined, oval mass • lobulated or smooth borders • low-level homogenous echotexture • not fixed • may or may not have through transmission <u>Doppler:</u> • color flow around periphery except in young people who can have color throughout them	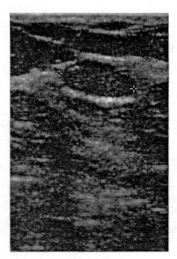

FIBROCYSTIC CHANGE
• composed of:
  1. cyst formation
  2. fibrosis
  3. sclerosis adenomas (glandular proliferation)
  4. epithelial hyperplasia (this can be a precursor to malignancy)
• common benign condition although a patient with this has a increased risk of developing carcinoma
• etiology is thought to be a disturbance in estrogen–progesterone balance
 	
SS
• nodularity and pain related to multiple breast cysts
 	
US
• hyperechoic dense breast
• small simple cysts scattered throughout the breast
• large cysts may also be present—smooth margin
	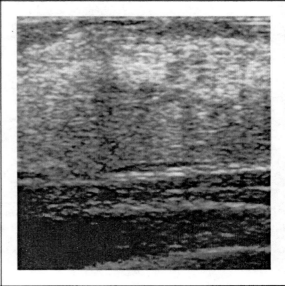

E) TECHNICAL FACTORS

TRANSDUCER	• high frequency > 7 MHz with a wide footprint to better visualize near-field • 5 MHz transducer might be necessary to visualize a large breast or the posterior part of an implant • stand-off pad may be required for placing the focal zone properly for superficial structures
INDICATIONS FOR BREAST ULTRASOUND	1. mammo with indeterminate lesion + no palpable mass 2. normal or abnormal mammo + palpable mass 3. no mammo + palpable mass (e.g., young or pregnant patient) BREAST ULTRASOUND SURVEY IS NOT RECOMMENDED i.e., no mammo + no palpable mass 4. guidance of breast intervention procedures
SCAN PLANES 	O'clock scan planes • transducer is oriented so that breast is viewed in sections from nipple outward • use a clockwise approach keeping the base of the transducer next to the nipple area and rotate other end of transducer around the breast in a circular pattern 12 o'clock—transducer will be in a longitudinal position 5 o'clock—transducer will be in a trans. oblique position 9 o'clock—transducer will be in a transverse position

PATIENT POSITION	SUPINE
	• contralateral posterior oblique position to minimize breast thickness
	ERECT
	• used if unable to locate mass seen on mammogram
	• use this technique to duplicate the mammographic position
	  • sit patient facing you
	  • support breast by placing one hand under breast
	  • use firm pressure with transducer to compress breast and scan from superior surface of breast in area of interest

DOCUMENTATION	• focal sonographic lesions are seen as disruption of normal breast architecture
	• document:
	  size, shape, and location of lesion
	  sonographic echotexture and characteristics
	  differentiate cystic from solid
	• with newer higher frequency probes, mammographic calcification can be documented on ultrasound
	• lymph node status—check drainage areas for lymph node enlargement

HELPFUL HINTS	• scan lightly over breast to avoid distorting breast architecture • small lesions < 1 cm may not be easily visualized because of wide beam width

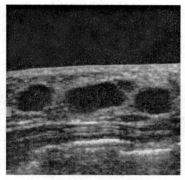

Breast cysts with stand-off pad

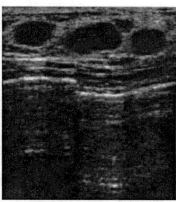

Same breast cysts without stand-off pad

OTHER PROCEDURES

CYST ASPIRATION WITH SONOGRAPHIC GUIDANCE/FINE NEEDLE ASPIRATION BIOPSY (FNAB)	• any lesion that does not have all the diagnostic criteria for cysts should be aspirated • removal of fluid or tissue from a mass with a small gauge needle • technique depends on type of transducer, sonologist's experience, and cyst features • principles for FNAB are the same as for cyst aspiration • document presence of needle in lesion
PRESURGICAL NEEDLE • Hookwire localization	• sonographic guidance is helpful when mass is in periphery of breast where mammographic guidance may be difficult
CORE BIOPSY	• using a larger bore biopsy needle to obtain histologic specimens from the breast • this is done using ultrasound guidance
STEREOTACTIC BREAST BIOPSY	• combines mammography and computer-assisted needle biopsy equipment • two stereo x-rays (images of same area from different angles) are taken • the computer determines the exact positioning of the biopsy needle from these images

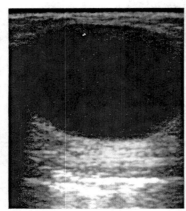 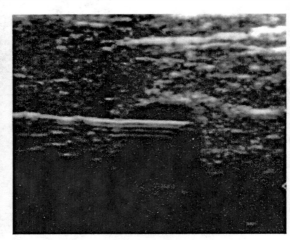 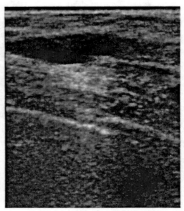

Large breast cyst   Needle within cyst during aspiration   Same breast cyst after aspiration

CRITERIA FOR INTERPRETATION OF LOCAL BREAST ULTRSOUND LESIONS

• none of these indicators can be used to absolutely distinguish benign from malignant, which must be done by histologic examination of the mass	PROBABILITY (↑ increased or ↓ decreased)	
	MALIGNANCY	BENIGN
MARGINS		
1. indistinct jagged	↑ ↑	
2. indistinct smooth	↑	
3. sharp jagged		↑
4. sharp smooth		↑ ↑
RETRO MASS ACOUSTIC CHARACTERISTICS		
1. posterior shadow	↑	
strong	↑ ↑	
moderate	↑	
light	↑	
2. enhancement		↑
3. no change		↑ ↑
INTERNAL ECHO PATTERN	few echos nonhomogenous	anechoic homogenous
ECHOGENICITY	solid hypoechoic lesion with echogenic rim	hypoechoic (fibroadenoma, sebaceous cyst) hyperechoic (hemorrhagic cysts, fibrocystic change) anechoic (cysts)
COMPRESSION	no change in shape	shape distorts
COMPRESSION'S EFFECT ON INTERNAL ECHOS	no change	becomes more homogenous
SHAPE	vertical shape taller than wide perpendicular to skin (long > trans)	horizontal shape wider than tall perpendicular to skin (trans > long)

DOPPLER	Resistive index (RI) and pulsitivity index (PI)
	  • using RI and PI to characterize masses is not advised
	  • results are controversial and not consistent and at this time there are no absolute criteria
	Presence of flow
	  • cysts will not have flow within them	

CHAPTER 4 - GALLBLADDER

A) NORMAL ANATOMY AND SONOGRAPHIC APPEARANCE

DEFINITION	• small, muscular, pear-shaped sac that is the reservoir for bile

STRUCTURE

1. FUNDUS
• rounded interior portion
a) Phrygian cap
• GB fundus is folded inward on itself
• most common anomaly of GB

2. BODY
• middle portion of GB
a) Infundibulum/Hartmann's pouch
• situated between the body and neck that portion of GB that tapers toward neck closet to cystic duct
• stones tend to accumulate at this point
b) Junctional fold
• fold(s) or kink(s) between the body and infundibulum of GB

3. WALL
• thinner than wall of intestine because lacks circular and transverse muscle layer and submucosa
  inner wall—mucosa: epithelial lining
  middle wall—lamina propria: smooth muscle layer
• contraction of this muscle by hormonal stimulation ejects contents of GB into cystic duct
• outer coat is the visceral peritoneum

4. NECK
• superior tapering portion of GB
• tapers into cystic duct
• curves medially toward the porta hepatis
• contains spiral folds around its lumen
• fixed in its position at the main lobar fissure

5. CYSTIC DUCT
• joins CHD 1–2 cm above the duodenum to form CBD
• superior to GB neck
a) Spiral valve of Heister/spiral part of cystic duct
• not a true valve but a tortuous area of cystic duct at its junction with the neck of GB

6. COMMON HEPATIC DUCT
• portion of bile duct above insertion of cystic duct

7. COMMON BILE DUCT
• runs downward in the right free margin of the lesser omentum, enters the pancreas to join the main pancreatic duct at the hepatopancreatic ampulla

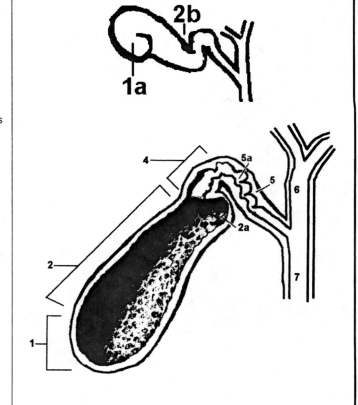

NORMAL ANATOMY

SHAPE	• pear-shaped saccular organ that has much variation in size and shape • variations in shape include ovoid, spherical, elongated	
SIZE	Normal Fasting Range of Adult Measurements:	
	Length	7–11 cm
	Widest cross-sectional diameter	1.5–4 cm
	Volume	30–50 cc [$\pi/6$ (LxWxH)]
	Wall thickness	1–3 mm (measured parallel to sound beam adjacent to liver)
LOCATION	• under visceral surface of liver adjacent to the interlobar fissure • situated along the junction of the medial segment of the left lobe and right lobe • intraperitoneal • body and fundus are extremely variable in position, but neck is fixed **Sonographic Locator:** Main lobar fissure • echogenic linear structure along same path as middle hepatic vein • GB lies posterior and caudal to main lobar fissure	

NORMAL SONOGRAPHIC APPEARANCE

• fluid-filled ellipsoid structure adjacent to and indenting the inferior-medial aspect of the right lobe of the liver
• smooth wall that is normally not measurable

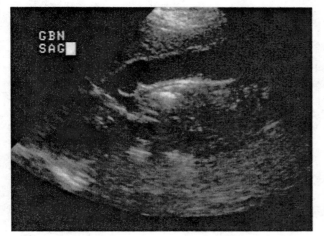

Sagittal scan of GB

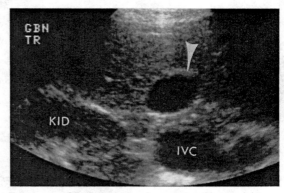

Transverse GB (arrow) showing relationships to right kidney (kid) and IVC

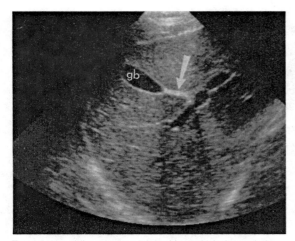

Transverse oblique scan plane with cephalad angulation shows the relationship between the main lobar fissure (arrow) and gallbladder (gb)

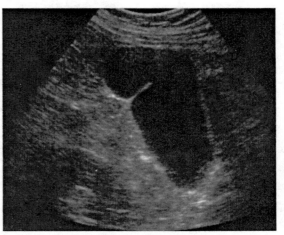

Phrygian cap: longitudinal scan plane

(continued)

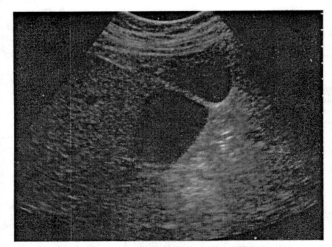

Appearance of Phrygian cap with transverse scan plane

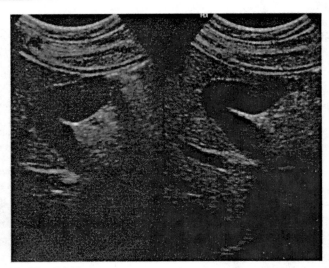

Junctional fold

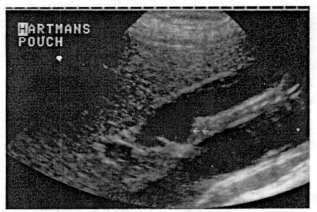

Hartman's pouch (arrows)

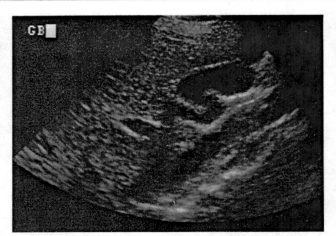

Normal GB with many folds

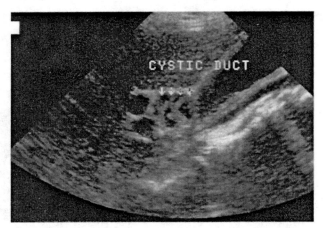

Dilated cystic duct (arrows): although not normally seen, this scan was included to demonstrate the tortuous nature of the duct

SONOGRAPHIC APPEARANCES OF GALLBLADDER

CONTRACTED GALLBLADDER

- nonfasting
- double concentric structure with three layers:
  1. echogenic outer layer
  2. middle anechoic area
  3. hypoechoic inner layer

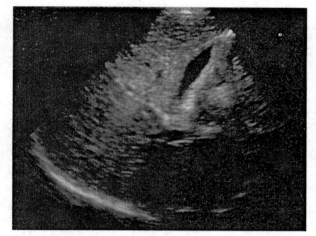

Longitudinal

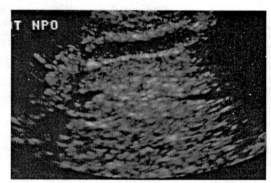

Transverse

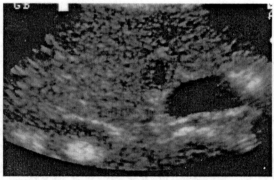

Transverse

ERROR IN VISUALIZATION

- GB mistaken as bowel:
  small stones
  contracted GB
  anomalous GB location
  stones in cystic duct/GB neck

- Other areas mistaken as GB
  gas-filled duodenum
  air in biliary tree
  cystic mass in liver, kidney, pancreas, adrenal gland
  tortuous vessels

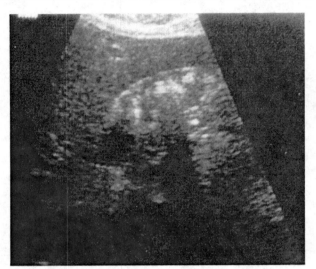

This GB affected with chronic cholecystitis, stones, and adenomyomatosis could be mistaken as bowel

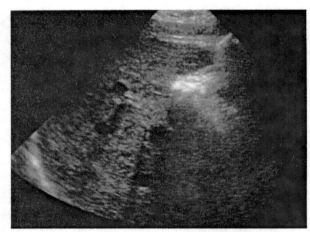

Gas in the duodenum should not be mistaken as stone-filled GB

"WES" TRIAD/"DOUBLE ARC" SIGN

- strong broad acoustic shadowing from or near the GB fossa seen sometimes with chronic cholecystitis
- recognizing this sign will help differentiate a stone-filled GB from bowel

WES TRIAD:
  W: the wall (hypoechoic)
  E: the stone(s) (echogenic)
  S: the shadow (hypoechoic)

DOUBLE ARC:
- two parallel arcuate lines separated by an anechoic space (bile)
  1. proximal curvilinear line = wall of GB
  2. distal echogenic curvilinear line = surface of gallstones
- second arc is followed by acoustic shadowing
- can be mimicked by barium-filled bowel, calcified GB wall, air in the biliary tree

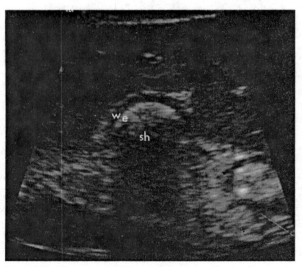

W = GB wall; e = echo/stone; sh = acoustic shadow

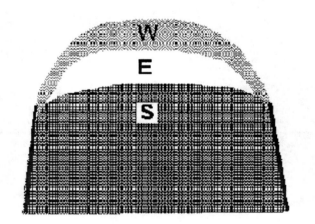

B) PHYSIOLOGY

GALLBLADDER AND BILE FUNCTION	
BILE	• bile salts are formed in hepatic cells from cholesterol • 1–1.5 liters produced daily as a direct secretory product of liver • stored in GB
CONTENT	• water, bile salts, bilirubin, cholesterol, fatty acids, lecithin, electrolytes (e.g., sodium, potassium) • water and electrolytes are reabsorbed by the GB in the concentration process, which causes the bile to become highly concentrated
FUNCTION OF BILE	• aids in digestion by: accelerating the action of pancreatic enzymes breaking up or emulsifying large particles of fatty acids, monoglycerides, cholesterol, and other lipids into smaller globules in the small intestine
CHANGES IN BILE	sludge • occurs when bile crystallizes in GB due to an upset in biologic chemical balances stones • can form within bile
FUNCTION OF GB	1. CONCENTRATION OF BILE • water and salt ions are absorbed by GB mucosa • bile concentrates mostly by the active transport of sodium through the GB epithelium • bile is normally concentrated about 5-fold to a maximum of 12–20-fold 2. STORAGE OF BILE • bile is secreted continually by liver cells and is normally stored in the GB until needed in the duodenum • when small bowel is empty, the ampulla of Vater closes and the backed up bile overflows into the cystic duct and GB 3. DISBURSING BILE • high concentration of fats or partially digested proteins stimulates the intestinal mucosa to secrete the hormone cholecystokinin (CCK) • GB contracts in response to CCK • when fat is not in the meal, the GB empties poorly • CCK is responsible for: contraction of the GB muscularis to force bile into CBD relaxation of the sphincter of Oddi/hepatopancreatic ampulla increasing bile flow from liver

C) LAB TESTS

PRINCIPLE	INTERPRETATION	
BILIRUBIN • is the end product of the natural breakdown of red blood cells (RBCs) • measurement of concentration of bilirubin, which is the predominant pigment in bile	DIRECT INCREASED VALUES • extrahepatic obstruction (e.g., gallstones, carcinoma of GB, bile duct or pancreas, biliary fistula) • bile duct disease • intrahepatic disruption (e.g., hepatitis, cirrhosis)	INDIRECT INCREASED VALUES • hemolysis • RBC degradation • abnormal hepatocellular uptake (e.g., hepatitis)
LEUKOCYTES (White Blood Cell [WBC] Count) • measures reaction of body to infection	INCREASED VALUES • acute and chronic cholecystitis • injury to bile ducts • internal biliary fistula or retained bile duct stones	
ALKALINE PHOSPHATASE (ALP) • enzyme produced in liver and secreted through bile ducts	INCREASED VALUES • biliary obstruction	

D) ANOMALIES

GALLBLADDER ANOMALY	US APPEARANCE

CARCINOMA OF GALLBLADDER
 	
1. <u>PRIMARY CARCINOMA</u>
• GB carcinoma is most common biliary tree malignancy (although cancer of pancreas is most common tumor to obstruct biliary system)
• most common site is fundus and neck
• can be associated with stones, calcified GB wall
• chronic cholecystitis may lead to GB carcinoma
• more frequently seen in elderly women
 	
SS
• asymptotic or
• nausea, vomiting, intolerance to fatty foods
 	
2. <u>METASTATIC DISEASE TO GB</u>
• focal GB wall thickening in association with nonshadowing intraluminal soft tissue masses
• primaries that metastasize to GB are:
  direct: stomach, pancreas, bile ducts
  indirect: lung, kidneys, esophagus, melanoma (most common)
 	
SS
• RUQ pain, anorexia, nausea, vomiting
• obstructive jaundice when infiltration of biliary ducts occurs
• cholangitis
 	
US FOR CARCINOMA
• findings depend on the size, character of tumor, and extent of spread
• gallstones within a mass are suspicious of carcinoma of GB
 	
<u>Early Findings:</u>
• loss of smooth border of GB
• cholelithiasis (in primary carcinoma)
  Infiltrating type:
   • localized or diffuse GB wall thickening
  Fungating type:
   • polypoid lesion with irregular borders growing into lumen
 	
<u>Later Findings:</u>
• complex, echogenic solid mass filling GB with no bile filling lumen
• mass that shadows, but is not mobile
• diffusely irregular GB wall
• infiltration of liver by tumor
	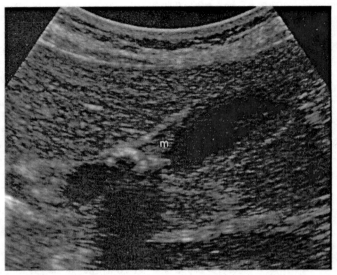
	Stones adjacent to GB mass (m)
	
	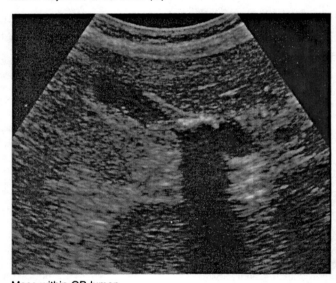
	Mass within GB lumen

US APPEARANCE

Doppler:
• infiltration of the tumor into the portal trunk causes a high-velocity, turbulent Doppler signal

Diff. Dx.: Tumors versus sludge
• lack of blood flow does not completely help the differential because no flow can occur in hypovascular tumors and in tumefactive sludge

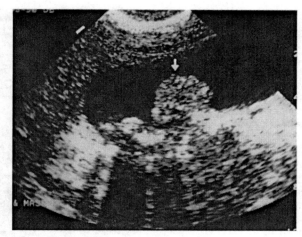

Primary carcinoma (arrow) in GB

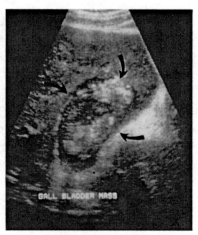

Heterogeneous mass representing GB carcinoma

GALLBLADDER ANOMALY	US APPEARANCE

CHOLECYSTITIS
• acute or chronic inflammation of GB

ACUTE
1. ACALCULOUS CHOLECYSTITIS (5% of acute cholecystitis)
• represents acute or chronic GB inflammation in the absence of stones
• thought to develop because of ischemic compromise to GB
• causes include infection, pancreatic reflux, trauma, sepsis
• many untreated cases progress to gangrene and GB rupture

SS
• positive sonographic Murphy's sign (when the probe is directly over the GB the patient has the most tenderness)
• nonvisualization of GB on nuclear medicine lidofenin (HIDA) scan
• usually occurs in critically ill patients

US
• enlarged GB with diffuse or focal wall thickening
• focal hypoechoic regions in wall
• sludge and debris with **no** calculi
• pericholecystic fluid

2. CALCULOUS CHOLECYSTITIS (95% of acute cholecystitis)
• acute inflammation of the GB caused by obstruction of the GB neck or cystic duct by a stone
• acute onset is usually precipitated by a meal containing fat, when the GB, which is contracting vigorously, expels a stone into the cystic duct

SS
• positive sonographic Murphy's sign (focal tenderness over GB to transducer pressure)
• RUQ pain radiating to shoulder, nausea, vomiting, leukocytosis, mild fever, anorexia

US
• tense, rounded, enlarged GB (transverse diameter > 5 cm)
• subserosal edema creating a halo sign (inner hyperechoic layer of lamina propria muscle + hypoechoic outer layer of edema in subserosa)
• pericholecystic fluid
• thickened GB wall (> 4–5 mm)
• cholelithiasis/sludge/echogenic bile (pus and fibrin)
• stone impacted in cystic duct or neck of GB

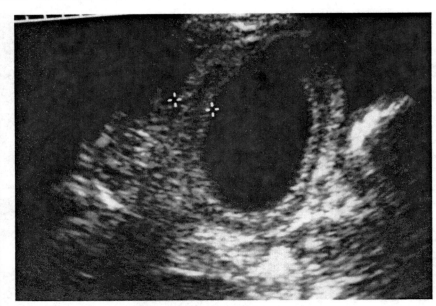

Acalculous cholecystitis: thick wall between calipers

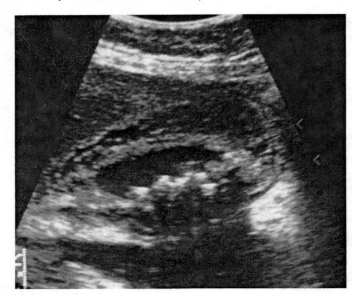

Acute cholecystitis

ANOMALY	US APPEARANCE
CHRONIC • inflammation over a longer period of time with or without repeated bouts of acute cholecystitis • associated with gallstones 90% of time SS • intolerant to fatty foods, nausea, belching, epigastric distress • GB is not usually tender US • GB can be contracted, normal or enlarged in size • thickened GB wall, but usually less than 5 times normal size • Rokitansky-Aschoff sinuses showing ringdown artifact are seen • 90% have stones	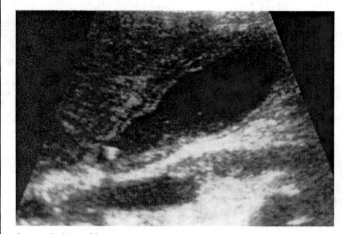 Acute cholecystitis 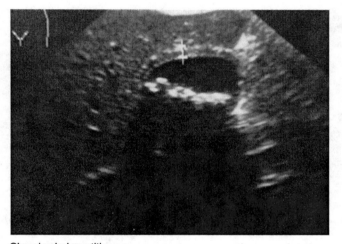 Chronic cholecystitis
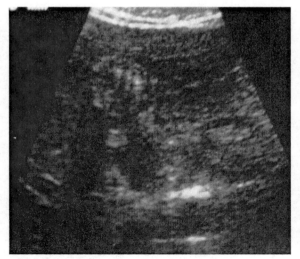 Chronic cholecystitis	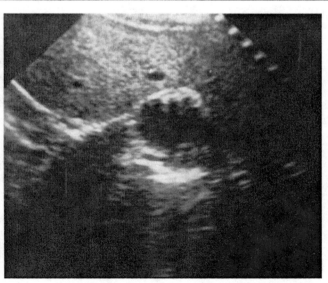 Rokitansky-Aschoff sinuses showing ringdown artifact are seen

COMPLICATIONS OF CHOLECYSTITIS	DESCRIPTION	US FINDINGS
EMPHYSEMATOUS CHOLECYSTITIS	• caused by ischemia and occurs more often in diabetics • tends to occur in elderly men or debilitated people • not associated with gallstones • gas develops because of infection with gas-forming organisms • can occur in lumen or wall • can perforate	• acoustic shadowing from gas/air in GB wall • rare findings include gas bubbles arising from GB wall • may have ringdown artifact • gas in bile ducts
EMPYEMA	• GB that becomes more pus filled • complication of acute cholecystitis • leads to pericholecystic abscess • usually have gallstones • 75% progress to gangrene and 25% perforate	• GB wall markedly thickened • edema, fluid exudate, hemorrhage surrounding GB • echogenic debris within GB
GANGRENOUS CHOLECYSTITIS	• wall undergoes hemorrhage, necrosis and develops microabscesses • ulcerations perforate wall causing abscess and/or generalized peritonitis SS • RUQ pain, tenderness, fever, leukocytosis, palpable GB	• patchy, necrotic appearance of wall • pericholecystic abscess • thickened GB wall • stones or fine gravel
PERFORATION	• occurs in 8%–12% of patients with acute cholecystitis • common site is fundus • occurs due to obstruction of the cystic duct, which produces mucosal injury, edema, congestion and circulatory compromise of the wall, which leads to gangrene and perforation	• pericholecystic abscess/fluid collection seen as: encapsulated abscess—a well defined band of low-level echos around GB extensive abscess—poorly defined hypoechoic mass surrounding an indistinct GB
PERICHOLECYSTIC ABSCESS	• serious complication of cholecystitis • develops after GB perforation • associated with acute symptoms	• anechoic to complex collection encircling GB which may contain air/gas
PORCELAIN GALLBLADDER	• extensive calcification of GB wall • associated with cholelithiasis and chronic inflammation • etiology is controversial with several theories in literature • ASSOCIATED WITH SIGNIFICANT RISK OF GB CARCINOMA	• echogenic walls with shadow • hyperechoic semilunar structure with a posterior acoustic shadow in the GB fossa

COMPLICATIONS OF CHOLECYSTITIS (*Continued*)	DESCRIPTION	US FINDINGS
XANTHOGRANULOMATOUS CHOLECYSTITIS	• rare condition • shrunken, nodular GB • chronically inflamed with focal areas of necrosis and hemorrhage	• differential includes carcinoma of GB • small irregularly shaped inhomogenous GB

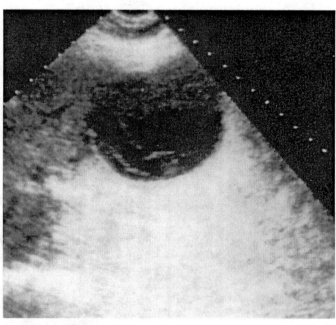

Gangrenous GB

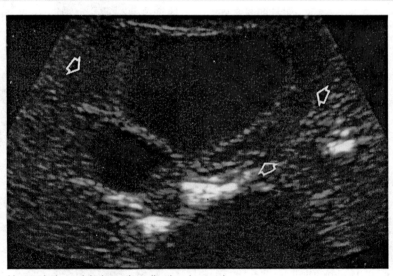

Hypoechoic pericholecystic collection (arrows)

GALLBLADDER ANOMALY	US APPEARANCE

CHOLELITHIASIS (GALLSTONES)

- stones form when cholesterol concentrations in GB are greater than the ability of bile to make them soluble
- cholesterol can crystallize and coalesce into stones
- important factors affecting gallstone formation are:
  abnormal bile composition
  stasis
  infection
  hypersecretion of biliary cholesterol
- types and composition:
  cholesterol stones: cholesterol
  pigment stones: bilirubin calcium salts
- high association with carcinoma of GB
- increased prevalence with age and for women
- for women risk factors include age, weight, number of children

SS
- can be asymptomatic
- RUQ pain ("colic") occurs because of obstruction of the gallstones in the biliary tree or GB

Treatment
- medications, shock wave lithotripsy, cholecystectomy

US
- echogenic focus with acoustic shadow
- if > 3 mm will cause acoustic shadowing
- stone should be gravity dependent
- WES sign (see section F)

Pitfalls:
1. stone does not move:
   impacted stone in neck will have no apparent change in its position
2. Other causes of acoustic shadowing in GB:
   spiral valves of Heister
   edge effect artifact at periphery of wall due to refraction of sound
   junctional fold
   loop of bowel
3. Other intraluminal echos without shadow:
Mobile:
   viscous bile, sludge, blood, pus, ascaris
Not mobile:
   polyps, tumor, GB folds, cholesterosis, adenomyomatosis
4. Causes for low-level echos in GB
   sludge
   cholesterol crystals
   multiple small stones
   pus, mucus
   parasites

Helpful Hints:
- to be almost 100% accurate for stones, make sure that the echogenic foci with shadow within the GB are imaged in two planes at right angles to each other
- look for "clean" shadow from the foci, compared to shadow from bowel gas, which contains reverberation echos
- turn and scan the patient erect to visualize gallstones that can lie hidden in a dependent portion of the GB
- having the patient cough can help make stones roll into a more visible area

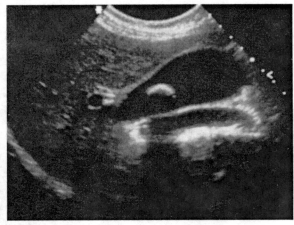

Single stone with shadow

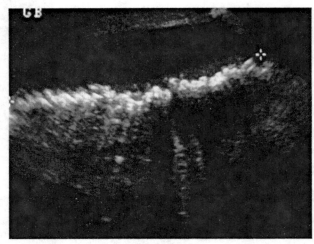

Sagittal GB: multiple stones with shadows

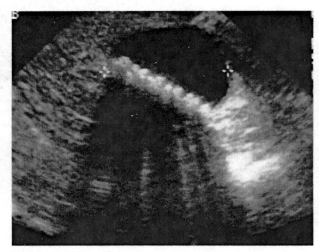

Transverse GB: multiple stones

US APPEARANCE

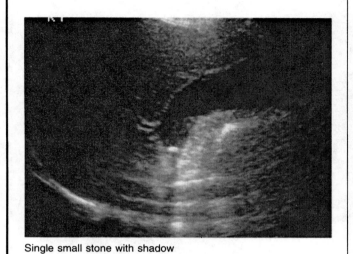

Single small stone with shadow

Single large stone filling GB lumen

GALLBLADDER ANOMALY	US APPEARANCE

CONGENITAL ANOMALIES
- many types with varied clinical significance:
  atresia
  total reduplication (duplicated/bifid GB)
  partial subdivision
  diverticula of GB

US
duplicated GB appears as two parallel pear-shaped cystic structures in GB fossa

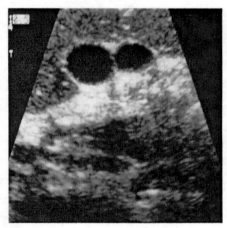

Transverse

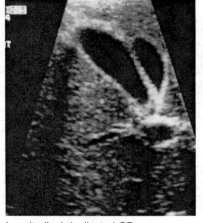

Longitudinal duplicated GB

GALLBLADDER ANOMALY	US APPEARANCE

ENLARGED GALLBLADDER

1. COURVOISIER'S GB
- obstruction of CBD by pressure from outside of the biliary system
- produces a distended GB
- caused by such pathology as pancreatic carcinoma

SS
- painless jaundice
- palpable GB due to acute distention

2. HYDROPIC GB
- complete blockage of cystic ducts causes hydrops or mucocele of the GB
- trapped bile is absorbed and replaced with a clear mucinous secretion from the lining of the GB

SS
- asymptomatic or
- epigastric pain, discomfort, nausea, vomiting
- palpable mass in RUQ

US
- dilated, tense GB, thin wall

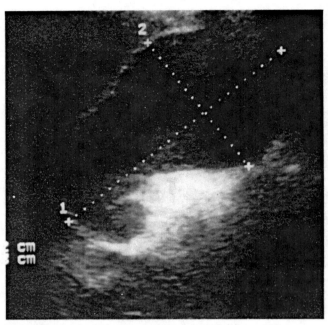

Enlarged GB measuring 12 cm in length

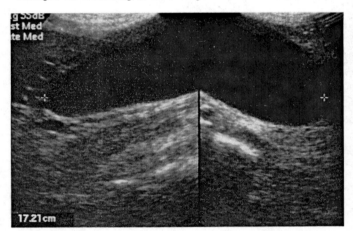

Enlarged GB: imaged using split screen gives an approximate length of 17 cm

GALLBLADDER ANOMALY	US APPEARANCE

SLUDGE

- echogenic bile
- stasis of bile in GB creates sludge
- no clinical significance
- occurs with:
  long periods of fasting
  alcoholism
  biliary obstruction
  patients receiving hyperalimentation

<u>1. PSEUDOSLUDGE</u>
- artifact created by beam averaging effect or partial volume phenomenon at diverging portion of ultrasound beam
- occurs usually in posterior GB and is difficult to distinguish from true sludge

<u>2. SLUDGE</u>
- nonshadowing low-amplitude echos that layer in the dependent part of the GB
- creates a fluid-fluid level

<u>3. SLUDGE BALLS/TUMEFACTIVE SLUDGE</u>
- echogenic sludge forms in the shape of a ball, stone, or mass
- occurs with long duration obstruction
- can resemble tumors
- lack of blood flow does not help the differential because no flow can occur in hypovascular tumors and in tumefactive sludge

US
- nonshadowing low-amplitude echos that layer in the dependent portion of the GB
- forms fluid-fluid layer that moves slowly when the patient changes position

<u>Helpful Hint:</u>
- sludge should be described as "viscous bile" in the absence of any sonographic evidence of a disease process

<u>Diff. Dx.:</u>
hematobile, blood, stone, tumor, polyp

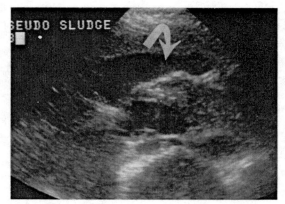

Pseudosludge (arrow)

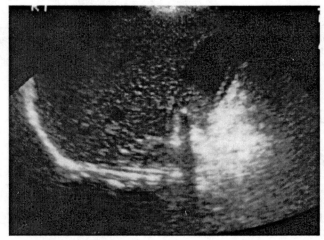

Sludge (stone within it)

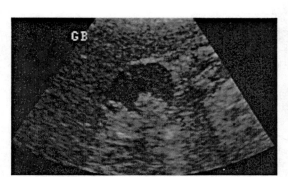

Tumefactive sludge

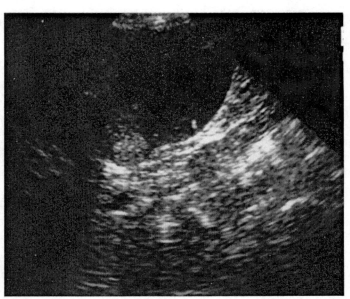

Sludge ball

GALLBLADDER WALL ANOMALY wall thickness varies with transducer placement and angulation	US DESCRIPTION
ADENOMA • benign epithelial tumor • histologically similar to bowel wall polyp	• pedunculated or sessile less than 1 cm diameter • are not mobile, and do not create a shadow <u>Diff. Dx.:</u> • carcinoma
ADENOMYOMATOSIS (HYPERPLASTIC CHOLECYSTOSES) • hyperplasia of epithelial and muscular layers of GB wall • outpouching of mucosa that extend into underlying connective tissue and sometimes into muscular layer • types: diffuse—entire GB involved segmental—proximal, middle, or distal third involved localized—most common type where it is confined usually to fundus SS • asymptomatic	• nonspecific focal or diffuse GB wall thickening • focal thickening occurs most commonly at the fundus • can get ringdown artifact from wall secondary to glandular elements in the muscle
CHOLESTEROLOSIS/CHOLESTEROL POLYP • a disturbance in cholesterol metabolsim causes an accumulation of triglycerides and cholesterol in lamina propria of GB wall • cholesterol nodules give GB strawberry appearance (not seen sonographically) causing multiple thickened mucosal plaques • can break off and become a nidus for stones • collection of cholesterol-filled macrophages can cause an elevation called a cholesterol polyp	Diffuse: • generally not seen on ultrasound Focal: • individual polyps, which are club shaped, and may be projecting into lumen of GB • usually have no shadowing
GENERALIZED WALL THICKNESS • wall thickness has been noted with many pathologies such as cholecystitis, hepatitis, ascites, alcoholic liver disease, hypoproteinemia, hypoalbuminemia, heart failure, renal disease, GB carcinoma	• increase in thickness of GB wall $\geq$ 4 mm

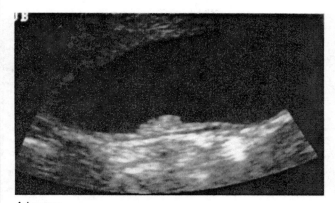

Adenoma

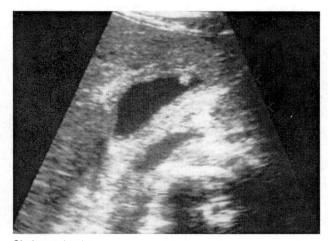

Cholesterol polyp

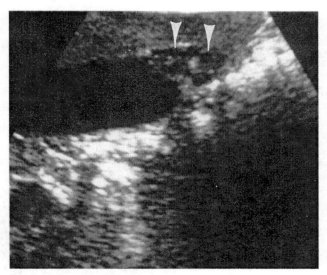

Focal adenomyomatosis

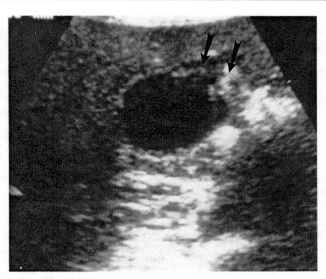

Focal adenomyomatosis in transverse GB

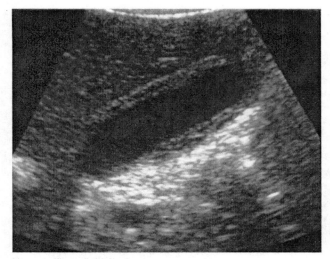

Nonspecific wall thickening

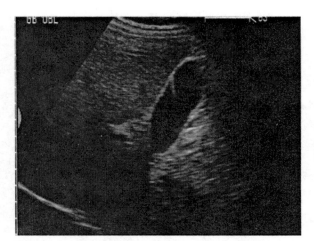

Comet-tail artifact emanates from possible cholesterol crystals in wall of GB (Courtesy of Chedoke-McMaster Hospital, Hamilton)

GALLBLADDER APPEARANCE DIFFERENTIAL

GALLBLADDER SIZE	TOO LARGE	TOO SMALL
	prolonged fasting IV hyperalimentation obstruction of cystic duct obstruction of distal CBD (Courvoisier's GB)	nonfasting GB congenital hypoplasia chronic cholecystitis biliary obstruction at level of CHD hepatitis
THICK GALLBLADDER WALL (> 3 mm)	BILIARY	NONBILIARY
	adenomyomatosis AIDS cholangiopathy carcinoma of GB cholecystitis contracted normal GB GB torsion GB tumor sclerosing cholangitis	ascites cirrhosis (ETOH disease) congestive heart failure hepatitis hypoproteinemia (hypoalbuminemia) infectious mononucleosis lymphatic obstruction multiple myeloma pancreatitis portal hypertension renal disease technical (inappropriate time-gain compensation [TGC] settings)
NONVISUALIZATION OF GALLBLADDER	calcification of the GB wall (porcelain GB) carcinoma of GB cholecystitis: emphysematous/gangrenous chronic cholecystitis filled with stones contracted nonfasting GB	ectopic: superficial/congenital absence obscured by bowel gas postcholecystectomy technical factors (obese, immobile patient)
DIFFERENTIAL FOR GALLBLADDER MASSES	COMMON	UNCOMMON
	adenomyomatosis GB carcinoma polyps tumefactive sludge	metastases chronic cholecystitis
GALLBLADDER FOSSA SHADOWING	air in biliary tree and/or GB wall bowel loop overlapping cholelithiasis edge artifact	GB wall abnormalities liver pathology junctional folds/spiral valves of Heister porcelain GB
CAUSES OF PERICHOLECYSTIC FLUID	abscess acute cholecystitis AIDS	ascites pancreatitis peritonitis
STRUCTURES MIMICKING GALLBLADDER	cysts: hepatic, omental, choledochal, renal enlarged cystic duct fluid-filled bowel loops	

E) TECHNICAL FACTORS

TRANSDUCER	3.5–5 MHz
PATIENT PREPARATION	• essential that patient fasts Infants and neonates: 4-hour fast Children: 6-hour fast Adults: 8-hour fast • contraction and collapse of the GB after eating makes it difficult to localize and evaluate sonographically
SCAN PLANES	• longitudinal and transverse scan planes • patient in supine, lying on left side, upright • several scan planes are obtained of the GB and bile duct system • full arrested inspiration can help bring the GB into view Patient positions: • GB should be examined in more than one patient position for many reasons: so that stones that are "hiding" can roll into view can help distinguish pseudo from real sludge check stone's mobility (see below) move bowel gas from region of GB
MINIMUM PROTOCOL	• regions of neck and fundus of GB • GB wall thickness • presence or absence of intraluminal foci • CBD
HELPFUL HINTS	Acoustic shadowing: • stone will not shadow if ultrasound beam is larger than stone • to demonstrate shadow try the following: decrease gain or power adjust focus to area of interest increase transducer frequency change position of patient so stones can gather together increasing the reflective surface Nonmobile stones: • several different approaches must be tried before documenting a stone nonmobile • have patient move from supine into several different positions such as both decubitis and upright • sometimes the stones move very slowly, so make sure you allow sufficient time • have the patient cough a few times as that can help to move the stone

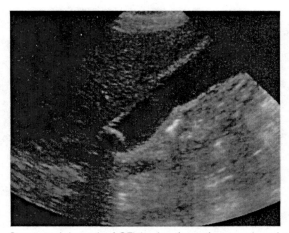 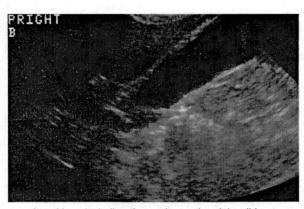

Stone stuck in neck of GB: having the patient cough and move into several positions including the supine and upright, did not dislodge the stone from the neck of the GB

CHAPTER 5 - GASTROINTESTINAL TRACT
A) NORMAL ANATOMY AND SONOGRAPHIC APPEARANCE

DEFINITION	• alimentary tract begins at the gastroesophageal junction and ends at the rectum • consists of the esophagus, stomach, small and large bowel

STRUCTURE

1. ESOPHAGUS
• hollow, highly distendible mainly muscular tube that extends from the pharynx to the gastroesophageal junction
• lined with squamous epithelium centrally

STOMACH
2. CARDIA
• surrounds lower esophageal sphincter

3. FUNDUS
• rounded portion superior and to left of cardia

4. BODY
• large central portion below fundus
a) Lesser curvature
• concave medial border of stomach
• two layers of visceral peritoneum (serosa) come together here and extend upward to liver as lesser omentum
b) Greater curvature
• convex lateral border of stomach
• two layers of visceral peritoneum (serosa) come together here and continue downward as greater omentum hanging over the intestines

5. PYLORUS
• distal aspect of stomach

SMALL BOWEL
6. DUODENUM
• shortest, widest and most fixed part
• originates at pyloric sphincter and merges with jejunum
  Segment 1—pylorus to superior duodenal flexure (cap)
  Segment 2—superior to inferior duodenal flexure
• major and minor papilla insert at this location
  Segment 3—horizontal inferior aspect
• Segment 4—ascending portion to ligament of Treitz

7. JEJUNUM
• extends from the small bowel at the region of the ligament of Treitz to the ileum

8. ILEUM
• longest portion of small bowel
• joins large intestine at ileocecal sphincter

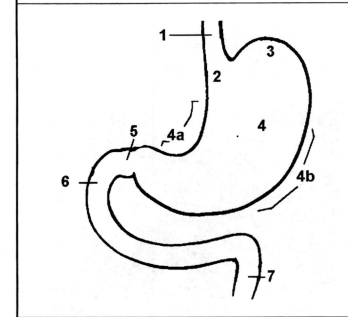

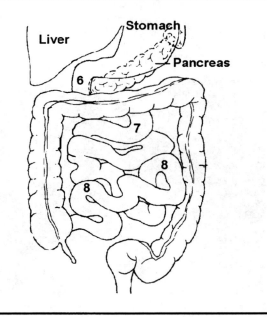

56

STRUCTURE

LARGE BOWEL AND APPENDIX
• 1.5 meters long from ileum to anus

1. ILEOCECAL SPHINCTER
• fold of mucous membrane that acts as a valve allowing materials from the small intestine to pass into the large intestine

2. CECUM
• blind pouch of bowel hanging below ileocecal valve

3. APPENDIX
• tubular structure attached to cecum

4. MESOAPPENDIX
• visceral peritoneum of appendix that attaches it to the inferior part of the ileum and posterior abdominal wall

5. ASCENDING COLON
• colon that ascends on the right side of abdomen

6. HEPATIC FLEXURE
• point at which at underside of liver colon turns abruptly to the left

7. TRANSVERSE COLON
• colon across the abdomen

8. SPLENIC FLEXURE
• point at which transverse colon curves to pass downward

9. DESCENDING COLON
• colon that descends on left side of abdomen

10. SIGMOID COLON
• begins at left iliac crest and projects inward to midline and terminates as the rectum

11. RECTUM
• last 20 cm of colon ending in anal canal

12. HAUSTRA
• series of pouches created by contractions of muscular wall give the colon its puckered appearance

13. ANAL CANAL
• terminal 2–3 cm of rectum

14. MESOCOLON
• also known as colonic mesentery

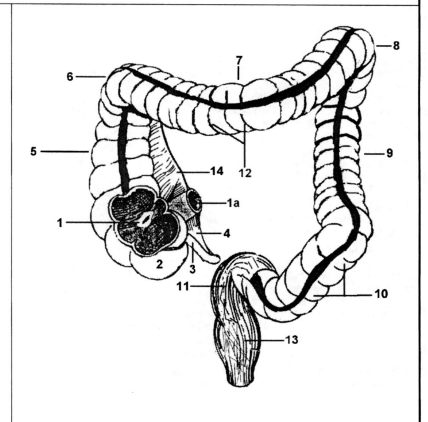

INTESTINAL WALL

• 4 layers in GI tract

1. MUCOSA/MUCOUS MEMBRANE
• inner linning
a) Epithelium lining
• glands that are in direct contact with contents of GI tract that protect and secrete
b) Lamina propria
• an underlying loose connective tissue that supports the epithelium and provides it with blood and lymph supply
c) Muscularis mucosa
d) Plicae circulares/circular folds/rugae of mucosa
• numerous folds or ridges in mucosa that further increase surface area
• flatten when gut is distended
• extend from pylorus to ileocecal valve

2. SUBMUCOSA
• loose connective tissue that binds mucosa to muscular layers
• contains blood vessels, lymphatics, nerve fibers and glands

3. MUSCULARIS PROPRIA
• smooth muscle found in two sheets
a) inner layer of circular fibers
b) outer layer of longitudinal fibers
• stomach has third sheet called the:
c) inner oblique layer (circular layer becomes the middle layer)
• when it contracts it breaks down food physically, mixes it with digestive secretions, and propels it through the tract
• contains major nerve supply to alimentary tract

4. SEROSA/ADVENTITIA/VISCERAL PERITONEUM
• outermost layer of serous membrane composed of connective tissue and epithelium
• forms portion of peritoneum

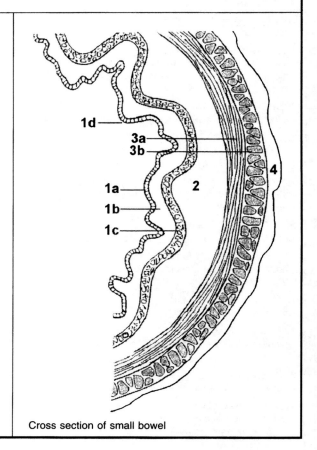

Cross section of small bowel

SIZE AND LOCATION

WALL SIZE	• measured from innermost echogenic layer to outermost echogenic layer			
	STOMACH	SMALL BOWEL	APPENDIX	LARGE BOWEL
Distended	3–5 mm	≤ 3 mm	< 2 mm	≤ 5 mm
Nondistended	3 mm	5 mm		
LOCATION	• directly under diaphragm in epigastric, umbilical, and left hypochondriac regions	• begins at pyloric sphincter of stomach, coils through the central and lower part of the abdominal cavity and opens into large intestine	• right iliac fossa	• extends from ileum to anus • attached to posterior abdominal wall by mesocolon of visceral peritoneum

SONOGRAPHIC ANATOMY

• normal bowel is compressible

GUT "SIGNATURE"

• usual appearance is that of a "bull's eye" or a echogenic mucosa and serosa surrounding the echolucent muscle

LAYER	POSITION	HISTOLOGIC LAYER	SONOGRAPHIC APPEARANCE
1	innermost layer closest to lumen	• superficial mucosa ± luminal content/mucosal interface	echogenic
2	↓	• deep mucosa + muscularis mucosa	hypoechoic
3	↓ central layer	• submucosa + submucosa/muscularis propria interface	echogenic
4	↓	muscularis propria	hypoechoic
5	outermost layer	• serosa + subserosal fat + marginal interface	echogenic

STOMACH	SMALL BOWEL	LARGE BOWEL

Esophageal gastric junction
• "target" or "bull's eye" structure lying anterior to aorta, caudal to diaphragm, and posterior to left lobe of liver
Gastric antrum
• target structure midline, inferior to liver
Gastric fundus
• round cystic structure in upper left quadrant
• can mimic cystic mass adjacent to spleen
  Layers
  Transabdominal scanning demonstrates 2 layers
1. mucosa and submucosa = inner echogenic layer
2. gastric muscle = outer hypoechoic layer
  Intraoperative high-frequency scanning demonstrates 5 layers of gut signature
 	
Reminder:
• not well seen unless distended with water or contrast agents
	• normally not well visualized sonographically
	• when fluid filled, appears as a tubular structure in long-axis view and as a target structure in cross section
	• peristalsis, air, or fluid content movement can be noted
	• normal loops are compressible
	• Duodenum
	  2nd portion—lateral to head of pancreas
	  3rd portion—anterior to aorta, IVC
	  4th portion—left to aorta adjacent to pancreas
		• haustral markings 3–5 cm apart
		• peristalsis can be noted
		• usually filled with gas and feces, which makes sonographic evaluation difficult
		• anterior aspect of bowel wall can often be seen and evaluated for thickness

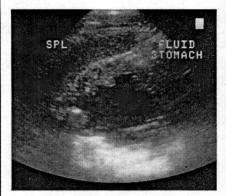

Left longitudinal scan showing the normal relationship of the spleen and stomach. The stomach contains fluid and some food giving it the appearance of a mass.

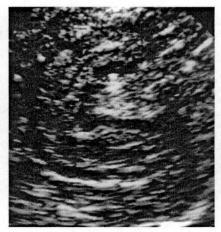

Normal bowel: note layers of bowel as described above

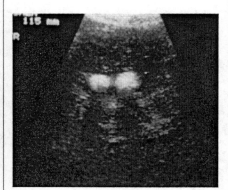

Fecaliths: incidental finding during abdominal sonogram; two fecaliths (fecal concretion) within fluid-filled loop of bowel

B) PHYSIOLOGY

DIGESTION	• all the chemical and mechanical phases from the mouth to small intestine are designed toward altering food into forms that can advance through the epithelial cells of the mucosa into underlying blood and lymph vessels		
	STOMACH	SMALL BOWEL	LARGE BOWEL
PURPOSE	• storage of food until it is accommodated in the duodenum • mixing of food with gastric secretions until it forms a semifluid mixture called chyme • slow emptying of chyme into small intestine	• receives chyme from stomach and breaks it down further by mechanical and enzymatic digestion • absorption of nutrients	• absorption of water, minerals, vitamins that pass to liver via portal vein • formation and expulsion of feces
OPERATION MECHANICAL	• peristaltic movements (mixing waves) macerate and mix food with gastric gland secretions reducing food to chyme • secretes a compound that influences the absorption of vitamin B_{12} from small intestine • mixing waves force some of food through pyloric sphincter into duodenum	• two main types of movements: 1. Segmentation • mixing contractions in areas containing food, which pushes chyme in contact with mucosa for absorption • bowel's long length and circular folds provide a large surface area for digestion 2. Peristalsis • propulsion moves chyme onward through intestinal tract	• movements of colon begin when substances enter through ileocecal valve • two main methods: 1. Haustral churning • mixing movement that involves relaxation and contraction of the walls that squeeze the contents into the next haustrum 2. Propulsive (mass) movement • modified type of peristalsis that occurs only a few times each day
CHEMICAL	• secreted substances include: enzyme pepsin hydrochloric acid mucus hormone gastrin intrinsic factor gastric lipase	Absorption • intestinal juice (water, enzymes, and mucus) is rapidly reabsorbed by villi • substances from chyme are absorbed when they come in contact with villi • aided by secretions from pancreas and liver (via GB)	1. Absorption and secretion of water and electrolytes • chyme becomes solid to semisolid after 3–10 hours in colon secondary to water resorption 2. Secretion • mucus is secreted by colon glands 3. Bacterial action • bacteria digest small amounts of cellulose • involved in formation of vitamins and gases

C) LAB TESTS

BLOOD STUDIES
• damaged organs release specific and non-specific enzymes and products into the blood

GASTRIN
• measures the blood level of a hormone that stimulates intestinal movement and the secretion of digestive juices
• evaluates acute and chronic peptic ulcer disease

SERUM AMYLASE
• evaluates intestinal obstruction, perforated ulcers, pancreatitis

FECES
• examined chemically and microscopically for presence of blood, fat, bile, and parasites

FECAL BLOOD
• Upper GI tract
  ulcer, gastritis, esophageal varicies, esophagitis
• Small and large bowel
  Meckel's diverticulum, polyps, infectious diarrhea, inflammatory bowel diseases, diverticular disease, carcinoma, ulcers
• Rectum and anus
  hemorrhoids, anorectal fissure

FECAL FAT
• malabsorption
• pancreatitis

D) ANOMALIES

ANOMALY	US APPEARANCE

APPENDICEAL MUCOCELE
• accumulation of mucus within an abnormally distended appendix
• occurs from:
  1. mucosal hyperplasia
  2. mucinous cystadenoma (most common form)
  3. cystadenocarcinoma
• histologically these mimic their ovarian counterparts
• pseudomyxoma peritonei can occur with perionteal implants of mucinous adenocarcinoma, which can cause the peritoneal cavity to become distended
 	
US
• depends on internal characteristics of lesion
• vary from purely cystic to hypoechoic mass
 	
Pseudomyxoma Peritonei
• similar appearance to ascites but may have septations and complex echos within
• bowel loops depressed by mucus rather than floating in it
 	
Diff. Dx.:
• ovarian cysts and neoplasms
• inflammatory bowel disease
• small or large bowel neoplasm
• pelvic inflammatory masses
	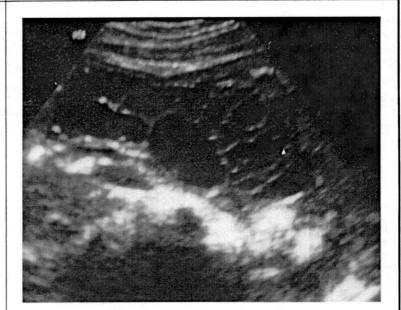
	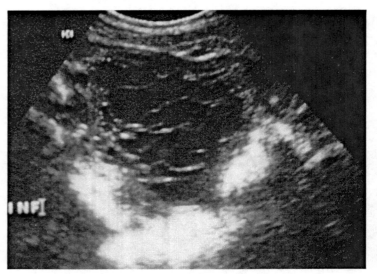

ANOMALY	US APPEARANCE

APPENDICITIS

- inflammation of the vermiform appendix due to obstruction of its lumen by fecal material, lymphoid hypertrophy, tumor, ascaris, appendicolith (stone)
- can occur at any age, but more prevalent in young adults
- if left untreated can result in edema, ischemia, gangrene, and perforation
- rupture causes peritonitis

SS
- pain: first periumbilical but then localizing to the right lower quadrant
- nausea or vomiting, mild fever, ↑ WBC

US
- same findings in children and adults
- total appendix measures > 6 mm in cross-sectional diameter
- wall thickness > 3 mm
- inflamed appendix appears as a:
  noncompressible, blind-end lumen arising from cecum
  target appearance in cross section
  nonperistaltic tubular structure
- may have small amount of periappendiceal fluid, mild cecal or terminal ileum thickening

<u>1. APPENDICOLITHS</u>
- calculi in the appendix
- they can obstruct the appendiceal lumen resulting in acute appendicitis

US
- appear as a persistent echogenic structure with shadowing within the appendix

<u>2. APPENDICEAL ABSCESS</u>
- perforation of an inflamed appendix occurs in almost half of cases
- results usually in a localized walled-off abscess
- free intraperitoneal spill can occur causing acute peritonitis

US
- complex mass in right iliac fossa area surrounded by enlarged appendix
- fecalith or gas bubbles contained within may cause echogenic echos with or without shadowing
- free fluid adjacent to cecum

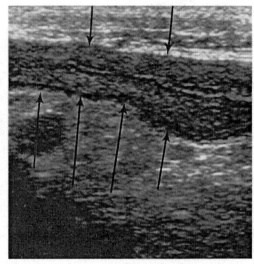

Inflamed appendix (Courtesy of Chedoke-McMaster Hospital, Hamilton)

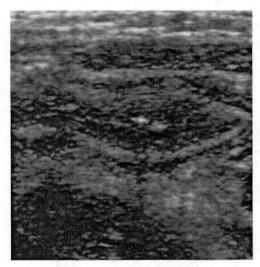

Appendicitis with shadowing appendicoliths

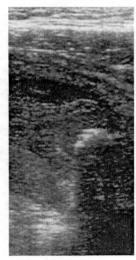

Inflamed appendix with fecolith

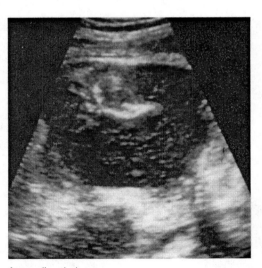

Appendiceal abscess

ANOMALY	US APPEARANCE

DIVERTICULAR DISEASE
- includes diverticulosis and diverticulitis
- condition of advancing years
- main cause is a low-fiber diet
- can occur anywhere in ailmentary tract, but this section will focus on the most common location, which is the colon

1. DIVERTICULA
- small saclike outpouchings occur in the wall of colon
- factors important in their development are areas where the muscularis has become weak and increased intraluminal pressure
- pouch becomes a permanent pocket protruding through colon wall
- they are elastic, compressible, and easily emptied of fecal material
- most are located in the sigmoid colon

2. DIVERTICULOSIS
- development of diverticula

SS
- most people remain asymptomatic
- 20% develop cramping, lower abdominal pain, constipation, distention, blood loss

3. DIVERTICULAR ABSCESS
- occasionally diverticuli can perforate and cause an abscess that is usually small and adjacent to bowel wall

4. DIVERTICULITIS
- inflammation within diverticula due to obstruction or perforation
- progression of an infection may lead to abscess formation, sinus tracts, and occasionally peritonitis

US
- not seen sonographically in absence of inflammation
- circumferential or asymmetric thickening of bowel wall
- gas-filled diverticular abscesses appear as focal echogenic areas adjacent to colonic wall
- edematous fat surrounding diverticulitis, which has a similar appearance to a "thyroid in the abdomen"

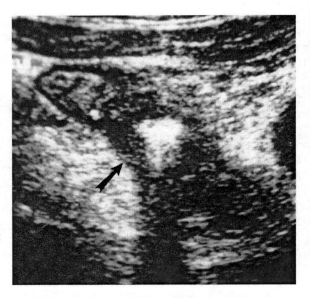

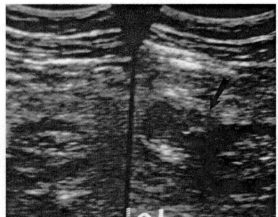

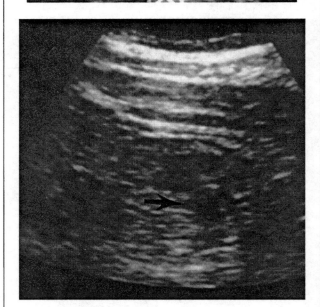

Diverticular abscess (arrows)

ANOMALY	US APPEARANCE

DUPLICATION CYSTS
 	
• uncommon
• occur anywhere along GI tract, but most common in distal ileum
• remnant defect of recanalization of GI tract or from faulty separation of primitive neurenteric canal during development
• do not communicate with bowel lumen but cause obstruction, usually within the 1st year of life due to compression of adjacent normal bowel
 	
SS
• abdominal mass
• nausea, vomiting, high intestinal obstruction
 	
US
• anechoic to relatively hypoechoic with low level echos or septations within
• small bowel duplication may be multiple
• 2 characteristic layers seen sonographically:
   echogenic mucosa
   echolucent muscular wall
• these two layers help to distinguish it from other types of cysts, such as omental and mesenteric cysts, which do not have this characteristic lining
• often occur on mesenteric border of bowel
 	
Diff. Dx.:
• GB, choledochal cyst, pseudocyst
	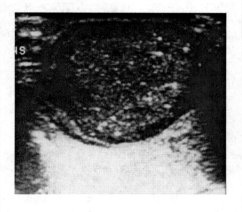

ANOMALY	US APPEARANCE
HYPERTROPHIC PYLORIC STENOSIS (HPS) • hypertrophy and hyperplasia of circular muscle, which causes the pylorus to elongate and constrict the pyloric canal • most common cause of gastric outlet obstruction in 1st month of life • congenital condition seen 3–4 times more commonly in males than females • familial tendency • acquired pyloric stenosis in adults is associated with chronic antral gastritis, peptic ulcers close to pylorus, inflammatory fibrosis, or malignant infiltration near pylorus **SS** • nonbilious, persistent, projectile vomiting in 2–3 week old infants • palpable abdominal mass (hypertrophied muscle) **US** • fluid distention of stomach, hyperperistalsis, poor stomach emptying • enlargement of the hypoechoic anteropyloric muscle (appears doughnut shaped) • failure of canal to distend to its normal caliber • peristaltic wave stops at pylorus Helpful Hints: • GB is a good landmark for pylorus location • HPS is unlikely with an empty stomach in the absence of vomiting or a nasogastric tube • a small amount of air or fluid can trickle through lumen, but it should never open up with HPS If negative: • if muscle measurement is normal, check position of superior mesenteric artery and vein for any malrotation • also check both kidneys for hydronephrosis • these two pathologies can cause similar symptoms to HPS Pitfalls: • overdistention of stomach increases patient discomfort and prevents optimal measurement of pylorus as it will displace the antrum and pylorus posteriorly • tangential scan planes may make the pyloric muscle appear artificially thickened Pseudothickening: • can occur related to antral pyloric spasm • wait and watch to see if it opens up • get image of pylorus while opening and take measurement from there • when wall measures in the borderline area of 2.5 mm this is often a cause Pylorus Specifications: • measure from base of echogenic mucosa to outer edge of muscle or serosal surface with transducer aligned on the long axis of the pyloric channel • suspect HPS when muscle > 3 mm or if pyloric channel is 17 mm or greater	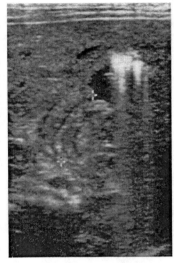 Length of pylorus at 16.6 mm 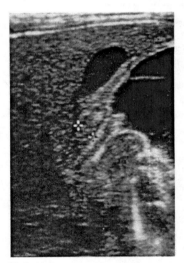 Wall thickness at 4 mm 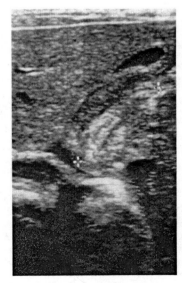 Length of pylorus at 22.5 mm

PARAMETER	NORMAL SIZE	ABNORMAL SIZE
Wall Thickness	< 3 mm	≥ 3 mm
Pyloric Length	≤ 16 mm	> 17 mm

ANOMALY	US APPEARANCE

INFLAMMATORY BOWEL DISEASE

- Etiology:
  idiopathic (Crohn's, ulcerative colitis, Bechet's disease)
  infectious
  iatrogenic (radiation)

1. CROHN'S DISEASE (ILEITIS/REGIONAL ENTERITIS/ GRANULOMATOUS ENTEROCOLITIS)

- recurrent inflammatory disease of bowel of unknown etiology
- creates granulomatous ulcers at any level of the alimentary tract
- prone to fistula and abscess formation
- complications include cholelithiasis, renal calculi, abscess collections, bowel obstructions, inflammation of adjacent abdominal organs (e.g., liver, ureters)
- occurs at any age, but peaks in the 2nd and 3rd decade of life
- females affected slightly more than males

SS
- diarrhea, abdominal cramps, rectal bleeding, fatigue, weight loss, low-grade fever
- these can be spaced by asymptotic weeks to months
- attacks may be precipitated by physical or emotional stress
- 20% of patients have an abrupt acute onset that may mimic acute appendicitis

US
- "donut sign" = thickened bowel wall that appears as a thick inhomogenous hypoehoic band (muscularis propria) surrounding an innermost echogenic core (air in compressed lumen)
- thickened small bowel or colonic wall appears hypoechoic due to edema
- matted bowel loops produce a large mass with irregular echos

Diff. Dx.:
- abscess
- tumor

2. ULCERATIVE COLITIS

- ulceroinflammatory disease limited to the colon
- chronic condition characterized by inflamed colon consisting of ulcerations, mucosal inflammation (not transmural), and microabscesses
- life-long condition that can range from mild to life-threatening
- more common among whites and females
- onset peaks between ages of 20 and 25
- can progress to carcinoma

SS
- relapsing disorder causing bloody mucoid diarrhea, lower abdominal pain, and cramps
- toxic megacolon (sudden cessation of bowel function with toxic dilatation) can occur in acute attacks
- often first attack is preceded by a stressful period in the patient's life and flare-ups may be precipitated by emotional or physical stress

US
- may have wall thickening
- wall stratification maintained compared to Crohn's

Diff. Dx.:
- bowel neoplasms

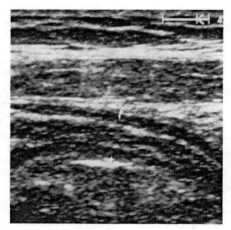

Thickened ileum (between calipers)

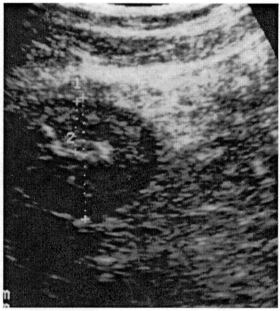

Thickened cecum

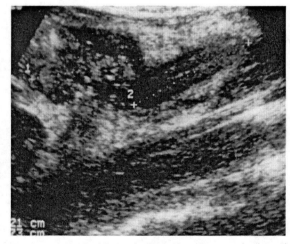

Thickened terminal ileum (caliper 2) and cecum (caliper 1)

COMPARISON OF CROHN'S DISEASE AND ULCERATIVE COLITIS

	CROHN'S DISEASE	ULCERATIVE COLITIS
BOWEL REGION	entire GI tract but most commonly involves terminal ileum and colon • small intestine alone 40% • small intestine & colon 30% • colon alone 30%	confined to colon
DISTRIBUTION	skip lesions (areas of normal mucosa between inflamed bowel) as different bowel segments may be affected	contiguous colonic involvement beginning in rectum to involve entire colon (pancolitis)
FISTULA	common	rare
RECTUM INVOLVEMENT	50%	95%
ANAL AREA	perianal fistulas and fissures	normal
TERMINAL ILEUM PROBLEMS	narrowed, inflamed, fissured	dilated and open
RESPONSE TO SURGERY	fair/poor and may worsen disease	removal cures disease
RISK FOR CANCER	no increase	high risk

MALIGNANCIES

- abdominal sonography is not the method of choice when investigating suspected bowel masses, although GI tumors can be visualized occasionally
- endoscopic US aids in prognosis due to its ability to establish depth of invasion

CARCINOMA

1. GASTRIC CARCINOMA

- most common gastric malignancy is adenocarcinoma
- factors associated with increased incidence are diet (e.g., consumption of nitrites), genetics, and host factors such as chronic gastritis or gastric adenomas
- prognosis depends on depth of invasion and extent of nodal and distant metastasis

SS

- generally asymptomatic until late in its course
- weight loss, abdominal pain, anorexia, vomiting

2. COLORECTAL CARCINOMA

- 98% of cancers in the colon are adenocarcinomas
- peak incidence is 60–70 years
- dietary factors that are predisposing to a higher incidence are low fiber, high carbohydrate and fat, and low intake of protective micronutrients
- spread by direct extension and by metastasis to lymph nodes, liver, lungs, and bones
- most important prognostic indicator is the extent at the time of diagnosis
- associated with chronic ulcerative colitis
- Location:
  30%—rectum
  25%—sigmoid
  10% each—descending, ascending, transverse colon, and cecum

SS

- can remain asymptomatic for years
- fatigue, anemia, occult bleeding, changes in bowel habits

3. SMALL INTESTINE CARCINOMA

- although it comprises 75% of the GI tract, tumors here account for less than 1% of malignant GI tumors
- frequency of malignant neoplasms are adenocarcinoma (45%), carcinoid (18%), sarcoma (18%), lymphoma (3%)

SS

- cramping pain, nausea, vomiting, weight loss

US

- the "bull's eye"/"typical target" sign used to describe sonographic appearance of bowel lesions consists of a thick hypoechoic rim with central echogenicity and can be associated with acoustic shadow due to bowel wall thickening or infiltration
- wall thickening is usually focal and irregular

LYMPHOMA

- 1–2% of all gastrointestinal malignancies
- diffuse infiltrating group of malignant solid tumors of the lymphoid tissue
  50%—gastric
  30%—small bowel, terminal ileum
  20%—large bowel
- incidence increased in age groups <10 years and >50 years
- occurs more frequently in patients with malabsorption syndromes, HIV, organ transplant with immunosuppression

SS

- vague or abdominal pain, anemia, weight loss, malabsorption, palpable abdominal mass

US

- densely reflective areas or target lesions caused by bowel wall thickened mucosal folds
- large, complex, irregular mass with internal echos due to necrosis
- decrease in peristalsis

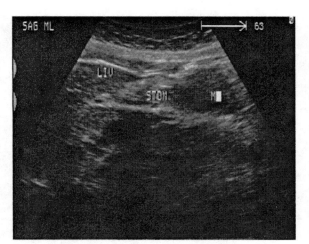

Sagittal midline scan: longitudinal scan plane of liver and stomach with mass (M) off inferior aspect—gastric carcinoma (courtesy of Chedoke-McMaster Hospital, Hamilton)

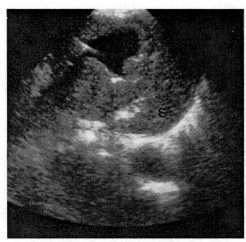

Gastroleiomyosarcoma adjacent to spleen (S)

US APPEARANCE

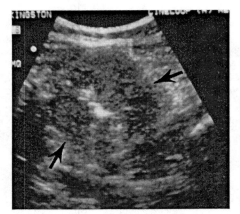

Large hypoechoic mass with central echogenic area right lower quadrant: carcinoma of bowel involving cecum and terminal ileum

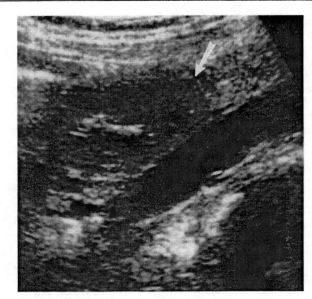

Carcinoma of bowel involving splenic flexure

METASTASES TO GI TRACT
- travel to GI tract by intraperitoneal spread, hematogenous dissemination or direct invasion
- common primaries include:
  malignant melanoma
  breast
  lung

1. STOMACH METASTASES
- unusual
- most common sources are leukemia and generalized lymphoma

2. COLON METASTASES
- uncommon

US
- most found by sonography are advanced and symptomatic
- hypoechoic, eccentric, short segment thickening
- target/focal mass that appears similar to a bull's eye or pseudokidney lesion
- other areas of metastases, lymphadenopathy

Early stages:
- high-resolution scanning can sometimes detect small hypoechoic mucosal elevations with preservation of wall layers

Later stages:
- diffusely thickened (may be focal) hypoechoic wall
- wall thickening causes "target" lesion
- rigid with no movement, suspect neoplasm
- evaluate for local adenopathy and distant spread

ANOMALY

OBSTRUCTION

- may occur at any level, but small intestine is most often involved due to small lumen
- two types:
1. mechanical (physical impediment)
- includes impaction (e.g., gallstones), tumors, adhesions (from previous surgery) and hernias
2. functional (paralytic ileus)
- when normal nervous stimulation that causes peristalsis is interrupted
- most common causes of obstruction are:
  children—intussusception, malrotation, meconium ileus
  adults—hernias, surgical adhesions

SS
- abdominal pain, vomiting, severe constipation, decrease in bowel sounds

GENERAL US FINDINGS
- multiple, tubular distended, fluid-filled loops of bowel
- distal to the site of obstruction there can be a sudden loss of definition of folds

COMMON CAUSES OF OBSTRUCTION

1. ADHESIONS
- fibrous bands secondary to previous surgery
- trauma, inflammation, and endometriosis can cause peritoneal inflammation and as this heals adhesions form between structures
- obstruction and strangulation of bowel can occur as with hernias

US
- not usually detected by ultrasound

2. HERNIAS
- weakness or defect in wall of peritoneal cavity
- common locations include inguinal and femoral canals, umbilicus, surgical scars
- most frequently small bowel protrudes, but omentum and colon may also protrude
- blood supply can become compromised causing stasis, edema, and eventually infarction

US
- abnormal location of bowel loops (e.g., femoral canal, scrotum)
- look for peristonalsis

3. INTESTINAL MALROTATION
- usually presents in 1st month of life with sudden onset of bilious vomiting
- symptoms are due to peritoneal bands or midgut volvulus

US
- dilated duodenum, dilated thick-walled bowel loops with peritoneal fluid
- mesenteric inversion (superior mesenteric vein [SMV] directly anterior or anterior and left of superior mesenteric artery [SMA])

4. INTUSSUSCEPTION
- slipping of one part of an intestine into another part just below it
- occurs when portion of gut (intussusceptum-inner) telescopes in an antegrade way into a more distal segment (intussuscipiens-outer)
- most common cause of obstruction between 3 months and 6 years of age

SS
- abdominal mass, pain, vomiting, rectal bleeding

US
- bowel mass with multiple concentric rings
- the many walls represent the returning and entering walls of the intussuseptum and the interface between them
- transverse scan plane: thick target or "donut" appearance on cross section with a central echogenic portion and a sonolucent outer rim or with multiple concentric layers
- longitudinal scan plane: "pseudokidney" appearance

5. SMA SYNDROME
- stomach and duodenum dilate to the point of the 3rd portion of duodenum
- superior mesenteric vessels indent the duodenum
- more commonly seen in very thin patients (anorexia nervosa), patients with severe trauma, anorexia

US
- dilated fluid-filled 2nd portion of duodenum
- compression of SMA

US APPEARANCE

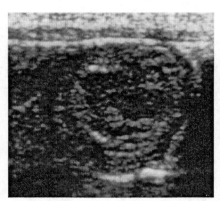

Intussusception: bowel mass with multiple concentric rings

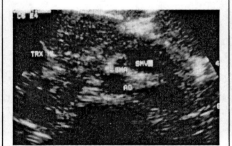

Intestinal malrotation: transverse scan through abdomen: note SMV to left of SMA

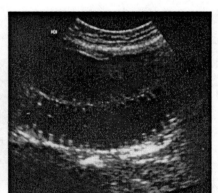

Dilated loops of small bowel

71

ANOMALY	US APPEARANCE

TYPHILITIS (NEUTROPENIC COLITIS/ILEOCECAL SYNDROME)
- necrotizing inflammation of cecum
- unknown etiology
- seen commonly with chemotherapy

US
- echogenic polypoid thickening of mucosa
- edema of cecal wall

Diff. Dx.:
- appendicitis
- inflammatory bowel disease
- tumor
- abscess

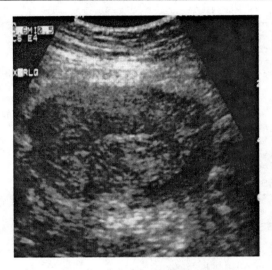

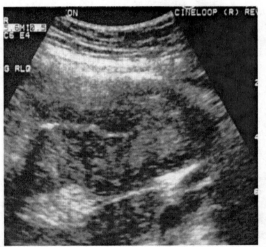

DIFFERENTIAL FOR NONSPECIFIC BOWEL THICKENING

abscess
diverticular mass/abscess
edma
hematoma, hemorrhage
infarction

infection (e.g., nectrotizing enterocolitis)
infiltrative process (e.g., amyloidosis)
inflammatory bowel disease
malabsorption
neoplasia (e.g., lymphoma, metastases)
radiation

• following are various US images of nonspecific bowel thickening

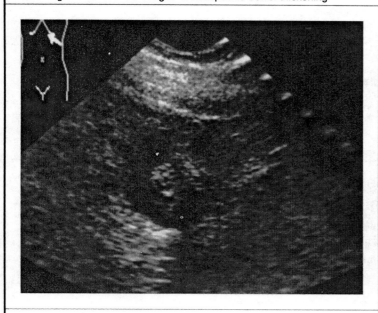
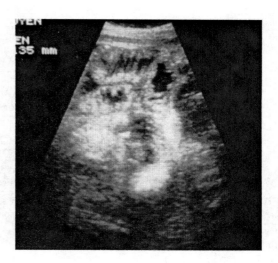
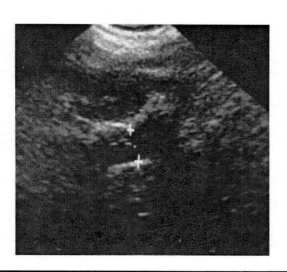
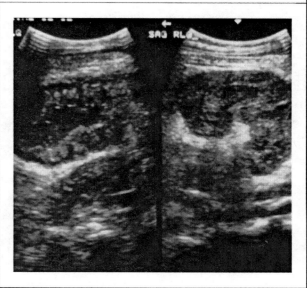

E) TECHNICAL FACTORS

TRANSDUCER **ABDOMINAL** **ULTRASOUND**	• high frequency (> 5 MHz) • linear or curvilinear array • decrease overall gain

ENDOSCOPIC
ULTRASOUND
	• requires expertise of an endoscopist and sonologist
	• 5–7.5 MHz, high-frequency transducer
	• direct visualization of esophageal, gastric, and duodenal wall
	• Advantages:
	  determine depth of invasion or known malignancy
	  detecting adjacent lymphadenopathy
	  detecting tumor recurrence

TECHNIQUE	• an initial survey of the abdomen is performed followed by a more focused study of the area of interest with a high-resolution linear or curvilinear transducer • gentle graded compression is applied and withdrawn • normal gut is compressible and normal peristalsis is noted • diligent, patient examination is needed to adequately examine the areas of interest
STOMACH	• oral contrast agents • intravenous (IV) glucagon given to induce gastric relaxation • fasting to avoid residual foods or foreign bodies that can appear as foreign bodies
PYLORUS	• high-frequency transducer • scan below xiphoid and to right of midline • scanned in long and short axes
SMALL AND LARGE **BOWEL**	• difficult due to bowel gas and/or mesenteric fat • note bowel peristalsis and bowel wall thickness
APPENDIX	• global survey of pelvis with 3.5 or 5.0 MHz transducer • graded compression at region of maximum tenderness indicated by patient

TECHNICAL
DIFFICULTIES OR
HELPFUL HINTS
	Compression
	• use graded compression
	• apply compression slowly and release slowly moving gently along abdomen
	• helpful to:
	  1. displace overlying bowel gas
	  2. decrease distance from transducer
	  3. localize area of tenderness
	
	Peristalsis
	• look for evidence of peristalsis to differentiate normal from abnormal loops of bowel

CHAPTER 6 - KIDNEYS
A) NORMAL ANATOMY AND SONOGRAPHIC APPEARANCE

DEFINITION	• paired glandular organs

STRUCTURE

1. MEDULLA (PYRAMIDS)
- triangular inner portion of kidneys that surrounds renal sinus
- represent collecting tubules and loops of Henle
- occupies inner 2/3 of parenchyma
- separated from each other by bands of cortical tissue called columns of Bertin

a) Apex—pointed toward central collecting system
b) Base—peripheral portion

2. RENAL CORTEX
- consists of glomerula complex
- occupies outer 1/3 of parenchyma

a) Column of Bertin
- cortica extend inward to renal sinus between pyramids
- hypertrophy of this area can create a mass effect

b) Cortical medulla junction (CMJ)
- can be seen on ultrasound due to the different echogenicity

3. COLLECTING SYSTEM
a) Minor calyces
- 7–13 per kidney
- adjacent to renal pyramid
- connects to an infundibulum

b) Major calyces (infundibulum)
- 2–3 per kidney
- funnel-shaped tube connecting minor calyx to renal pelvis

c) Papilla
- apex of pyramid that opens into minor calyx

d) Renal pelvis
- funnel-shaped sac located in renal sinus
- proximal expanded portion of ureter into which various major calyces drain

e) Ureter
- posterior to artery and vein

4. HILUM
- opens anterior and medial to kidney
- entrance to renal sinus
- renal vessels, ureter, lymphatics, and nerves enter and exit kidney here

5. RENAL SINUS
- collecting system, renal vessels, nerves, lymphatics, fat and fibrous tissue

6. UPPER POLE
- most superior border of kidney

7. LOWER POLE
- most inferior border of kidney
- more lateral than upper poles

8. KIDNEY LAYERS
a) Renal (true) capsule
- innermost smooth fibrous layer closely applied to renal cortex
- barrier against trauma, infection

b) Perinephric fat
- fatty tissue lying between the fascia and renal capsule (perinephric space)
- protects and fixes kidney position

c) Gerota's fascia (perinephric fascia)
- thin fibrous capsule of connective tissue continuous with peritoneum that surrounds fat and encloses kidney and adrenal gland

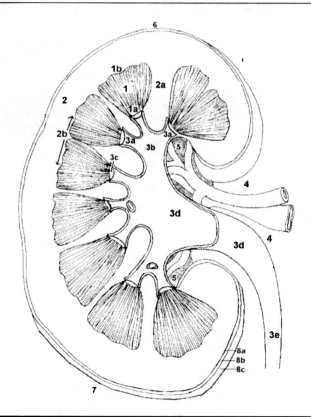

ANATOMY		
SHAPE	• bean or reniform shape • medial border: concave, hilum indents medial border • lateral border: convex	
SIZE	ADULT	CHILD
LENGTH	• 10–12 cm maximum midsagittal length • left kidney can be longer than right by 0.5 cm • kidneys should measure within 1 cm of each other • in normal conditions, therefore, the right can be 0.5 cm longer than left or left can be 1.5 cm longer than right	> 1 yr $= 6.79 + 0.22 \times$ age (years) < 1 yr $= 4.98 + 0.155 \times$ age (months)
WIDTH	4–5 cm	
THICKNESS (AP)	2–3.5 cm	
RENAL CORTEX	**Cortex Thickness** • use CMJ to distinguish between cortex from medulla • measured from margin of renal sinus to surface of kidney **Pyramids** • occupy 50% or less of parenchymal thickness • considered enlarged if their height is greater than overlying cortex	• accentuated CMJ up to 6 months of age • fetal lobulations are normal prominent indentations of the renal contour • by age 2 they become similar sonographically to adult kidneys
LOCATION	• located in perirenal space of the retroperitoneum, which is closed superiorly, laterally, and across midline, but is potentially open inferiorly to posterior perirenal space • embedded in fat and fibrous connective tissue on either side of the spine and the base of the ribs RIGHT—about 1 inch lower than left LEFT—slightly longer, narrower, and more superior than right	
	1. Fibrous capsule 2. Adipose/perirenal fat in Gerota's space 3. Perinephric fascia (Gerota's fascia) **a)** Anterior layer **b)** Posterior layer 4. Peritoneum 5. Pararenal fat 6. Extraperitoneal fascia	

REGIONAL ANATOMY OF KIDNEY

	RIGHT KIDNEY	LEFT KIDNEY
ANTERIOR	liver duodenum and small bowel hepatic flexure	stomach spleen tail of pancreas splenic flexure small bowel
POSTERIOR	diaphragm • muscle: psoas, quadratus lumborum, transversis abdominis • 11th, 12th ribs	
MEDIAL	right ureter IVC right adrenal gland exit of renal vein, entrance of renal artery	left ureter aorta left adrenal gland exit of renal vein, entrance of renal artery
SUPERIOR	right adrenal gland	left adrenal gland

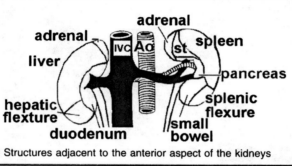

Structures adjacent to the anterior aspect of the kidneys

SONOGRAPHIC ECHOGENICITY

1. (Central) 2. Renal sinus	• central echodense zone made up of fibrofatty tissue • increasing echogenicity with age or lipomatosis • decreases in echogenicity in neonates or with reduced total body fat • Lateral scan plane = ovoid • Transverse plane = round	4. CMJ	• multiple, small echogenic specular echos that represent the arcuate vessels • marker for evaluation of cortical thickness
		5. Renal cortex	• homogenous low-level echos • iso- or hypoechoic to liver or spleen • uniform thickness except in neonates
3. Medulla/ medullary pyramids	• hypoechoic round blunted structures • 1.2–1.5 cm thick • between cortex and sinus • very prominent in newborns	6. Columns of Bertin	• cortical tissue extending into space between adjacent pyramids
		7. Renal capsule	• echogenic border surrounding the kidney • specular reflector
		8. Perirenal fat	• highly echogenic

Sagittal scan: adult right kidney

Transverse mid pole

Transverse upper pole

Transverse lower pole

2-day neonate kidney

3-month-old kidney

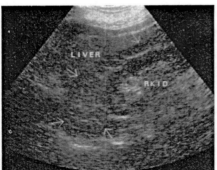

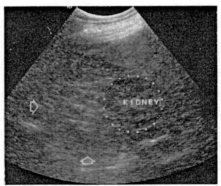

Pitfall: Note prominent perinephric fat (between arrows) adjacent to kidney; not to be mistaken for neoplasm

B) VASCULATURE

RENAL BLOOD FLOW PATTERN

Left Renal Vein + joins Left Testicular/Ovarian Vein → IVC
              ↗
Aorta → Renal Arteries → Kidney
                    ↘
Right Renal Vein → → → → → → → → IVC

DOPPLER

Arterial:
- persistent antegrade flow throughout cardiac cycle
- resistive index < 0.7

Venous:
- continual flow throughout cardiac cycle, which may vary slightly with respiration

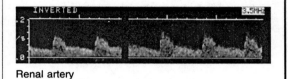

Renal artery

ANATOMY (veins run parallel to arteries)

1. RENAL ARTERY (MAIN)
- renal vein lies anterior to renal artery
- divides in hilum to form several pairs of segmental arteries
- Right
  longer than left
  passes behind IVC and right renal vein
- Left
  lies posterior to renal vein, body of pancreas, splenic vein
  inferior mesenteric vein crosses it anteriorly

2. SEGMENTAL ARTERIES
- located in hilum
- each supplies one segment of kidney
- branch in renal sinus to form interlobar arteries

3. INTERLOBAR ARTERIES
- run in parenchyma between pyramids

4. ARCUATE ARTERIES
- arise from interlobar arteries
- run between cortex and medulla and create high-level specular echos over medulla

5. INTERLOBULAR (CORTICAL) ARTERIES
- arise from arcuate and interlobar arteries and supply cortex
- Microscopic level:
  AFFERENT ARTERIOLE
    feeds glomerulus
  EFFERENT ARTERIOLE
    contains blood from glomerulus
    opens into network of capillaries entwined about convoluted tubules and collecting ducts

6. INTERLOBULAR VEIN

7. ARCUATE VEIN

8. INTERLOBAR VEINS
- drain area around the capillaries and collecting ducts in the medulla

9. MAIN RENAL VEIN
- Right
  short, lies in front of renal artery
  has no extrarenal tributaries
- Left
  longer than right, crosses anterior side of aorta below SMA
  tributaries: left inferior phrenic, internal spermatic, and adrenal

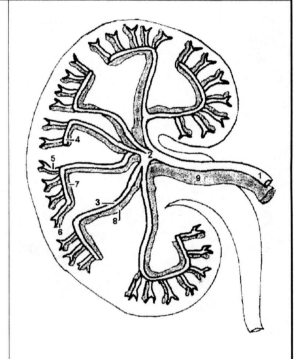

RELATIONSHIP BETWEEN RENAL VESSELS

1. AORTA
2. LEFT RENAL ARTERY
3. RIGHT RENAL ARTERY
4. SMA
5. IVC
6. LEFT RENAL VEIN
7. RIGHT RENAL VEIN

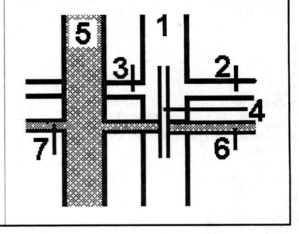

C) PHYSIOLOGY

FUNCTION

1. FLUID REGULATION
- 25% of blood pumped from heart flows through kidneys
- kidneys process (refines and reabsorbs) about 45 gallons of water a day
- fluid not reabsorbed continues through tubular network to make about 2 quarts of urine a day
- benefits:
  - filters and cleanses blood of toxic wastes, excess water, and salts, thereby regulating water, electrolyte, and acid–base (pH) content of blood
  - excretion of inorganic compounds (Na^+, K^+, Ca^{++})
  - excretion of organic compounds (creatinine)

2. ENDOCRINE FUNCTIONS
- skeletal development (vitamin D and Ca^{++} metabolism) helps to metabolize vitamin D, which strengthens bones
- blood pressure regulation manufactures renin, which helps regulate blood pressure
- RBC production (erythrocyte volume regulation) manufactures erythropoietin, which regulates RBC count

OPERATION

THE NEPHRON
- each kidney consists of millions of these functioning units
- form urine by glomerular filtration, tubular reabsorption, tubular secretion

1. INTERLOBULAR ARTERY

2. AFFERENT ARTERIOLE

3. EFFERENT ARTERIOLE

4. GLOMERLUS
- each nephron has this double-walled cup that contains a filtering knot of capillaries

a) Capsular spaces
- plasma passes through pores of glomerulus into this space then into the proximal tubule

5. TUBULES
- each has convoluted and straight part

a) Proximal
- closest to glomerulus

b) Loop of Henle
- increases the concentration of urine by drawing water out of tubule and into tissue

c) Distal
- along with collecting duct absorbs the remaining water
- only 1% of original filtrate passes into minor calyces

6. COLLECTING DUCT
- distal aspect of nephron, which empties into the minor calyces

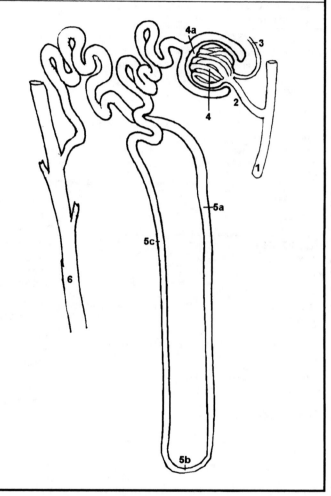

D) LAB TESTS

TEST	INTERPRETATION	
	ELEVATED	DECREASED
BLOOD STUDIES • renal function failure causes the accumulation of waste products in the blood		
BLOOD UREA NITROGEN (BUN) • urea is the waste product of protein metabolism normally filtered out of the blood by the kidneys • reflects protein and excretory capacity of kidneys	• renal dysfunction (kidney disease, failure, obstruction) • dehydration	• hepatic damage • malnutrition • overhydration
CREATININE • by-product of muscle catabolism that is filtered out of the blood by the kidneys • levels are proportional to body's muscle mass and remain fairly constant, so any increase usually indicates diminished renal function	• renal failure • chronic nephritis • urinary tract obstruction	N/A
ELECTROLYTES • kidney plays a major role in regulation of the toxicity, volume, and acidity of body fluids • e.g., chloride (Cl), bicarbonate (HCO_3), potassium (K), sodium (Na)	• acute renal failure (Cl, K) • renal tubular acidosis (Cl) • glomerulonephritis (K)	• chronic renal failure • acute renal failure (Na, HCO_3) • renal tubular acidosis (HCO_3, K, Na)
PHOSPHORUS • involved in body functions such as bone formation and carbohydate metabolism • also abnormal when there is a malfunctioning parathyroid gland or abnormal vitamin D levels	• chronic nephritis	• renal tubular acidosis
URINALYSIS • volume and content of urine is determined		
BACTERIA	• urinary tract infections (UTIs) in kidney and/or bladder • acute pyelonephritis	N/A
HEMATURIA • RBCs of casts in urine • any amount in urine is abnormal	• acute and chronic pyelonephritis • inflammation • tumor	N/A
pH • screening test for renal and respiratory diseases and some metabolic disorders • important with patients with calculi as the formation of calculi depends on the pH of the urine	pH > 7 ALKALINE URINE • UTIs • chronic renal failure • pyloric obstruction	pH < 7 ACIDIC URINE • uncontrolled diabetes • pulmonary emphysema • dehydration
PROTEINURIA • presence of protein in urine • any amount above a trace is abnormal	• nephritis • polycystic disease • stones • carcinoma	N/A
URINE UREA NITROGEN		• obstructive uropathy • chronic glomerulonephritis
URINE VOLUME 1,200–1,500 mL/day = normal	POLYURIA • diabetes • chronic glomerulonephritis • chronic pyelonephritis	OLIGURIA • renal failure • acute and chronic glomerulonephritis
WHITE BLOOD CELLS	• infection	

ANOMALY	US APPEARANCE
BENIGN TUMORS **1. ANGIOMYOLIPOMA** • most common benign solid tumor • overgrowth of normal tissue (fat, muscle, and blood vessels) • more common in women • usually unilateral (usually right side), may be multiple • associated with tubular sclerosis SS • usually asymptomatic • if ruptures can cause flank pain, hematuria US • homogenous well defined cortical mass • hyperechoic (due to high fat content) well defined mass • size varies from 1–20 cm **2. ONCOCYTOMA** • uncommon, usually benign tumors • occur in middle to old age • more common in males • usually single, can be multiple and bilateral • may grow up to 12 cm SS • asymptomatic • pain, hematuria US • well defined, smooth margins • homogenous low-level echos • often has a central stellate fibrotic scar Diff. Dx.: • renal cell carcinoma	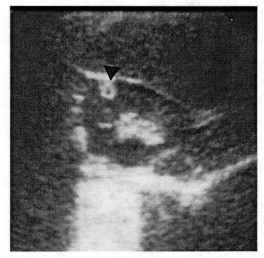 Transverse scan: small angiomyolipoma (arrow) 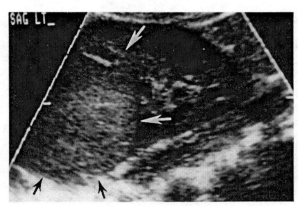 Sagittal scan: moderate size angiomyolipoma in upper pole of kidney (between arrows) 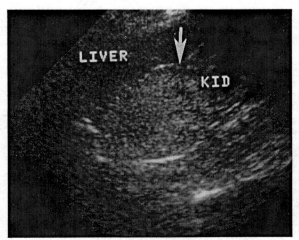 Sagittal scan: large angiomyolipoma almost filling kidney fossa (arrow)

ANOMALY	US APPEARANCE

CALCIFICATION

1. NEPHROCALCINOSIS
- calcium deposits within renal parenchyma
- can occur in medulla, renal cortex, or both
- implies metabolic or renal abnormality

i) Cortical calcinosis
- sequella of acute cortical necrosis (rare form of acute renal failure with sparing of medulla, which is thought to result from disseminated intravascular coagulation), chronic glomerulonephritis, dialysis patients

US
- punctate or linear calcification around renal margin

ii) Medullary calcinosis
- implies disorder that produces hypercalcemia (e.g., multiple myeloma, hyperparathyroidism, metastatic bone disease, prolonged adrenocorticotropic hormone therapy, Cushing's syndrome, hyperparathyroidism, oral pharmocologic doses of vitamin E and calcium)

US
- echogenic medullary pyramids that <u>may</u> shadow
- normal cortical echogenicity

2. NEPHROLITHIASIS (renal stones/calculi)
- formation of stones anywhere within the collecting system
- primarily unilateral
- 3-fold increase in incidence in males
- commonly cause obstruction in the three most narrow areas of the ureter (UPJ, pelvic brim, UVJ)
- form more commonly within renal calyces and pelves (nephrolithiasis)
- tend to be small (2–3 mm)
- may pass into ureters producing pain (colic)
- staghorn calculi are large stones in center of kidney
- larger stones tend to remain silently within kidney

SS
- renal colic if stone is obstructing flow
- hematuria, pyuria

US
- appearance depends on size of stone
- highly echogenic focus/foci with acoustic shadowing

Diff. Dx.:
- refractive shadowing from renal sinus
- renal vessel calcification (usually do not shadow)

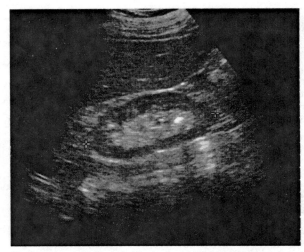

Single echogenic focus with shadow in lower pole

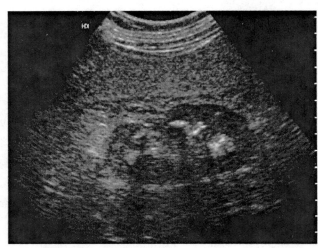

Multiple echogenic foci with shadow

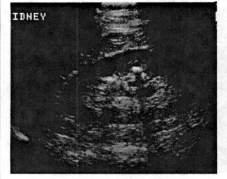

Multiple echogenic foci with shadow

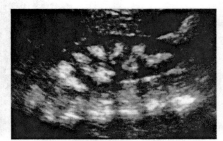

Medullary calcinosis

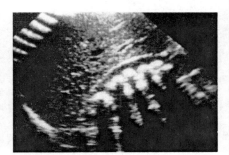

Medullary calcinosis

ANOMALY	US APPEARANCE

CYSTIC DISEASE

1. ADULT POLYCYSTIC KIDNEY DISEASE (APKD)

- multiple renal cysts that arise from tubules of the nephrons
- autosomal dominant of 100% penetrance but variable expression
- can be latent for many years and present in adult life
- slow progressive condition that can lead to chronic renal failure after age 40
- 40% have polycystic liver disease
- can also have cysts in spleen, pancreas, and lungs
- berry aneurysms are associated with APKD

SS
- asymptomatic until indications of renal insufficiency
- hypertension, palpable mass, urinary tract infection, polyuria, hematuria, flank pain, renal calculi
- increased serum creatin

US
- bilateral, very large kidneys with indistinct margins
- randomly placed multiple cortical cysts that vary in size
- some may contain internal echos that can represent hemorrhage or infection
- also scan liver, pancreas, and spleen for cysts

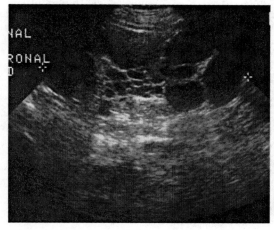

APKD

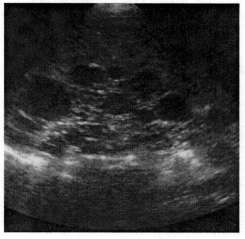

APKD

ANOMALY	US APPEARANCE

2. INFANTILE POLYCYSTIC KIDNEY DISEASE (IPKD)

- bilateral, rare autosomal recessive trait more common in females
- dilated renal collecting tubules that appear as multiple tiny 1–2-mm microcysts
- variable degree of genetic expression and outcome
- 4 subcategories depending on time of presentation and liver involvement
- Newborn (1. Perinatal and 2. Neonatal)
  present at birth
  may have rapid renal failure that leads to death in infancy
  on obstetric scan there will be marked oligohydramnios
  nephromegaly
- Childhood (3. Infantile and 4. Juvenile)
  survive infancy and occurs between the ages 3 and 5
  largely affects liver with hepatic fibrosis
  in older children the hepatic features are clinically more important than renal findings

US
- bilateral, enlarged, reniform-shaped diffusely echogenic kidneys
- individual cysts tend not to be resolved with ultrasound
- loss of CMJ definition
- liver is echogenic and also contains multiple liver cysts

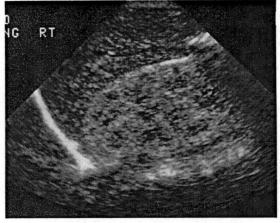

Sagittal scan: IPKD in 5 month old

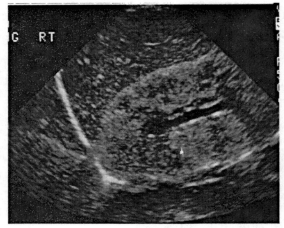

IPKD

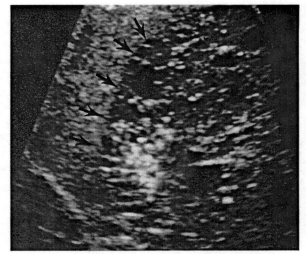

Sagittal scan of IPKD: arrows are demarcating the liver/ kidney interface

ANOMALY	US APPEARANCE
3. MEDULLARY CYSTIC KIDNEY **i) Medullary sponge kidney** • multiple cystic dilatations of the collecting ducts in the medulla • usually needs small calculi within these collecting ducts to make the diagnosis • presents usually in adults • benign process where renal function usually remains normal SS • can lead to medullary calculi with secondary hematuria, infection, and pain US • rarely medullary cysts seen • normal cortical echogenicity • normal or increased echogenicity of pyramids due to areas of echogenic foci that may not shadow **ii) Uremic medullary cystic disease** • rare, bilateral • usually onset of symptoms is in children (autosomal recessive) or young adults (autosomal dominant) • variable number of cysts in medulla • cortical tubular atrophy and interstitial fibrosis that lead to chronic renal failure in 5–10 years SS • renal failure US • definite, small cystic areas in medullary and CMJ portions of both kidneys • small kidneys with echogenic parenchyma and loss of corticomedullary differentiation	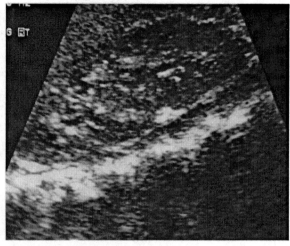 Medullary cystic disease 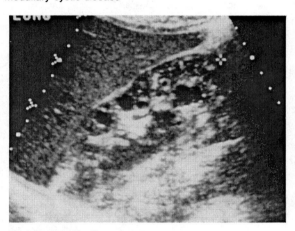 Medullary cystic disease

ANOMALY	US APPEARANCE

4. MULTICYSTIC DYSPLASTIC KIDNEY/CYSTIC RENAL DYSPLASIA (MCDK)

- sporadic disorder
- disturbance of ureteral branching causes terminal portions of collecting tubules to develop into cysts
- varying degrees of severity but usually involves entire kidney
- males affected more often than females
- associated with UPJ obstruction, ureteral agenesis, or atresia
- Unilateral
  75%
  most common cause of abdominal mass in newborn
  may be some renal function on affected side, but usually not
  normal serum creatine when unilateral
  unaffected kidney appears normal but can be enlarged due to compensatory hypertrophy
- Bilateral
  may result in renal failure

US
- abnormal kidney contains multiple cysts of varying size and shape
- cysts do not communicate
- absence of identifiable renal sinus and of renal parenchyma surrounding cysts
- kidney maintains its reniform shape

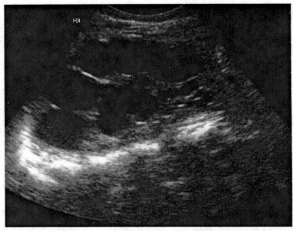

Longitudinal scan: multicystic dysplastic kidney (note how the reniform shape of the kidney has been mostly maintained)

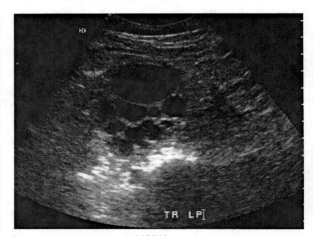

Transverse scan through MCDK

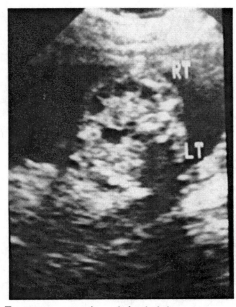

Transverse scan through fetal abdomen showing the early development of multicystic dysplastic kidney

ANOMALY

CYSTS

1. HEMORRHAGIC/INFECTED CYSTS
- bleeding into cystic mass caused by trauma or infection

SS
- flank pain with an acute bleed into cyst, hematuria
- infected cyst may cause fever and ↑ WBC in urine
- large hemorrhage may cause ↓ hematocrit

US
- cyst contains echogenic material that may be free floating
- slightly thickened walls
- hemorrhagic cysts have an echo pattern dependent on stage of hemorrhage
- do not meet classical sonographic criteria for a cyst; therefore subject to further investigation as differential can include neoplasms

2. PARAPELVIC/PARARENAL CYSTS
- see section later in chapter

3. SIMPLE CORTICAL CYST
- lined by tubular epithelium
- benign and generally of no clinical significance
- not common in children therefore suspect resolved hematoma
- solitary or multiple 1–5 cm in size (can reach up to 10 cm)
- can be multiloculated, but usually unilocular, but can have thin septations and still be considered benign

SS
- none unless they are large enough to palpate or compress collecting system

US CRITERIA FOR SIMPLE CYST
- anechoic lumen with smooth borders
- no measurable wall thickness
- sharp back wall echos
- increased through transmission with acoustic enhancement
- *any cystic area that does not meet these criteria is subject to follow-up or further investigation with computed tomography (CT) or MRI*

4. DIALYSIS-ASSOCIATED CYSTS
- usually simple cysts lined by tubular epithelium
- can contain calcium oxalate crystals
- renal cell carcinoma can occur in the wall of these cysts
- can hemorrhage
- patients with renal failure who are on dialysis can get cysts

US
- multiple sonolucent areas scattered throughout cortex and medulla, 1–2 cm in size in small kidneys
- meets all basic cystic criteria

Diff. Dx.:
- renal artery aneurysm, hydro/pyonephrosis, prominent renal pyramids, abscess, tumor, urinoma, lymphoma, hematoma

Helpful Hint:
- make sure "cyst" does not communicate with collecting system, which would indicate a hydronephrosis

US APPEARANCE

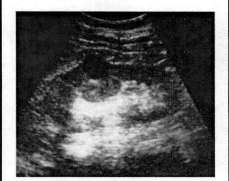

Single simple cyst

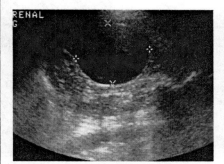

Large simple cyst

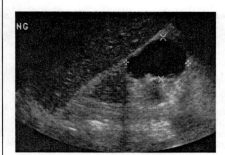

Irregularly shaped simple cyst

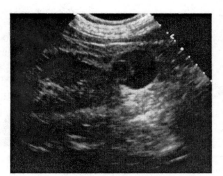

Complex cyst that should have follow-up

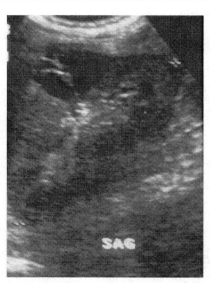

Septated cyst

ANOMALY	US APPEARANCE

HEMATOMA
 	
• causes:
  trauma (blunt or penetrating)
  postsurgical
 	
SS
• correlate with the severity of the trauma
 	
US CRITERIA FOR HEMATOMAS
• echogenicity varies with the clotting stage of the hemorrhage with the acute and chronic ones being more anechoic and the intermediate ones complex
 	
1. SUBCAPSULAR
• hematoma is adjacent to the kidney in a subcapsular location
 	
US
• capsular echogenic line is absent
• kidney appears flattened due to pressure of hematoma
• crescentric hypoechoic-anechoic area under renal capsule
 	
2. PARENCHYMAL
• hematoma within kidney
 	
US
• focal mass of variable echogenicity
• can simulate a renal neoplasm or abscess
 	
3. PERINEPHRIC
• bleeding into the perinephric (retroperitoneal) space
• usually located posterior-medially and will extend above and below the level of the kidney
 	
US
• tends to be thin and elongated conforming to outline of perinephric space
• difficult to visualize sonographically
	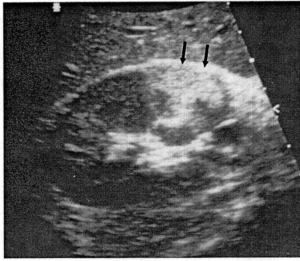
	Transverse kidney: resolved parenchymal hematoma (arrows)
	
	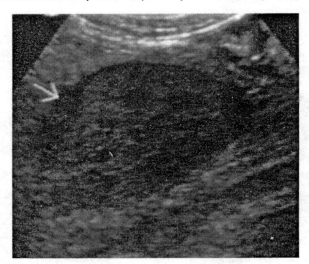
	Sagittal scan through lateral aspect of kidney shows collection (arrow) within perinephric space
	
	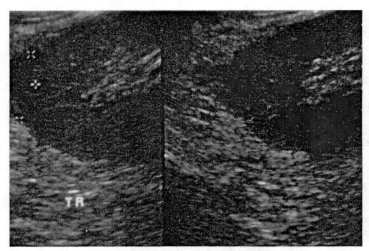
	Transverse scan of perinephric collection (calipers)

ANOMALY	US APPEARANCE

HYDRONEPHROSIS
- dilation of the renal collecting system due to obstruction of urine flow
- variable pattern of severity that depends on parameters such as duration, renal output, spontaneous collecting system decompression

1. MILD
- slight dilatation of collecting system

2. MODERATE
- further separation of renal pelvis by lucent mass, which appears as a cauliflower shape and not associated with any cortical thinning

3. SEVERE
- gross dilatation producing one large lucent mass within a small rim of renal tissue

Common specific types:
- Pyelocaliectasis
  dilatation of kidney pelvis and calyces
  not necessarily a type of hydronephrosis as it can be secondary to physiologic changes such as overhydration
- UPJ obstruction
  can be congenital (no single cause has definitely been established—rare other causes crossing blood vessels, fibrous bands, ischemia, mucosal folds, aortic aneurysm, renal cysts)
  will not present with dilated ureter

SS
- can be asymptomatic and depends on etiology
- renal stones cause flank pain, hematuria
- prostatic enlargement causes bladder symptoms

US
- visible renal parenchyma surrounding central cystic component
- small peripheral cystic areas (calyces) budding off a large central anechoic area (pelvis)
- cystlike (anechoic) areas that are relatively the same size and communicate with each other
- dilated ureter (depending on site of obstruction)

Doppler:
- use to distinguish prominent renal vessels from dilated renal collecting system

UNILATERAL MILD HYDRONEPHROSIS
- urinary tract obstruction results in increased intrarenal vascular resistance
- measurement and comparison of the resistive index (RI) can differentiate between significantly obstructed and nonobstructed dilatation of intrarenal collecting system in the absence of renal medical disease
- RI decreases following relief of obstruction or when the intrarenal collecting system returns to normal. Indications for obstruction:
1. Obstructed Kidneys RI > 0.70
   Nonobstructed Kidneys RI < 0.70
2. Obstruction is suggested when:
Resistive Index Ratio (RIR) > 1.1

$$RIR = \frac{RI \text{ of dilated kidney}}{RI \text{ of contralateral nonobstructed kidney}}$$

Helpful Hints:
- do postvoid scans for any hydronephrosis as pseudohydronephrosis can appear secondary to overfilling of the bladder
- should be able to trace the collecting system path by connecting the cystic areas to each other in hydronephrosis

PYONEPHROSIS
- pus in collecting system
- serious complication of hydronephrosis
- develops as a direct consequence of urinary stasis and secondary infection
- pus is unable to drain and fills renal pelvis, calyces, and ureter
- decreases renal function
- treatment must be prompt with drainage of affected area

SS
- fever, flank pain

US
- persistent dependent internal echos within a dilated collecting system
- shifting urine-debris level
- organisms can form gas that can cause prominent echos

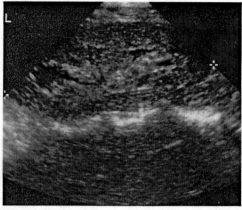
Mild hydronephrosis

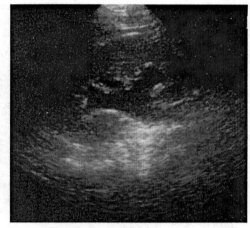
Moderate hydronephrosis

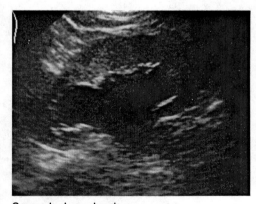
Severe hydronephrosis

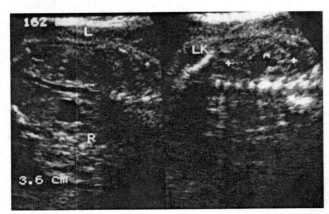

Fetal hydronephrosis: coronal scan through fetal abdomen showing bilateral dilated collecting systems (between calipers is total length of left kidney)

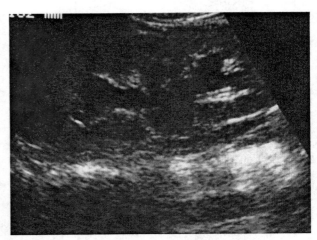

Maternal hydronephrosis: mild-moderate hydronephrosis can occur during pregnancy; caused by physiologic relaxation of smooth muscle or pressure on ureters at pelvic brim from enlarging uterus

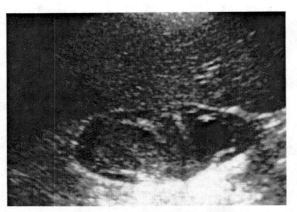

Pyonephrosis: echogenic debris within the collecting system

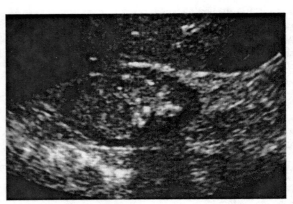

Sagittal scan: pyonephrosis

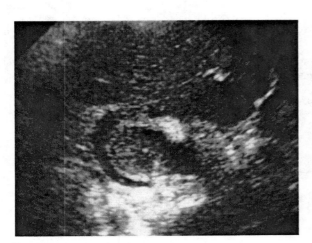

Transverse: pyonephrosis

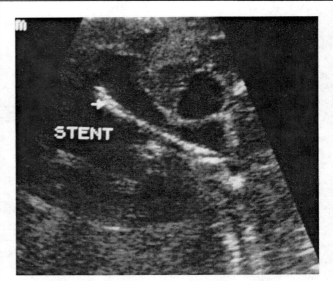

Stent (arrow) in collecting system to drain kidney collection when ureter is obstructed

TYPES AND CAUSES OF HYDRONEPHROSIS

OBSTRUCTIVE LESIONS					
RENAL PELVIS	**URETER INTRINSIC**	**URETER EXTRINSIC**	**BLADDER**	**PROSTATE**	**URETHRA**
calculi tumor ureteropelvic stricture	calculi tumor clot inflammation	pregnancy gynecologic masses retroperitoneal fibrosis/tumor/ hematoma	calculi tumor neurogenic bladder ureterocele	hyperplasia carcinoma prostatitis	posterior urethra valve urethral strictures bladder neck obstruction (BPH)

NONOBSTRUCTIVE LESIONS	CONGENITAL ANOMALIES
distended urinary bladder overhydration medications (diuretics) diabetes insipidus congenital megacalyces postobstructive dilatation chronic reflux acute pyelonephritis	ectopic ureterocele posterior urethral valves retrocaval ureter UPJ obstruction or narrowing urethral strictures meatal stenosis bladder neck obstruction severe vesicoureteral reflux

FALSE POSITIVE FOR HYDRONEPHROSIS	FALSE NEGATIVE FOR HYDRONEPHROSIS
extrarenal pelvis parapelvic cyst renal sinus lipomatosis renal cystic disease	severe dehydration nephrolithiasis with obstruction staghorn calculus that obscures dilatation acute renal obstruction numerous cysts that obscure obstruction misinterpretation as cystic disease or as large lucent pyramids technical factors (e.g., obese patient)

ANOMALY	US APPEARANCE

INFLAMMATORY DISEASE (Continued)

1. ACUTE LOBAR NEPHRONIA
(Acute Focal Bacterial Nephritis)
- focal bacterial nephritis
- inflammatory mass without drainable pus

SS
- fever, chills, flank pain

US
- poorly defined area containing echos of a lower amplitude and normal renal cortex
- disruption of CMJ

Diff. Dx.:
- abscess, tumor

2. FUNGUS BALLS
- caused by candida
- occurs in patients with low resistance to disease such as people with diabetes or malignancy or neonates
- renal involvement is secondary to systemic infection

SS
- flank pain, fever, chills

US
- echogenic nonshadowing mass in collecting system

Diff. Dx.:
- blood clot, tumor, pyogenic debris

3. GLOMERULONEPHRITIS
- inflammation of glomeruli
- Primary glomerulonephritis
  kidney is the only or predominant organ involved
- Secondary glomerulonephritis
  glomerulonephritis is part of a larger systemic disease such as immunologic (e.g., lupus), vascular (e.g., hypertension), metabolic (e.g., diabetes) or hereditary (e.g., Fabry's disease) disorders

Acute
- caused by many types of glomerulonephritis such as poststreptococcal, crescentric (rapidly progressive), or membranous

SS
- oliguria, edema, ↑ BUN, ↑ creatinine, ↑ potassium, hematuria, hypertension, nausea, vomiting, fever, recent infection

US
- initially kidney may appear normal or enlarged
- progresses with an increasing echogenicity of cortex
- medullary pyramids well visualized secondary to edema

Chronic
- end stage of specific types of acute glomerulonephritis
- common cause of renal failure
- can cause end stage fibrosis, which can lead to distortion of renal outline

SS
- nonspecific symptoms (e.g., vomiting, weakness)
- oliguria, polyuria, proteinuria, hypertension

US
- bilateral small echogenic kidneys
- scarring seen as echogenic bands that can distort renal outline

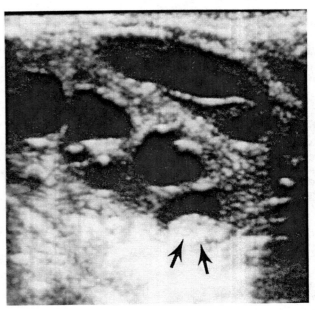

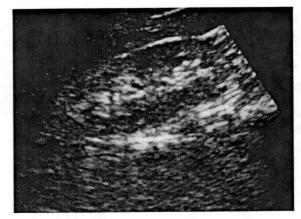

Fungus ball (arrow)

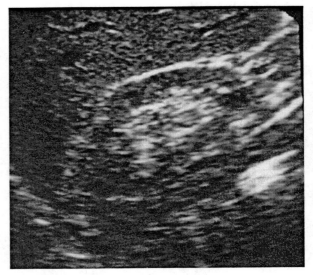

Acute pyelonephritis

Acute pyelonephritis

ANOMALY	US APPEARANCE

INFLAMMATORY DISEASE (*Continued*)

4. PYELONEPHRITIS
- an inflammation of one or both kidneys involving the nephrons and renal pelvis
- most common disease of urinary tract system
- pathways of renal infection are:
  ascending = bladder infection + vesicoureteral and intrarenal reflux
  bloodstream = bacteremic spread (less common)

Acute
- most common type of renal infection
- more common in females due to the shorter urethral path for bacteria
- associated with urinary obstruction, reflux, pregnancy, diabetes mellitus, immunosuppression, immunodeficiency, pre-existing renal lesions

SS
- dysuria, frequency, fever, chills, ↑ WBC, bacteruria, back pain

US
- normal size or enlarged, hypoechoic kidney due to edema
- possible calculi
- may have mild hydronephrosis
- CMJ area is enlarged and more hypoechoic due to small abscess and areas of necrosis

Chronic
- bacerial infection is the primary cause, but other factors such as obstruction and reflex are also involved
- scar tissue can form in kidneys, which severely impairs its function

SS
- proteinuria, chronic UTIs, hypotensive, dysuria, frequency, polyuria

US
- increased echogenicity of medulla and cortex of kidney due to fibrosis
- normal to small kidney size
- focal or multifocal loss of parenchyma
- areas of scarring usually at poles, which are associated with an underlying blunted calyce

Diff. Dx.:
- glomerulonephritis, but with that disease the scarring will be more diffuse and kidneys will be symmetrically involved

5. XANTHOGRANULOMATOUS PYELONEPHRITIS
- rare form of chronic pyelonephritis in patients with obstruction uropathy secondary to long-standing calculi
- creates multiple inflammatory masses that often simulate renal carcinoma

SS
- malaise, flank pain, mass, weight loss, chronic UTIs

US
- varies with pattern of involvement
- Diffuse
  parenchyma replaced with multiple sonolucent areas (debris-filled calyces and/or focal parenchymal destruction)
  echogenicity of masses depend on how much debris and necrosis is within them
  diffuse parenchymal calcifications, often with an obstructing pelvocalyceal stone
  enlarged kidney
- Focal
  one or more masses (anechoic to hypoechoic) surrounding a single calyx that contains a calculus

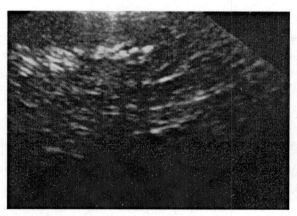

Chronic pyelonephritis with urolithiasis

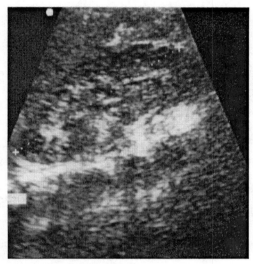

Chronic pyelonephritis

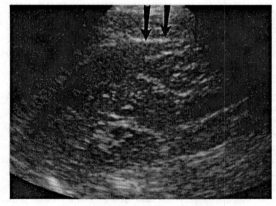

Chronic pyelonephritis has caused scarring along outer renal margin (arrows)

ANOMALY	US APPEARANCE

MALIGNANCY OF KIDNEYS

1. LYMPHOMA
• malignant neoplasms of lymphoid tissue
• kidneys are rarely a site of primary lymphoma but are a common metastatic pathway in patients with disseminated lymphomatous malignancies

SS
• gross hematuria, fever, weight loss

US
• usually bilateral
• may present as:
solitary or multiple nodule: homogenous hypoechoic mass with poor through transmission
diffuse infiltration: renal enlargement with diffuse decreased renal echogenicity

Diff. Dx.:
• renal cysts

2. METASTASES
• due to the large volume of blood flowing through the kidneys it is a frequent site of metastases but not usually detected clinically or sonographically
• common primaries include lung, breast, GI, prostate, pancreas, and melanoma

US
• heterogeneous mass that is attenuating

3. RENAL CELL CARCINOMA
(Adenocarcinoma, Hypernephroma)
• most common renal malignant neoplasm
• frequently seen in older population, 3:1 frequency in males
• increased incidence among smokers
• encapsulated, firm solid mass that may undergo necrosis
• smaller adenocarcinomas (< 3 cm) are known as adenomas because they very rarely metastasize
• invades renal vein, IVC, and into right side of heart
• metastasizes (often before giving symptoms) to lungs (50%), bone (33%), lymph nodes, liver, adrenals, contralateral kidney, brain

SS
• hematuria (can be only intermittent and microscopic)
• pain, fever, palpable mass, weight loss

US
• unilateral (99%), single, well-encapsulated mass with irregular margins with no acoustic enhancement
• inhomogeneity due to hemorrhage, necrosis, or cystic degeneration
• usually iso- or hypoechoic to normal kidney parenchyma
• check IVC and renal vein for tumor thrombus and contralateral kidney for extension of tumor

Doppler:
• hypervascular (higher doppler peak-systolic frequency shifts)
• contains numerous arteriovenous shunts
• can invade renal veins and IVC
• tumor thrombus:
often isoechoic with primary tumor
distends veins (bland thrombus which does not contain malignancy, does not distend the vein)
demonstrates neovascularity

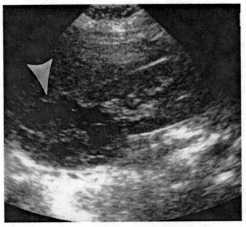

Renal cell carcinoma (arrow) in upper pole of kidney

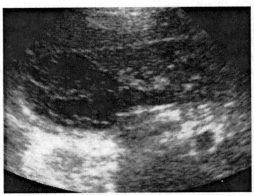

Renal cell carcinoma

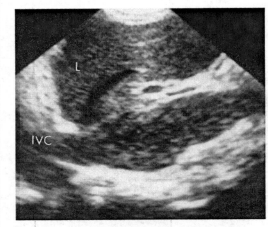

Sagittal scan: tumor extension fills IVC; liver (L)

ANOMALY	US APPEARANCE

4. TRANSITIONAL CELL CARCINOMA
- arises from transitional epithelium that lines the collecting system (renal pelvis, ureter, and bladder)
- occurs more frequently in men after the age of 50
- most common site is the bladder
- tend to be multiple along the urinary tract

SS
- gross hematuria

US
- solid homogenous discrete mass within renal pelvis
- not well defined or encapsulated
- isoechoic to renal parenchyma
- also see Chapter 14—Urinary Bladder under anomalies

5. WILMS' TUMOR
- see "Pediatric Neoplasms" in this chapter

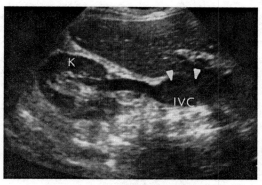

Transverse scan: tumor extension into renal vein and IVC; kidney (K)

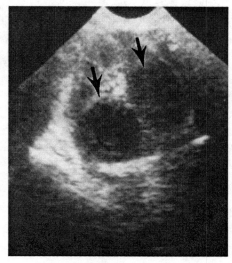

Transverse left kidney with two hypoechoic masses: renal metastases (arrows)

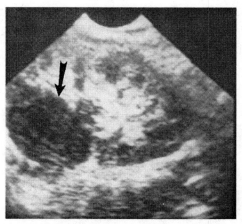

Hypoechoic mass in kidney: renal metastasis (arrow)

ANOMALY

PARAPELVIC/PARARENAL CYSTS

- not true cysts as they arise in renal sinus from lymphatics or other nonrenal parenchyma tissue
- located in hilum next to calyces and do not communicate with collecting system
- frequently bilateral

SS
- usually asymptomatic

US
- characteristics of a simple cyst within renal hilum
- circular appearance in transverse and longitudinal scan planes
- may displace pelvocaliceal complex
- difficult to differentiate from hydronephrosis, may need contrast study to distinguish such as intravenous pyelogram (IVP) or CT scan
- do not communicate with each other or with a dilated renal pelvis

US APPEARANCE

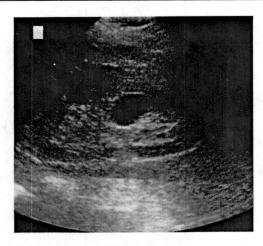 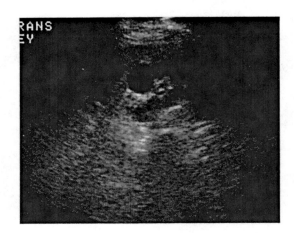

ANOMALY	US APPEARANCE

PEDIATRIC NEOPLASM

1. <u>MESOBLASTIC NEPHROMA</u> (Fetal Renal Hamartoma)
- benign neoplasm
- most common solid renal mass found in the first 3 months of life
- rare in older children and adults

SS
- asymptomatic abdominal mass, hematuria, hypertension

US
- preservation of reniform shape of kidney until tumor becomes very large
- evenly echogenic with low-level echos
- hemorrhage, necrosis, and cyst formation can be seen in larger masses

2. <u>NEPHROBLASTOMA</u> (Wilms' Tumor)
- most common renal malignancy in children
- more commonly occurs in young children (90% under 5 years of age)
- may be bilateral (5%–10%) and multiple
- may be associated with congenital anomalies in other organs

SS
- flank mass, hypertension, nausea, hematuria, fever, weight loss, anemia

US
- well encapsulated large mass that compresses renal tissue
- appearance varies according to amount of necrosis and/or hemorrhage that has occurred
- homogenous unless necrotic, then can be complex
- examine contralateral kidney, renal vein, and IVC for tumor spread

<u>Diff. Dx.:</u>
- neuroblastoma (adrenal): usually quite heterogeneous with irregular hyperechoic areas intermixed with less echogenic areas

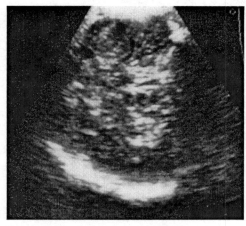

Large irregular heterogeneous mass in mid-upper pole of kidney

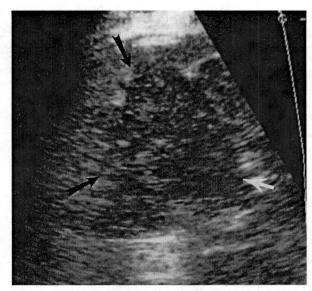

Sagittal upper pole of kidney, arrows indicating large mass

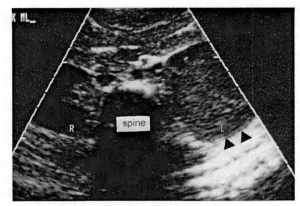

Transverse pediatric abdomen showing tumor in left kidney (arrows); right kidney (R)

ANOMALY	US APPEARANCE

PERINEPHRIC COLLECTIONS

• retroperitoneal fluid collections may develop in any potential space near the kidney

1. ABSCESS (can occur in kidney as well)
• extension of suppurative inflammation through renal capsule into perinephric tissue

SS
• flank pain, fever, chills, ↑ WBC

US
• well marginated anechoic/complex mass
• thickened, irregular wall
• may contain debris (internal echos)
• acoustic enhancement
• gas can cause highly echogenic echos

2. HEMATOMA/HEMORRHAGE
• see previous specific section on hematomas

3. LYMPHOCELE
• localized collection of lymphatic fluid caused by damaged lymphatic channels

US
• well defined cystic area with or without septations
• hypoechoic to anechoic
• may contain echos if accompanied by a hemorrhage

4. PANCREATIC PSEUDOCYST
• encapsulated collections of pancreatic juices
• body walls off contents of pancreatic leakage, which may break through to collect in the lesser sac or anterior pararenal space

US
• sharply defined uni- or multiloculated masses with echogenic, thick smooth walls
• may contain internal echos and septations

5. URINOMA
• encapsulated collection of extravasated urine
• caused by renal injuries, surgery (transplants), infection, tumor, calculus erosion, ureteral obstruction

US
• anechoic unless the collection is infected
• can contain septations

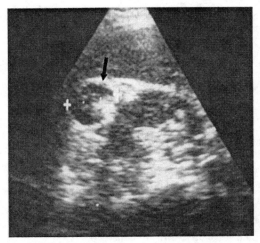

Transverse kidney with abscess demonstrated between calipers

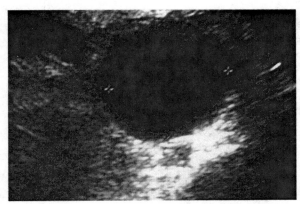

Lymphocele

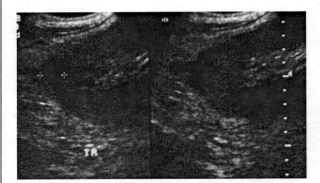

Fluid collection in perinephric space

US APPEARANCE OF PERINEPHRIC COLLECTIONS

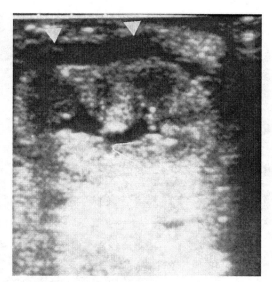

Anechoic fluid collection in perinephric space

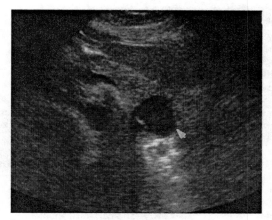

Pancreatic pseudocyst between tail of pancreas and left kidney

POSTOP MASSES	WHEN USUALLY OCCURS	SONOGRAPHIC APPEARANCE
ABSCESS	2 months average 6 days to 4 months	• variable location • echo free to complex echo pattern
HEMATOMA	< 4 days average 4 days to 4 months	• acute and chronic phase = anechoic • intermediate phase = complex
LYMPHOCELE	5 weeks average 10 days to 2 years	• anechoic with or without septations well defined • usually larger in size than abscess or urinoma
URINOMA	< 3 days average 1 day to 3 weeks	• hypoechoic to anechoic mass with possible septations • most located near lower pole of kidney

ANOMALY	US APPEARANCE

RENAL FAILURE
- deterioration of renal function that is frequently reversible and can be acute or chronic in nature
- caused by:
  i) Prerenal causes
- poor perfusion secondary to a systemic cause
  low blood volume
     may result from occlusion or renal artery stenosis
  decreased cardiac output
     congestive heart failure may cause renal hypoperfusion
  ii) Renal medical disease
- Acute tubular necrosis
  most common cause of acute renal failure
  reversible disease that is caused by ischemia due to major trauma, massive hemorrhage, compartmental syndrome, septic shock, transfusion reaction, pancreatitis
- Pyelonephritis
  an inflammation of one or both kidneys involving the nephrons and renal pelvis
- Immunological disease
- Metabolic disorders
  diabetes mellitus, amyloidosis, nephrocalcinosis, gout
- Polycystic disease
- Infection
- Chronic nephrotoxicity
  exposure to toxic substances such as drugs, heavy metals, radiation
  iii) Postrenal causes
- due to outflow obstruction
- urinary tract obstruction

1. ACUTE RENAL FAILURE
- acute suppression of kidney function and urine flow
- caused by:
  vascular obstruction
  severe glomerular disease
  acute tubulointerstitial nephritis
  massive infection
  urinary obstruction
  acute tubular necrosis

SS
- ↑ serum creatinine

US
- can have a normal appearance
- kidney may be normal or enlarged in size
- echogenicity of kidney increases as renal failure progresses from acute to chronic
- medulla well visualized due to edema

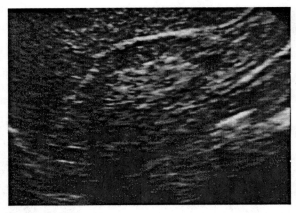
Acute renal failure

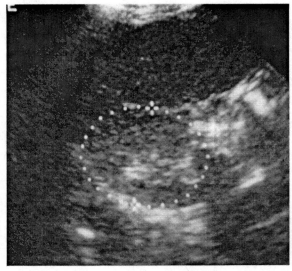
Ellipse tracing echogenic kidney in transverse scan plane

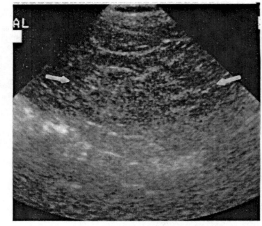
Sagittal scan of echogenic kidney between arrows

ANOMALY	US APPEARANCE

2. CHRONIC RENAL FAILURE (RENAL INSUFFICIENCY)
- develops over months to years
- progressive and generally irreversible decline in glomerular filtration rate (GFR) that is described in 3 stages:

<u>1st Stage</u>
- can be asymptomatic even with diminished renal reserve

<u>2nd Stage</u>—renal insufficiency
- decrease GFR and 75% of nephrons lost

<u>3rd Stage</u>—end-stage renal failure (uremia)
- 90% of nephrons lost
- blood levels of nitrogenous wastes and creatine increase further

US
- kidney may be normal or small in size
- increased echogenicity of kidney
- poor correlation between kidney size, echogenicity, and how well the kidney is functioning in the normal range (e.g., a normal-appearing kidney can have poor function)

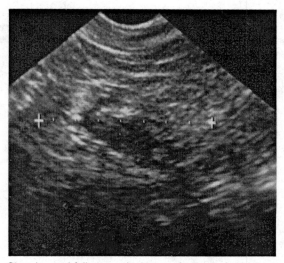

Chronic renal failure: sagittal scan of echogenic kidney

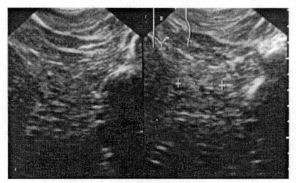

Chronic renal failure: transverse kidney

RENAL SINUS LIPOMATOSIS (FIBROLIPOMATOSIS)
- parenchymal atrophy with fatty tissue in real sinus, hilum, and perinephric space
- common in older patients
- linked to obesity

SS
- asymptomatic or
- may have chronic calculus disease and inflammation

US
- large echogenic renal sinus
- kidneys may be enlarged

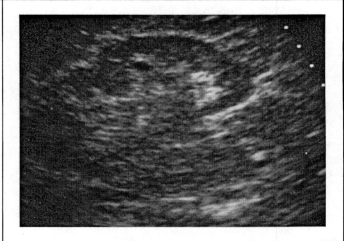

ANOMALY	US APPEARANCE

TRANSPLANTATION

- when the kidneys can no longer maintain homeostasis, during chronic renal failure, patient must undergo dialysis and/or renal transplant
- native kidneys and ureters are usually not removed and transplanted kidney is placed within the ileopelvic region

Anastomoses:
- renal artery is anastomosed to hypogastric artery or external iliac artery
- renal vein is anastomosed to external iliac vein

US ROLES

Pretransplant: rule out anomalies in donor kidney such as:
- outflow tract obstruction
- calculi (renal and occasionally GB)
- neoplasm

Posttransplant: document and evaluate:
- size and position
- Doppler flow studies (see below)
- echogenicity: CMJ contrast and echogenicity of renal parenchyma
- any obstruction: check collecting system and urinary bladder
- any extrarenal fluid collections

Types of Peritransplant Fluid Collections: small peritransplant collections are common and are not significant unless infected or if they compress the new kidney:
- hematoma or seroma (common in first 2 weeks)
  larger hematomas can compress causing obstruction
- urinoma (first 2 postoperative weeks)
  urine extravasation early posttransplant
  can be serious complication
- abscess
  difficult to distinguish from other fluid collections
- lymphoceles (first 1–3 weeks)
  often a delayed finding caused by damage to lymphatics in transplant bed
  can cause hydronephrosis

Doppler Flow Studies:
- sonographic routine should evaluate:
  1. main renal artery
     pulsed doppler recording RI (normal RI = 0.5–0.7)
  2. interlobar of arcuate arteries
     pulsed doppler recording RI in upper, middle and lower poles
  3. evaluate overall distribution of flow within kidney
     want to see good flow throughout diastolic phase
     absence of flow in diastole, rejection or ATN are to be considered
  4. anastomosis sites of main renal artery and vein

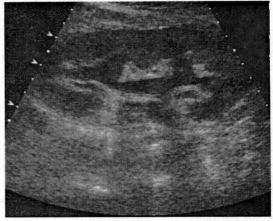

Longitudinal scan through normal renal transplant

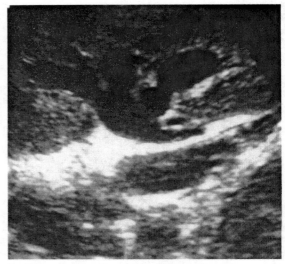

Sagittal scan through renal transplant with mild hydronephrosis

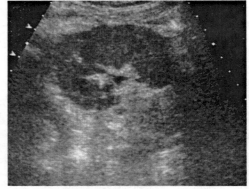

Transverse scan through normal renal transplant: note how the renal pelvis is orientated posteriorly

104

US APPEARANCE OF TRANSPLANTATION

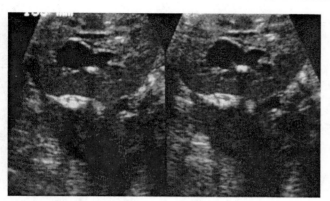

Transverse transplant kidney with small calculi

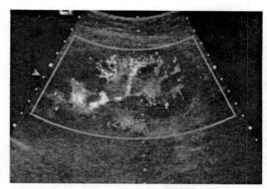

Doppler flow of transplanted kidney showing good diastolic flow

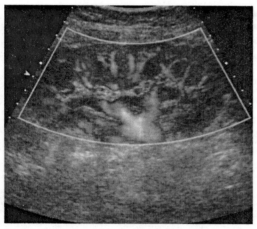

Power Doppler showing excellent vascular perfusion through entire kidney

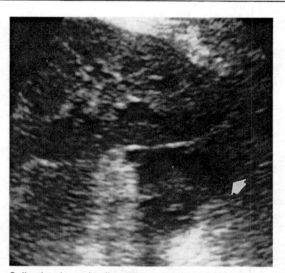

Collection (arrow) adjacent to transplanted kidney; differential diagnosis includes hematoma, urinoma, lymphocele

TRANSPLANT FAILURE CAUSES

Other causes for acute posttransplant renal failure are:
renal vein thrombosis
ureteric obstruction
pyelonephritis
cytomegalovirus infection

CAUSE	US FINDINGS
ACUTE TUBULAR NECROSIS • result of ischemia • most common cause of acute posttransplant renal failure SS • ↑ creatine, low urine output	• usually normal sonogram • renal sinus may show decreased echogenicity • absence of blood flow in diastole
ACUTE RENAL ARTERY OCCLUSION • endovasculitis narrows vessels leading to occlusion and ischemia • cellular or interstitial rejection causes edema, which impairs circulation	• normal sonographic anatomy with absence of arterial flow to the kidney
ACUTE REJECTION • most common cause of renal failure after the 1st week SS • fever, graft tenderness, oliguria Doppler: • decreased blood flow due to decreased renal function • increased capillary resistance often due to external compression of vessels • decreased diastolic flow, absence of flow throughout diastole	i) Acute • increased cortical thickness • enlarged hypoechoic pyramids • decreased renal sinus echos • enlarged kidney with distortion of renal outline • irregular sonolucent areas in cortex • indistinct CMJ • perirenal fluid ii) Cortical/Ischemia • focal edema, hemorrhage, infarction
GRAFT RUPTURE • occurs scondary to acute rejections • hemorrhage occurs along lateral border of kidney SS • tachycardia, hypotension, oliguria, ↓ hematocrit, pain, tenderness, swelling	• fluid collection adjacent to kidney Pitfall: • make sure an overdistended bladder is not mistaken for an extrarenal collection

ABNORMAL DOPPLER FINDINGS IN TRANSPLANTED KIDNEYS

HIGH RI VALUES • biopsy is the only definitive procedure for identifying the cause of rejection • acutely the differential is between acute rejection or acute tubular necrosis	• acute rejection • acute tubular necrosis • renal vein thrombosis • drug toxicity • renal compression • pyelonephritis • obstruction
ARTERIAL OCCLUSION	• absence of arterial signals in main, segmental, and interlobar arteries
VENOUS THROMBOSIS (OCCLUSION)	• markedly increased arterial resistance • reversal of early diastolic flow
VESSEL STENOSIS (KINKS)	• bruits and turbulence • main renal artery peak systolic velocities > 250 cm/sec
ARTERIOVENOUS (AV) FISTULAS	• decreased RI • increased systolic and diastolic velocity • arterialization of draining vein's waveform

RENAL MEDICAL DISEASE

TYPE	ACCOMPANIED BY	US APPEARANCE
RENAL CORTICAL DISEASE		
TYPE 1 CORTICAL DISEASE • due to glomerular infiltrate	acute and chronic glomerulonephritis acute lupus nephritis hypertensive nephrosclerosis nephritis renal transplant rejection	• increased cortical echogenicity more than liver and spleen • increase in CMJ differentiation • kidneys decrease in size as disease progresses
TYPE 2 CORTICAL DISEASE • due to focal lesions	cysts abscesses hematomas bacterial nephritis IPKD, APKD chronic pyelonephritis (UTI) chronic glomerulonephritis renal artery aneurysm	• depends on etiology
RENAL MEDULLARY DISEASE		
RENAL PAPILLARY NECROSIS • present in variety of pathologic conditions	diabetes obstructive uropathy sickle cell pyelonephritis acute tubular necrosis renal vein thrombosis	• multiple round cystic spaces in medulla around renal sinus • specular reflections from arcuate vessels are noted at periphery of these spaces
RENAL SINUS DISEASE		
CALYCEAL DIVERTICULI CALCIFICATION • Wolffian duct remnants that may develop stones		• gravity-dependent echogenic debris within a cystic structure
COLLECTING SYSTEM CALCIFICATION • uric acid lithiasis	ileostomy patients myeloproliferative disorders gout	• echodense calculi with acoustic shadow
CORTICAL CALCIFICATION • can be focal or diffuse	renal tubular disease enzyme disorders hypercalcemic states parenchymal disease idiopathic malignant neoplasm	• classic distribution is along CMJ
MEDULLARY NEPHROCALCINOSIS • calculi within the renal pyramids	distal tubular acidosis prolonged ACTH therapy hyperparathyroidism Cushing's syndrome	• normal cortical echogenicity • focal areas of increased echogenicity corresponding to renal pyramids
NEPHROLITHIASIS • calculi within the kidney	hyperparathyroidism hypervitaminosis D renal tubular acidosis medullary sponge kidney	• calculi
RENAL SINUS LIPOMATOSIS • excessive deposit of fat in renal sinus, hilum, and perinephric space	obesity parenchymal atrophy normal variant	• enlarged kidney • fat in renal sinus is larger than usual and may be hypoechoic
RENAL VASCULAR CALCIFICATION • calcification in renal arterial vessels	diabetes hypertension atherosclerotic vascular disease	• echogenic foci with shadow in area of renal sinus

COMMON DIFFERENTIALS IN KIDNEY SONOGRAPHY

ENLARGED KIDNEY	UNILATERAL	BILATERAL
	• compensatory hypertrophy (hypoplasia or agenesis of opposite side) • cross-fused ectopic • duplex collecting system • hydronephrosis • multicystic renal dysplasia • neoplasm • pyelonephritis • pyonephrosis • renal neoplasm • xanthogranulomatous pyelonephritis	• acromegaly • acute disease (glomerulonephritis, arteritis, tubular necrosis, uric acid nephropathy) • Beckwith-Wiedemann syndrome • cysts and cystic disease • duplex collecting systems • hydronephrosis • leukemia, lymphoma • myeloma • renal neoplasm • xanthogranulomatous pyelonephritis
KIDNEY DIFFICULT TO IMAGE	• kidney tissue replaced by tumor or other infiltrative processes • pseudokidney (bowel in renal fossa) • renal agenesis, ectopic or other deformities (horseshoe kidney) • small hypoplastic kidney (chronic renal failure)	
BILATERAL SMALL KIDNEYS	• chronic renal diseases (e.g., pyelonephritis, reflux, glomerulonephritis) • diabetic nephropathy • hyperparathyroidism • hypertensive nephropathy	• ischemic atrophy • medullary cystic disease • normal aging • obstructive atrophy
CYSTIC AREA AT HILUM	• abscess • adrenal pathology • extrarenal pelvis • hematoma • hydronephrosis	• lymph nodes • parapelvic cyst or other cyst • renal vessel pathology (arterial aneurysm, vein thrombus)
MULTIPLE CYSTIC STRUCTURES	• APKD • hydronephrosis • MCDK	• multiple simple cysts • uremic disease
SOLID MASS	• angiomyolipoma • column of Bertin • focal pyelonephritis • lymphoma	• metastases • oncocytoma • renal cell carcinoma • transitional cell carcinoma
COMPLEX CYSTIC MASS	• abscess • cystic renal cell carcinoma • hematoma • hemorrhagic cysts	• infected cyst • multiseptated cyst • multilocular cystic nephroma
CALCIFICATION	• calcification in cyst wall or tumor • cortical nephrocalcinosis (with severe calcification most of kidney can be obscured) • medullary nephrocalcinosis (pyramids are hyperechoic relative to cortex/sometimes shadowing) • nephrolithiasis (highly echogenic foci in collecting system area with shadow)	

RENAL VARIANTS OF NORMAL AND CONGENITAL ANOMALIES

ANOMALY	US APPEARANCE
ABNORMAL AMOUNT OF RENAL TISSUE 1. AGENESIS • occurs as a result of failure of ureteric bud to develop and grow into metanephric mass of mesoderm • Bilateral agenesis (Potter's syndrome) associated with oligohydramnios, pulmonary hypoplasia and is not compatible with life • Unilateral agenesis associated with congenital uterine and vaginal anomalies contralateral kidney may become enlarged as it undergoes compensatory hypertrophy US • bowel in renal fossa • no kidney in renal fossa (check for ectopic, crossed renal ectopia, or fused kidney) 2. HYPOPLASIA • failure of the kidney to develop to normal size • most commonly unilateral Pitfall: • normally placed kidney with echogenic renal cortex, which makes it difficult to visualize sonographically	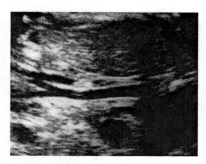 Potter's syndrome 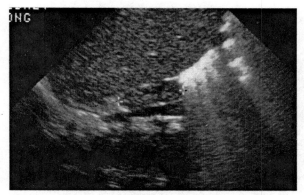 Hypoplastic kidney: 2 cm size kidney seen in 3 month old indicating renal atrophy

COLUMN OF BERTIN/RENAL COLUMN HYPERTROPHY	US APPEARANCE

COLUMN OF BERTIN/RENAL COLUMN HYPERTROPHY

- common anomaly
- inward extensions of the cortex between pyramids
- created by the cortex between the pyramids hypertrophying causing the renal column to be thicker than normal

US
- isoechoic to renal cortex
- creates mass effect and indents the renal sinus laterally
- clearly defined from renal sinus
- continuous with renal cortex

Diff. Dx.:
- neoplasms

US APPEARANCE

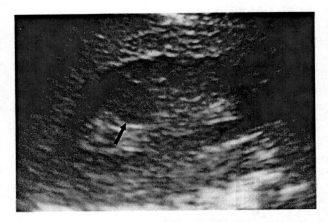

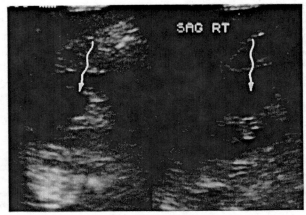

DUPLICATION OF COLLECTING SYSTEM	US APPEARANCE

DUPLICATION OF COLLECTING SYSTEM

- occurs in up to 4% of population and is the most common major genitourinary (GU) anomaly
- can be complete or partial
- ureters develop from separate ureteric buds that have grown from single Wolffian duct
  lower pole ureter—enters bladder at trigone, but has a shorter course and is prone to reflux
  upper pole ureter—enters bladder below this point and can be ectopic inserting into the urethra, vagina, or uterus, seminal vesicles
    upper pole more commonly dilated secondary to obstruction
  ureteroceles—cystlike dilatation of ureter near its opening into the bladder associated with duplication of ureters
    usually results in hydroureteronephrosis of affected ureter and associated pole of kidney

US
- kidney that can be larger than normal in length
- 2 distinct hyperechoic renal sinus areas on a longitudinal scan
- dilated ureter should be followed and searched for ureterocele

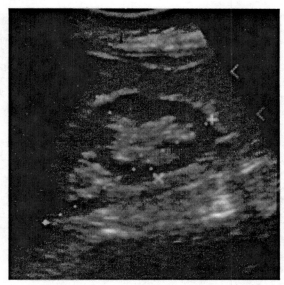

Sagittal kidney: cortical tissue through middle of kidney

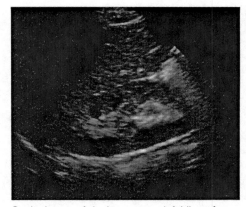

Sagittal scan of duplex system: infolding of cortical tissue in the kidney with two separate renal sinuses

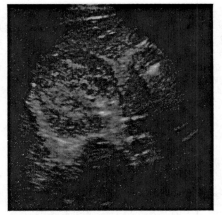

Duplex system transverse scan through the cortical tissue at mid pole

ANOMALY	US APPEARANCE

ECTOPIC KIDNEYS
- failure of one or both kidneys to ascend from their embryologic pelvic position into the abdomen
- the abnormal position may create kinking in the ureters, which can cause obstruction
- can be malformed due to lack of pressure from adjacent organs during growth

1. CROSSED RENAL ECTOPIA
- both kidneys are on same side and ascend into one renal fossa

2. UNILATERAL FUSED KIDNEY
- fused form of above, which forms on large renal mass of tissue
- more common

Diff. Dx.:
- single kidney with duplicated system
- mass within a kidney

3. PELVIC KIDNEY
- one kidney fails to ascend to the normal position and remains in the pelvis
- kidney locates adjacent to bladder, anterior to sacrum
- may mimic unilateral agenesis
- can be associated with other anomalies

SS
- palpable mass but usually none as mostly seen as an incidental finding and therefore clinically insignificant

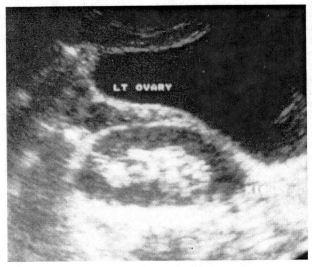

Kidney adjacent to bladder (b) and left ovary in pelvis

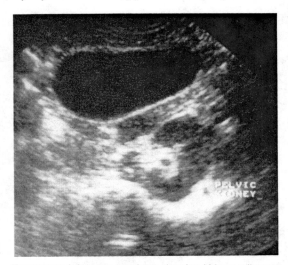

Transverse left lower quadrant showing kidney adjacent to bladder

EXTRARENAL PELVIS
- normal variant of renal anatomy
- a significant portion of renal pelvis lies outside renal contour
- key to diagnosis is its medial location
- clinically significant as can simulate hydronephrosis

SS
- none

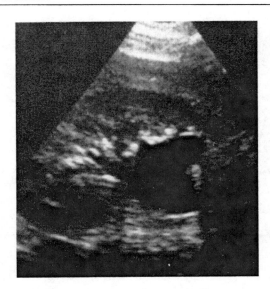

HORSESHOE KIDNEY	US APPEARANCE

HORSESHOE KIDNEY

- fusion of upper (10%) or lower poles (90%) of kidneys producing a horseshoe-shaped structure
- normal ascent is stopped by mesenteric vessels, therefore are found lower in the abdomen than normal
- may be malrotated
- ureters pass anteriorly to lower poles

SS
- none or can present as a pulsatile mass

US
- fused kidneys lying lower in abdomen anterior to great vessels
- lower pole of kidney is medial and very anterior, which causes the kidneys to have more of a vertical axis than normal

Helpful Hint:
- both kidneys appear lower than normal
- lower poles lie more medial
- ill-defined lower poles

Pitfall:
- renal tissue (isthmus) crosses midline fairly anteriorly and can be obscured by bowel gas

US APPEARANCE

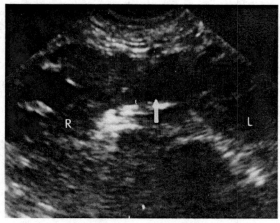

Kidney tissue across midline (arrow) joining the right (R) and left (L) kidneys

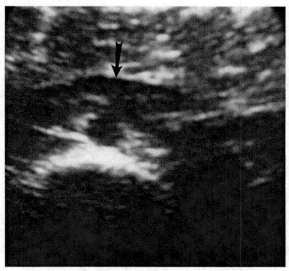

Transverse scan of abdomen showing fused kidneys (arrow)

ANOMALY	US APPEARANCE

JUNCTIONAL PARENCHYMAL DEFECT

- deep focal interlobular groove in which hyperechoic perinephric fat can extend caused by an incomplete embryologic fusion of the upper and lower poles
- communicates with renal sinus medially

US
- wedge-shaped hyperechoic defect (arrow) in the anterior aspect between the upper and middle thirds of the kidney

Pitfall:
- can be mistaken for a neoplasm or scar
- differentiated from above, because of its typical triangular shape and its location

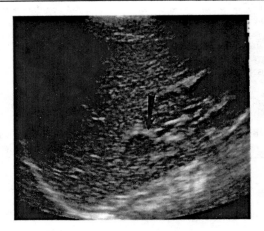

PSEUDOKIDNEY

- not a renal pathology, but can cause confusion when trying to locate a kidney
- it is a false image of a kidney created by the ascending and descending colon
- muscle wall is hypoechoic and the lumen is echogenic, so stool-filled colon can appear as a kidney
- to avoid this artifact, care must be taken to image the kidney through its entirety in both planes

Diff. Dx.:
- this appearance can also occur with colonic pathology that has wall thickening (e.g., ischemia or hemorrhage of bowel)

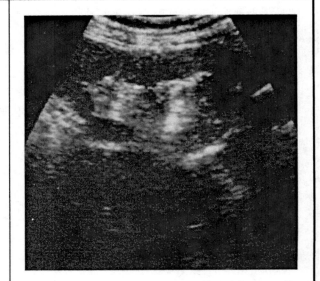

SPLENIC HUMP (DROMEDARY HUMP)

- normal variant of contour created by the spleen indenting the upper outer aspect of left kidney
- should not be mistaken with a mass protruding from the border of the kidney
- to rule out that the 'hump' is not a kidney mass, make sure that the CMJ is visualized within hump

US
- smooth bulge protruding from lateral mid portion of left kidney

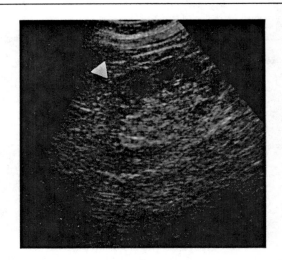

F) TECHNICAL FACTORS

TRANSDUCER	• highest frequency transducer will allow proper penetration Adults 3.5–5 MHz Children 5–7.5 MHz	
PATIENT PREPARATION	• none required, but generally done as part of a general abdominal US examination where the patient is fasting • if bladder or ureteral pathology is to be excluded as well, the patient should drink water to fill the urinary bladder	
TECHNIQUE	RIGHT KIDNEY	LEFT KIDNEY
	• right kidney best visualized with the patient supine or in the left lateral decubitus position using the liver as an acoustic window • scan in the anterior axillary line • can be performed from a coronal right lateral approach	• spleen acts as an acoustic window • left kidney best visualized in either the right lateral decubitus position, using spleen or fluid-filled stomach as an acoustic window coronal scan plane intercostal • scan in the posterior axillary line
	• maximum length obtained during held maximum inspiration • renal parenchymal echogenicity should be compared to liver (if greater than liver at the same depth, the renal cortex is considered to be echogenic) • renal medullary pyramids and renal CMJ should be identified	
MINIMUM PROTOCOL	• transverse and longitudinal* images to demonstrate the kidney's: size, shape, and contour position echogenicity • assess perirenal spaces for fluid collections and masses (* make sure that the true long axis of kidney is obtained so that renal size is accurate)	
DOPPLER	• 3–5-MHz transducer • sample volume small (2–5 mm) • low wall filter (< 50 Hz) • minimum frequency range (PRF) PROTOCOL • RI measurements of main, interlobar, and arcuate arteries • patency of main renal vein documented • several waveforms would be obtained for each vessel examined • both kidneys should always be examined	

HELPFUL HINTS	
PROBLEM	SOLUTION
PRONE POSITION • if patient can only be scanned in this position the paraspinal muscles may attenuate much of the sound beam and the ribs may create acoustic shadows leading to poor visualization	• place a bolster or rolled sheet under the patient's abdomen at the level of the kidneys • dorsal and ventral borders of kidneys are better seen in prone or supine positions
DIFFICULTY VISUALIZING ALL BORDERS OF KIDNEYS	1. Decubitus position • true frontal plane is obtained, which allows for better visualization of renal, perirenal and pararenal spaces • medial and lateral borders are best seen in this position 2. Coronal scan plane • allows easier differentiation between hydronephrosis and a parapelvic cyst
SUPINE POSITION • patient can only lie supine	• coronal scan plane through each flank is helpful

CHAPTER 7 - LIVER

A) NORMAL ANATOMY AND SONOGRAPHIC APPEARANCES

DEFINITION	• central organ of metabolism in body • 2% of body's weight, but receives 28% of cardiac output to accomplish its functions

STRUCTURE

• divided into three lobes
• liver is covered by a thin connective tissue layer called Glisson's capsule

1. RIGHT LOBE
• largest lobe and lies right of midline
a) Anterior segment
b) Posterior segment

2. LEFT LOBE
• lies in epigastrium and some partially on the left and right of midline
a) Medial (quadrate) segment
b) Lateral segment

3. CAUDATE LOBE
• smaller than right and left lobes
• lies posterior to medial segment of left lobe
• bordered:
  posteriorly by IVC
  laterally by ligamentum venosum
  anteriorly by left portal vein
• may receive branches of left and right portal veins
• has separate hepatic veins that drain directly into IVC

4. PORTA HEPATIS
• main vessels and biliary ducts leave and enter liver at this point

5. PORTAL TRIAD
• travel together throughout liver in a sheath formed by Glisson's capsule
a) Portal vein
b) Hepatic artery
c) Bile duct

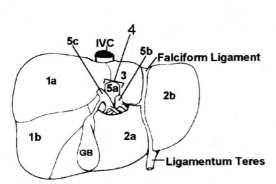

Posterior surface of liver

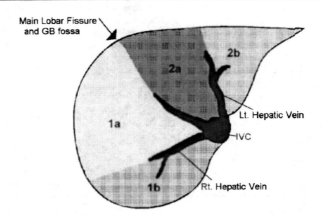

Transverse plane through liver

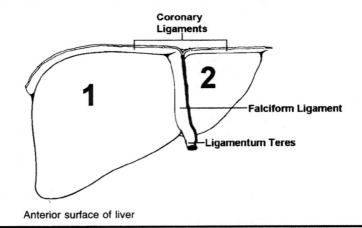

Anterior surface of liver

HEPATIC LOBAR ANATOMY

lobes are defined by the branches of portal venous branches that lead into center of them and by the hepatic veins that separate them
• ligaments, fissures, and GB are also important boundary landmarks

LOBE	SEPARATING LANDMARK	LOCATION
LEFT LATERAL/ LEFT MEDIAL	ligamentum teres	• embryologic remnant of obliterated umbilical vein that connected placental venous blood with left portal vein of liver • hyperechoic structure in left lobe of liver in caudad aspect of left intersegmental fissure
	umbilical segment of left portal vein—ascending	• turns anterior in middle aspect of left intersegmental fissure • runs in middle segment of left intersegmental fissure
	left hepatic vein	• runs in cranial aspect of left intersegmental fissure
LEFT LATERAL/ RIGHT ANTERIOR	interlobar fissure (main lobar fissure)	• extends from the long axis of GB (GB fossa) to the right portal vein and the IVC • sonographically seen as echogenic line extending from porta hepatis to neck of GB
	middle hepatic vein	• runs obliquely and vertically toward middle hepatic vein from GB fossa in main lobar fissure
RIGHT ANTERIOR/ RIGHT POSTERIOR	right hepatic vein	• courses between anterior and posterior branches of right portal vein • runs in right intersegmental fissure
CAUDATE LOBE/ LEFT LATERAL LOBE	fissure for ligamentum venosum	• contains hepatogastric ligament • anterior margin of caudate lobe between caudate lobe and lateral segment of left lobe of liver
	left portal vein—initial	• anterior margin of caudate lobe between caudate lobe and medial segment of left lobe of liver

RIGHT LOBE

Right Inter Segmental Fissure

Right Hepatic Vein

Posterior Segment

Anterior Segment

Main Lobar Fissure

through Gallbladder fossa + IVC

Middle Hepatic Vein

LEFT LOBE

Left Inter Segmental Fissure

Left Hepatic Vein

Medial Segment

Lateral Segment

HEPATIC LOBAR ANATOMY

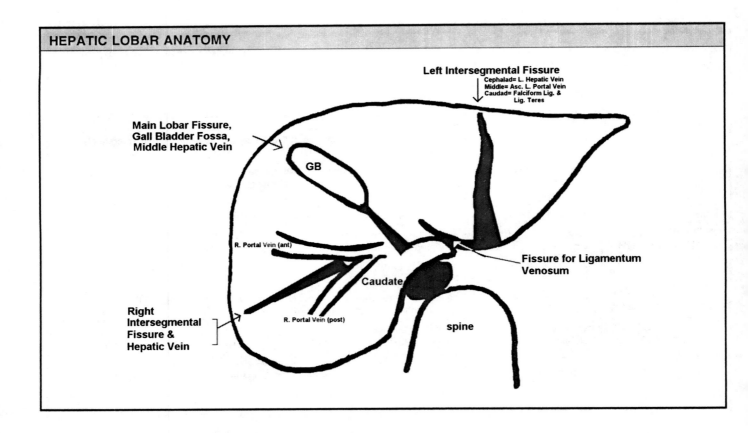

Left Intersegmental Fissure
Cephalad= L. Hepatic Vein
Middle= Asc. L. Portal Vein
Caudad= Falciform Lig. &
Lig. Teres

**Main Lobar Fissure,
Gall Bladder Fossa,
Middle Hepatic Vein**

GB

R. Portal Vein (ant)

**Fissure for Ligamentum
Venosum**

Caudate

**Right
Intersegmental
Fissure &
Hepatic Vein**

R. Portal Vein (post)

spine

HEPATIC SEGMENTAL ANATOMY
• division of lobes into separate segments
• useful to be aware of because surgeons use these segments when performing surgery on hepatic lesions
• each lobe of liver contains specific segments that are numbered counterclockwise 1–4 in left and 5–8 in right

CAUDATE LOBE
• Segment 1 = lower mid portion of liver
  separated from segment 4 by left portal vein
  separated from segment 2 by ligamentum venosum

LEFT LOBE
• Segment 2 = upper outer aspect left lobe
  left of umbilical portion of left portal vein, ligamentum venosum, falciform ligament
• Segment 3 = lower outer aspect left lobe
  left of umbilical portion of left portal vein, ligamentum venosum, falciform ligament
  falciform ligament separates segment 3 from 4
• Segment 4 (quadrate lobe) = upper mid left lobe
  right of umbilical portion of left portal vein and falciform ligament
  left of middle hepatic vein and main lobar fissure

RIGHT LOBE
• Segment 5 = lower mid right lobe
  bordered medially by GB and middle hepatic vein
• Segment 6 = lower lateral right lobe
  part of liver closest to kidney
• Segment 7 = upper lateral right lobe
  separated from segment 8 by right hepatic vein
• Segment 8 = upper mid right lobe

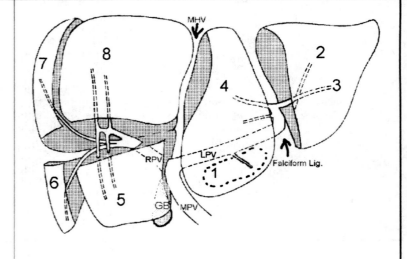

LIGAMENTS

1. CORONARY LIGAMENT
- peritoneal reflections around bare area
  Upper—continuous with right layer of falciform ligament
  Lower—continuous with right posterior triangular ligament and passes horizontal to the lower limit of posterior surface of right lobe
- upper and lower layer of peritoneum are continuous with right triangular ligament laterally

a) Left triangular ligament
- passes from upper surface of left liver upward and backward to under diaphragm
  Anterior: continuous with falciform ligament
  Posterior: continuous with lesser omentum
- continues with anterior layer of lesser omentum

b) Right triangular ligament
- short and V shaped
- most lateral portion of coronary ligament

c) Hepatorenal ligament
- caudal portion of coronary ligament reflected onto diaphragm and right kidney

2. BARE AREA
- liver is completely covered by peritoneum except for this small triangular area on posterior surface of right lobe
- the peritoneum reflects from the liver onto the diaphragm leaving this small area without peritoneal covering

3. FALCIFORM LIGAMENT
- sickle-shaped reflection of parietal peritoneum that connects the diaphragm to the superior surface of the liver
- conducts umbilical vein to liver during fetal development
- layers separate to form right and left layers when it reaches liver:
  Right layer—upper layer of coronary ligament
  left layer—upper layer of left triangular ligament

4. LIGAMENTUM TERES (ROUND LIGAMENT)
- lies in free border of falciform ligament in left intersegmental fissure
- extends from left portal vein through liver to umbilicus
- remains of obliterated fetal ductus venosus (umbilical vein)
- sonographically seen on transverse scan as a round hyperechoic density just to right of midline

5. LIGAMENTUM VENOSUM
- remnant of fetal ductus venosus that conducted blood from left portal vein to IVC
- sonographically seen on transverse and longitudinal scans as echogenic line extending transversely from porta hepatis

LESSER OMENTUM (6 + 7)
6. HEPATODUODENAL LIGAMENT
- peritoneal folds that contain the main portal vein, proper hepatic artery, and CBD at the porta hepatis

7. HEPATOGASTRIC LIGAMENT
- located in fissure for ligamentum venosum between the caudate lobe and the lateral segment of the left lobe

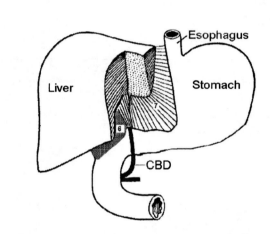

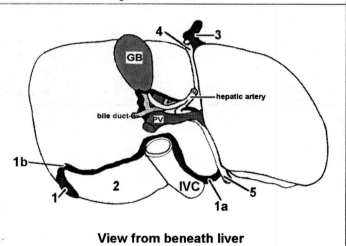

View from beneath liver

NORMAL ANATOMY		
SIZE	• difficult to measure accurately with real-time equipment because of limited field of view	
Methods of measure	• Craniocaudal length measure length of right lobe of liver in the right midclavicular line hepatomegaly usually present if length > 15.5 cm • Caudate/right lobe ratio caudate lobe can have a different appearance from rest of liver due to its dual blood supply measure ratio of caudate lobe/right lobe is a helpful indicator of cirrhosis normal ratio < 0.65 and cirrhosis if ratio > 0.65	
Indicators of hepatomegaly	• lower edges of liver become rounded as opposed to having a sharp wedge shape • extension of right lobe inferior to overlie a significant portion of the right kidney (must distinguish this from Reidel's lobe)	
SHAPE	Normal variants of shape • Reidel's lobe projection of inferior tip of right lobe that can extend below inferior pole of right kidney can be mistaken for a pathologic abnormality • Body shape various major types of body habitus can alter the shape of a normal organ	
LOCATION	• intraperitoneal (surrounded by peritoneum except for segment called the bare area posterior to dome of liver) • located under diaphragm in RUQ of abdomen • occupies most of right hypochondrium and part of epigastrium of abdomen	
RELATIONSHIPS	superior	diaphragm peritoneum (except bare area) base of right lung pericardium cardiac ventricles
	anterior	peritoneum (except falciform ligament attachment) diaphragm
	right surface	peritoneum
	posterior surface	bare area
	interior/visceral surface	porta hepatis

SONOGRAPHIC ECHOGENICITY

PARENCHYMA	• diffusely, uniform, homogenous fine-medium level echogenicity • in adults the liver is: minimally more echogenic or isoechoic to normal renal cortex less echogenic than spleen
FISSURES	• Longitudinal scan plane echogenic curvilinear lines • Transverse scan plane round hyperechoic structures

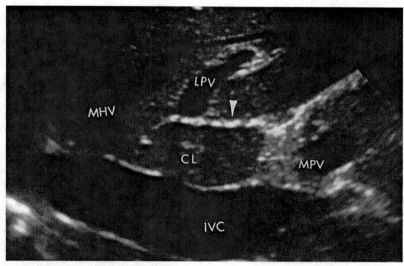

Sagittal: caudate lobe (CL): between IVC and fissure for ligamentum venosum (arrow); left portal vein (LPV); main hepatic vein (MHV)

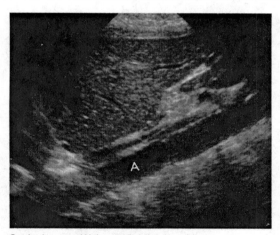

Sagittal: aorta (A) beneath left lobe of liver

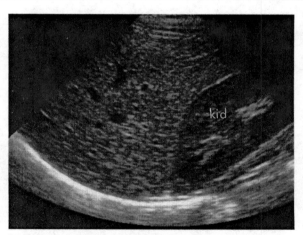

Sagittal: right lobe of liver/kidney interface

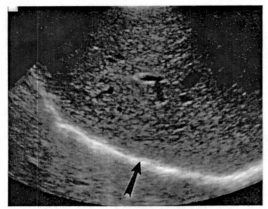

Sagittal superior aspect of right lobe showing diaphragm (arrow)

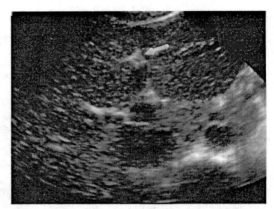

Transverse: left lobe of liver—ligamentum teres (arrow)

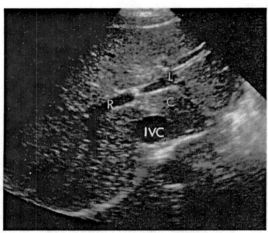

Transverse: middle aspect of liver—left (L) and right (R) portal venous system; caudate lobe (C)

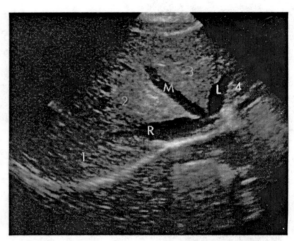

Transverse: hepatic veins emptying into IVC; 1, posterior segment right lobe; 2, anterior segment right lobe; 3, medial segment left lobe; 4, lateral segment left lobe

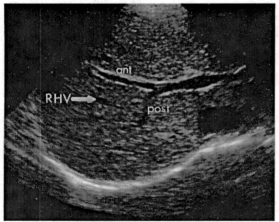

Transverse: right lobe with right portal vein coursing through it; anterior (ant) and posterior (post) right portal vein; right hepatic vein (RHV)

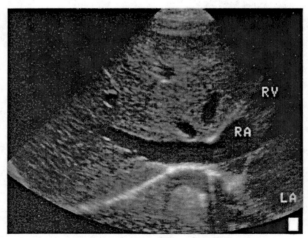

Transverse: superior aspect of liver showing the vena cava emptying into the right atrium (RA) of heart

B) VASCULATURE

COMPARISON OF HEPATIC VASCULATURE

	PORTAL SYSTEM	HEPATIC VEINS	HEPATIC ARTERIES
FUNCTION	• carries deoxygenated blood from spleen, pancreas, GB, and bowel to liver • 60%–70% of hepatic blood supply is portal	• carries deoxygenated blood from liver into IVC	• carries oxygenated blood from aorta to liver
DISTINGUISHING SONOGRAPHIC FEATURES	• **intra** segmental • originate from porta hepatis • caliber is greater nearer the porta hepatis • have echogenic reflective walls due to collagen within walls • branch horizontally	• **inter** lobar • **inter** segmental • drain toward right atrium • caliber increases as they approach the diaphragm and IVC • do **not** have reflective walls • branch longitudinally • caliber varies with respiration • with an oblique coronal subxiphoid view, they form a "W" or star shape with its base on the IVC	• very small, especially away from the porta hepatis
SCANNING TECHNIQUE	<u>Main Portal Vein and Left Portal Vein:</u> • best evaluated from anterior approach <u>Right Portal Vein:</u> • best from a right intercostal approach	• transverse scan plane • high in epigastrium	• anterior approach
DOPPLER FLOW PATTERN	• low-velocity continuous flow toward liver with mild undulations because of heartbeats • velocity of portal venous flow increased during inspiration and after meals	• blood flow toward IVC • characteristic triphasic curve, which reflects cardiac activity	antegrade flow in diastole • low resistance flow

Portal system

Hepatic veins

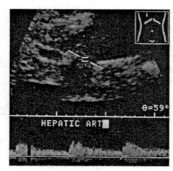

Hepatic arteries

BLOOD SUPPLY AND DRAINAGE TO LIVER

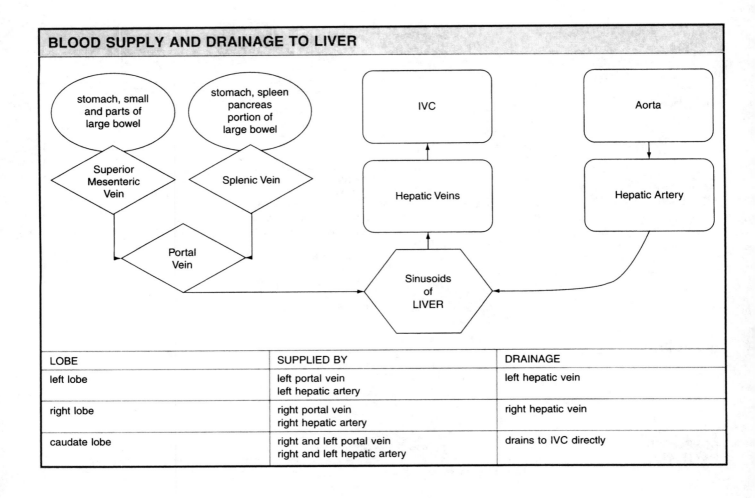

LOBE	SUPPLIED BY	DRAINAGE
left lobe	left portal vein left hepatic artery	left hepatic vein
right lobe	right portal vein right hepatic artery	right hepatic vein
caudate lobe	right and left portal vein right and left hepatic artery	drains to IVC directly

HEPATIC VESSELS AND THEIR ORIGINS

1. AORTA
2. CELIAC TRUNK
3. SPLENIC ARTERY
4. SUPERIOR MESENTERIC ARTERY
5. COMMON HEPATIC ARTERY
- divides below porta hepatis into right and left branches
- right branch passes behind common hepatic duct and gives off cystic artery, which can normally be found running to the GB in the triangle formed by the liver, CHD, and cystic duct
- many variations in arterial and duct systems

6. PROPER HEPATIC ARTERY
- common hepatic artery becomes the proper where the gastroduodenal artery branches off

7. RIGHT HEPATIC ARTERY
8. LEFT HEPATIC ARTERY
9. GASTRODUODENAL ARTERY
- branch of common hepatic artery

10. IVC
11. SUPERIOR MESENTERIC VEIN
12. SPLENIC VEIN
13. INFERIOR MESENTERIC VEIN
14. MAIN PORTAL VEIN
- contains deoxygenated blood and waste products from spleen, pancreas, stomach, intestines, GB
- 8 cm long
- Origin
  convergence of superior mesenteric vein + splenic vein behind neck of pancreas, anterior to IVC
- Path
  travels upward and to the right to become enclosed by the peritoneum that forms the right free margin of the lesser omentum, anterior to epiploic foramen
- runs alongside hepatic artery, anterior to IVC, cephalad to head of pancreas and caudal to the caudate lobe
  terminates at porta hepatis where it divides into right and left portal veins

15. RIGHT PORTAL VEIN
- runs centrally within right lobe of liver (intrasegmental)
- larger, more posterior and more caudal branch of main portal vein
- receives cystic vein
- divides into:
  Anterior branch
- lies centrally within the anterior segment of right lobe
  Posterior branch
- lies centrally within the posterior segment of right lobe

16. LEFT PORTAL VEIN
- enters left lobe where joined by paraumbilical veins and ligamentum teres
- smaller, more anterior and cranial branch by main portal vein
- runs centrally within left lobe of liver (intrasegmental) with exception of ascending portion, which runs in left intersegmental fissure and creates a division between the left medial and lateral segments of the left lobe

17. COMMON BILE DUCT
18. GALLBLADDER
19. HEPATIC VEINS
- Left, Middle and Right Hepatic veins drain into IVC
- contain no valves
- middle hepatic vein usually forms common trunk with left hepatic vein

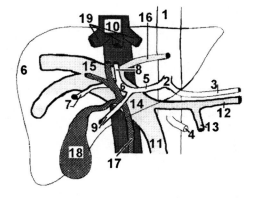

PORTAL SYSTEMIC VENOUS COLLATERALS

- an increase in portal venous pressure or portal hypertension is caused when portal blood cannot pass easily through the liver due to diseases such as cirrhosis
- portal systemic venous collaterals (varices) develop as alternate routes for the portal circulation to reach the heart
- common portosystemic collateral routes:
  paraumbilical veins drain the left portal vein to the umbilicus
  splenic vein into renal vein creating splenorenal collaterals
  left gastric (coronary) vein via esophageal varices to inferior esophageal vein
  others: pelvis, rectum, retroperitoneal region (spleen-kidney), renal fossae, GB bed

1. MAIN PORTAL VEIN
2. LEFT AND RIGHT GASTRIC VEINS
3. ESOPHAGUS VEINS
4. UMBILICAL VEINS (not usually patent except in extreme portal hypertension)
5. SUPERIOR MESENTERIC VEIN
6. INFERIOR MESENTERIC VEIN
7. SPLENIC VEIN
8. RIGHT AND LEFT GASTROEPIPLOIC VEINS (GASTRO-OMENTAL VEINS)
9. RECTAL VEINS
10. COMMON ILIAC VEINS
11. INTERNAL ILIAC VEINS
12. EXTERNAL ILIAC VEINS

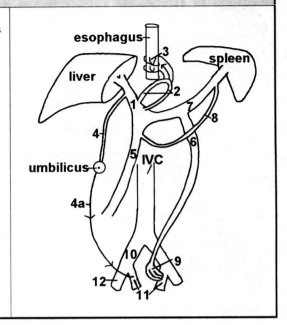

C) PHYSIOLOGY

FUNCTION
- maintains body's metabolic homeostasis by:
  processing amino acids, carbohydrates, lipids, vitamins
  phagocytosing particulate material in digestive system
  synthesizing proteins in blood
  altering circulating metabolites
  detoxifying and excreting waste products into bile

LOBULE
- liver made up of thousands of these 1–2-mm diameter hexagon-shaped functional units
- consists of cords of hepatic cells arranged in radial pattern around a central vein

1. CENTRAL VEIN (TERMINAL HEPATIC VENULE)
- blood enters periphery of lobule, travels toward center through sinusoids then exits through this vein
- terminal tributary of hepatic vein
- drains into sublobular veins, which unite to form the hepatic veins, which open into the IVC

2. SINUSOIDS
- vascular spaces between hepatocytes where blood passes through

a) Kupffer cells
  line the sinusoids
  part of reticulendothelial system
  perform phagocytic and degradative functions such as destroying worn out WBCs and RBCs and bacteria

3. HEPATIC PARENCHYMA

a) Cords of cells
- hepatocytes that radiate from central vein to periphery of lobule

b) Liver acinus
- alternate description of hepatic parenchyma, which describes a zonal distribution of hepatocytes based on their metabolic activity
- zone 1 is closest to vascular supply and zone 3 abuts the central vein

4. INTERLOBULAR VEINS
- branches of portal vein spread out between lobules

5. HEPATIC ARTERIOLE
- small branches of the hepatic artery that end in sinusoids

6. BILE CAPILLARY/CANALICULUS
- cells produce bile into these tiny lumens, which are really a continuous series of small spaces between two rows of liver cells
- merge to eventually form the right and left hepatic ducts

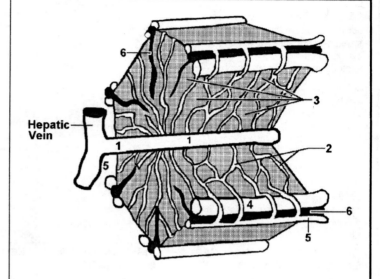

Hepatic Vein

D) LAB TESTS

PRINCIPLE	INTERPRETATION
• liver has a large reserve capacity; therefore, there can be significant hepatocellular loss before it shows clinically • enzyme tests show early change	
ALANINE AMINOTRANSFERASE (ALT) OR SERUM GLUTAMIC PYRUVIC TRANSAMINASE (SGPT) • specific indicator of liver damage	INCREASED VALUES • hepatocellular pathology (e.g., acute [viral] hepatitis, severe hepatotoxicity)
ALBUMIN AND GLOBULINS • comprises more than 50% of total serum protein • transports substances that are insoluble in water alone (e.g., bilirubin) • synthesized by liver, therefore decreased hepatic synthesis will decrease its level	INCREASED VALUES • multiple myeloma DECREASED VALUES • decreased liver function (i.e., cirrhosis of liver, acute liver failure) • lack of protein (severe malnutrition)
ALKALINE PHOSPHATASE (Alk Phos OR ALP) • produced by liver, bone, intestines, placenta • when disease causes destruction of liver cells, this enzyme seeps into the blood	INCREASED VALUES • bile duct pathology (i.e., biliary obstruction, atresia) • mildly increases with diffuse liver pathology • advanced pregnancy • bone disease
α-FETOPROTEIN (AFP) • is glycoprotein produced in rapidly multiplying hepatocytes in adults • used to monitor chemotherapy treatment • produced by fetal tissues and is used in prenatal diagnosis for neural tube defects	INCREASED LEVELS • hepatocellular carcinoma • testicular (germ cell) carcinoma
ASPARTATE AMINOTRANSFERASE (AST) OR SERUM GLUTAMIC OXALOACETIC TRANSAMINASE (SGOT) • enzyme found in high metabolic activity tissue, i.e., heart, liver, muscle, brain • released when there is cellular damage in the tissues where it is found • helpful in detecting acute hepatitis before jaundice occurs	INCREASED VALUES • hepatocellular pathology (e.g., acute [viral] hepatitis, severe hepatotoxicity) • myocardial infarction
BILIRUBIN • product of breakdown of hemoglobin in destroyed RBCs • measurement of concentration of bilirubin, which is the predominant pigment in bile 1. TOTAL BILIRUBIN VALUE • nonspecific finding, since hemolytic, medical, or obstructive jaundice can cause it to be elevated • normal = 1.6 1.6 = Direct (1.1) + Indirect (0.5) • abnormal > 2 (hyperbilirubinemia/jaundice) 2. INDIRECT (UNCONJUGATED) BILIRUBIN • normal = 0.5 • protein bound in serum • prehepatic, water-insoluble bilirubin • transported in plasma to liver cells where it is conjugated • if liver cells are damaged, indirect bilirubin increases 3. DIRECT (CONJUGATED) BILIRUBIN • normal = 1.1 • produced in liver by conjugating indirect bilirubin • transported to bowel by biliary ducts • water-soluble bilirubin	 1. INCREASED VALUES • hepatocellular diseases (metastases, hepatitis, cirrhosis) 2. INCREASED VALUES • hemolytic jaundice, secondary to RBC breakdown 3. INCREASED VALUES • extrahepatic bile duct obstruction • intrahepatic disruption (e.g., viral or alcoholic hepatitis) • bile duct disease
HEPATITIS TESTING • many tests are used to determine if a patient has been exposed to, is currently infected with, or is a carrier of viral hepatitis • tests can evaluate whether the genesis is hepatitis A or B, non-A, non-B	Hepatitis panel: antigen antibody testing for hepatitis and hepatitis B. Test includes: antibody to hepatitis A virus (anti-HAV) with IgM discrimination antibody to hepatitis B core antigen (anti-HC) with IgM discrimination hepatitis B surface antigen (HBsAg) hepatitis B surface antibody hepatitis C antibody

PRINCIPLE	INTERPRETATION
LACTIC ACID DEHYDROGENASE (LDH) • found in tissues of several systems (kidneys, heart, skeletal muscle, brain, liver lungs) • cellular death causes enzyme to increase • used usually to detect myocardial or pulmonary infarction	INCREASED VALUE • infectious mononucleosis • hepatitis • cirrhosis • obstructive jaundice
PROTHROMBIN (PT/PTT) • liver enzyme that is part of the blood clotting mechanism <u>PROTHROMBIN TIME (PT)</u> • measures the time required for a fibrin clot to form in a sample <u>ACTIVATED PARTIAL PROTHROMBIN TIME (PTT)</u> • measures the time required for the formation of a fibrin clot after the addition of an activator	INCREASED VALUE • extensive hepatic disease (causes decrease in clotting factors) • presence of heparin (anticoagulant therapy)
URINALYSIS URINE BILIRUBIN • test differentiates between complete and incomplete obstruction of ducts	INCREASED VALUE • hemolytic diseases • liver damage • severe infections

LIVER FUNCTION TESTS CONDENSED TABLE

X = elevation   XX = moderate elevation   XXX = severe elevation

	AFP	ALT/SGPT	AST/SGOT	BILIRUBIN INDIRECT	DIRECT	ALP
CARCINOMA	XXX	X	X			XX
CIRRHOSIS		X	X		XXX	X
HEMATOLOGIC DISEASE				XXX		
HEPATITIS		XXX	XX		XXX	X
OBSTRUCTIVE JAUNDICE		X	X		XXX	XXX

E) ANOMALIES

1) Diffuse Anomalies
2) Focal Anomalies
3) Vascular Anomalies

1) DIFFUSE ANOMALIES OF LIVER

DIFFUSE ANOMALY	US APPEARANCE

CIRRHOSIS

- fibrosis of liver, which can be classified as micro or macro nodular
- irreversible, chronic condition
- causes:
  alcoholism (Laennec's disease = cirrhosis + ETOH abuse)
  hepatitis B, C, postnecrotic
  primary biliary cirrhosis (destruction of intrahepatic bile ducts with resulting fibrosis from unknown etiology)
  hemochromatosis (excess accumulation of iron mainly within liver and pancreas)
  Wilson's disease (abnormality of copper metabolism)
  α_1-antitrypsin deficiency (low level of this serum protease inhibitor)

SS
<u>Late Cirrhosis</u>
- elevated AST (SGOT), ALT (SGPT)
- hyperbilirubinemia
- hypoproteinemia
- jaundice, ascites
- GI bleeding secondary to varices
- edema secondary to poor hepatic protein production

US
<u>Early Changes of Cirrhosis</u>
- enlarged liver, spleen (↑ caudate lobe/right lobe ratio > 0.65)
- increased echogenicity due to fatty change of the liver with patchy texture as liver regenerates
- increased attenuation
- vessels not well seen

<u>Late Changes of Cirrhosis</u>
- liver decreased in size (although liver can increase in size with hemochromatosis)
- lobular contour to liver
- increased echogenicity is mainly due to fatty change

<u>Complications of Chronic Cirrhosis</u>
- ascites
- portal hypertension with reversal of portal flow
- splenomegaly
- collaterals develop in portal venous system (varices)
- hepatoma

<u>Doppler:</u>
- hyperdynamic circulation due to the decrease in arterial resistance
- reduced pulsatility index of SMA
- paradoxical variations of portal flow during normal respiration

<u>Diff. Dx.:</u>
- heterogeneous appearance of liver can simulate diffuse primary or secondary carcinoma

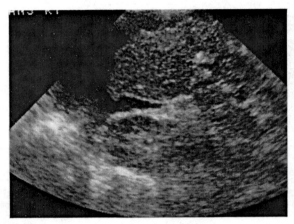

Transverse scan through late-stage cirrhosis

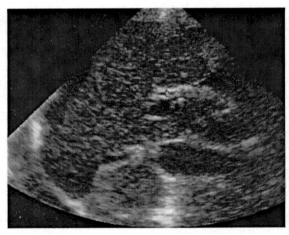

Small liver with surrounding ascites

DIFFUSE ANOMALY	US APPEARANCE

FATTY CHANGE

- reversible process
- accumulation of lipids in the hepatocytes due to a wide variety of etiologies which include:
  Toxic: ETOH abuse (most common), steroids, chemotherapy
  Nutritional: obesity, malnutrition
  Metabolic: diabetes, glycogen storage disease
  Other: ulcerative colitis, Crohn's disease, duodenal bypass

SS

- usually asymptomatic
- can rarely cause abnormal LFTs (↑ SGOT, SGPT, bilirubin)

US

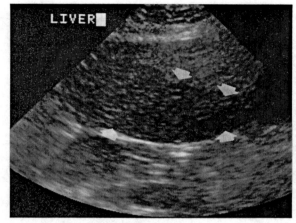

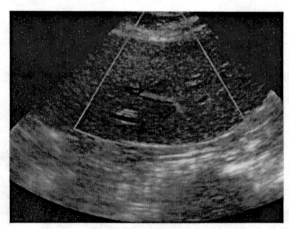

Area of fatty sparring (between arrows)

DIFFUSE APPEARANCE	FOCAL APPEARANCE
• fat increases liver echogenicity and ultrasound attenuation	• does not cause mass effect (nondisplaced portal vasculature)
Grade 1—Mild	• two types of focal processes:
• normal size liver	
• normal visualization of borders	1. Sparring
• lose visualization of portal tracts	• hypoechoic focal area of normal liver tissue in an otherwise fatty infiltrated liver
Grade 2	• usually found anterior to GB or portal vein in posterior portion of right or left lobe
• may have mild increase in size of liver	
• moderate diffuse increase in fine echos	2. Infiltration
Grade 3—Severe	• hyperechoic focal areas of fat in a liver with otherwise normal echo texture
• diaphragm becomes difficult to visualize due to attenuation	• can have an angular or bandlike appearance
• further increase in echogenicity	
• difficulty in visualization of deeper portions of liver	
• renal cortex appears more hypoechoic compared to liver in moderate to severe fatty change	

To prove it is an area of sparring versus mass, follow hepatic vessel through area in question: right portal vein traveling its normal course through hypoechoic region

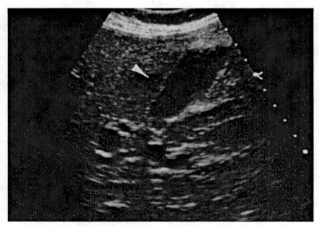

Fatty sparring adjacent to GB

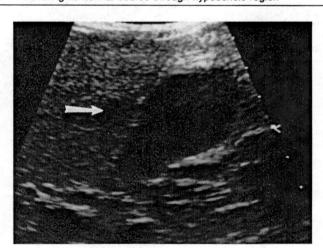

Focal fatty sparring in GB bed

(continued)

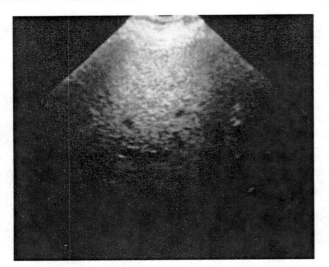

Fatty liver: gross attenuation

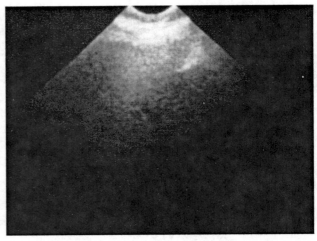

Fatty liver: transverse scan: vessels and diaphragm are not well visualized

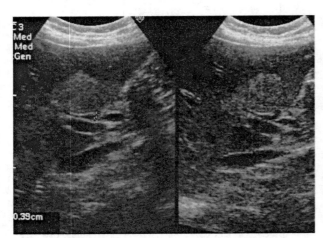

Focal fatty infiltration of liver: note how it does not displace adjacent structures

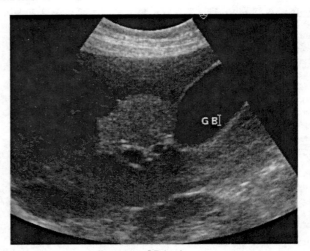

Focal fatty area adjacent to GB bed

DIFFUSE ANOMALY	US APPEARANCE

GLYCOGEN STORAGE DISEASE TYPE 1 VON GIERKE'S
- genetic disorder of carbohydrate metabolism
- excessive glycogen accumulates in hepatocytes
- increased incidence of adenomas

SS
- hypoglycemia
- decreased glucose-6-phosphatase

US
- hepatomegaly, renomegaly
- diffuse increased echogenicity of liver with increased attenuation
- associated with hepatic adenomas

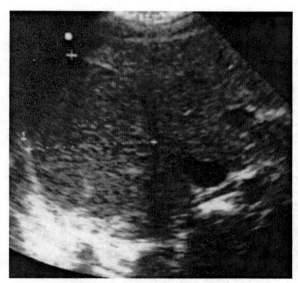

Glycogen storage disease: von Gierke's 1 with adenoma (between calipers)

DIFFUSE ANOMALY	US APPEARANCE

HEPATITIS

1. ACUTE HEPATITIS

- etiologies:

  Toxic: alcohol, drugs, toxins

  Infective: viral, bacterial, parasitic or secondary to toxic effects of infection elsewhere (e.g., cytomegalovirus, Epstein-Barr virus, herpes simplex virus, rubella, yellow fever)
- bilirubin increases due to hepatocellular damage and intrahepatic cholestasis
- Hepatitis A

  infectious hepatitis as it is easily spread by oral/fecal route

  short-lived, benign acute hepatitis that is not followed by chronic liver disease
- Hepatitis B

  serum hepatitis contracted through an infected person's body secretions such as blood

  may go on to chronic hepatitis and progress to cirrhosis

  predisposes to liver carcinoma
- Hepatitis C

  third viral group that has previously been included in the non-A and non-B hepatitis group caused by inoculations and blood transfusions

  more likely to cause chronic hepatitis and cirrhosis than hepatitis B

SS

- nausea, fever followed by jaundice
- hepatomegaly
- ↑ AST (SGOT) and ↑ ALT (SGPT), ↑ serum bilirubin, ↑ ALP

US

- hepatosplenomegaly
- increased echogenicity of portal triads (periportal brightness/"starry sky")
- normal appearance or overall decreased echogenicity of liver
- thickened GB wall

2. CHRONIC HEPATITIS

- is continuing acute hepatitis for more than 6 months
- usually caused by hepatitis viruses, but may also be caused by

  Wilson's disease

  α_1-antitrypsin deficiency

  alcohol

  drugs

SS

- fatigue, mild jaundice

US

- coarse liver echo pattern
- decreased echogenicity of portal triads to periportal fibrosis

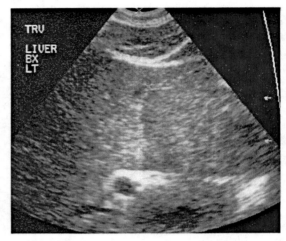

Normal-appearing liver, but on biopsy patient was diagnosed with chronic mildly active hepatitis

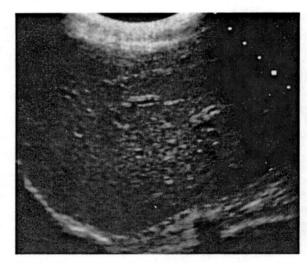

Periportal brightness in hypoechoic liver

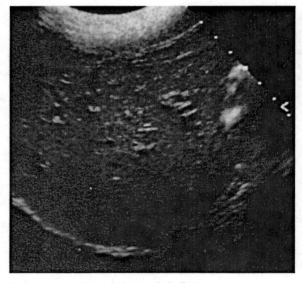

Periportal brightness in hypoechoic liver

COMMON DIFFERENTIALS WITH DIFFUSE SONOGRAPHIC FINDINGS

ECHO PATTERN	DIFFERENTIAL	
HOMOGENOUS, BUT DIFFUSELY "BRIGHT"	• technical fault (overall increase in gain) • normal variant • carcinoma (hepatocellular and diffuse secondary) • granulomas • tuberculosis • multiple tiny cysts of congenital cystic disease—previous hydatid cysts • parenchymal fibrosis (cirrhosis, chronic hepatitis, glycogen storage disease)	

DISCRETE BRIGHT ECHOGENIC FOCI (FOCUS)	• air in liver
	  1) biliary = from surgery, ERCP (papillotomy)
	  2) portal = necrotizing endocarditis
	• calcified granulomas (TB, histoplasmosis)	

DIFFUSE HYPOECHOIC	• amyloidosis • acute hepatitis • technical fault (too low a gain)	
ENLARGED LIVER—HEPATOMEGALY	• abscess • cirrhosis • congenital (anemia, cystic fibrosis) • congestive failure • cyst (hydatid) • elevated venous pressure	• fatty infiltration • hemochromatosis • hepatitis (viral, infectious, and serum) • metastases • neoplasm

2) FOCAL ANOMALIES OF LIVER

FOCAL ANOMALY	US APPEARANCE

ABSCESS/INFLAMMATORY LESIONS

1. AMEBIC
- parasitic
- common worldwide, but less common in United states
- 40% of cases involve liver with usually solitary or rarely multiple abscesses
- colonic amebiasis causes dysentery (bloody diarrhea associated with abdominal pain and fever)

US
- variable appearance
- round or oval hypoechoic mass
- contains homogeneous, low-level echos
- well defined, smooth thin walls
- acoustic enhancement

2. PYOGENIC
- most common type of abscess
- rarely occurs as a presenting lesion because it usually occurs as a complication of some other disease usually in older or ill patients
- multiple in 50%–70% of patients
- right posterior lobe most frequently involved
- causes include ascending cholangitis, trauma, surgery, portal phlebitis, infarction

SS
- fever, pain, chills, normal LFTs, ↑ WBC
- hot hepatic focus on gallium scan corresponding to abscess

US
- varied appearance, but predominantly fluid filled with enhancement
- primarily hypoechoic but can have echogenic areas
- irregular borders
- walls become thicker and more irregular with time
- may contain debris, gas, or calcification that can shadow

3. CANDIDA
- fungal infection that can vary from superficial lesions in healthy people to disseminated infections in immunocompromised patients
- candida can be introduced into blood via IV lines, catheters, peritoneal dialysis, surgery, drug abuse

US
- target hypoechoic lesions with target hyperechoic center

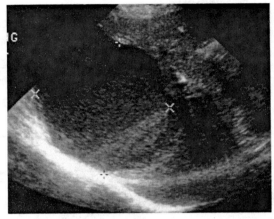

Liver abscess between calipers

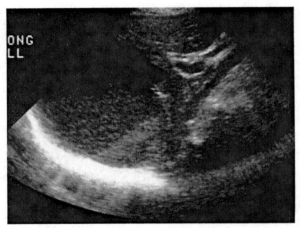

Liver abscess

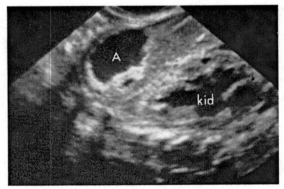

Sagittal liver with large hepatic abscess (A) and note of kidney with hydronephrosis (kid)

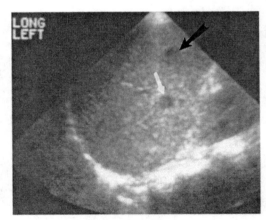

Candida: target lesions (arrow)

FOCAL ANOMALY	US APPEARANCE

CYSTS

True:
• fluid-filled space having a thin epithelial lining
False:
• abscesses, parasitic cysts, posttraumatic cysts, necrotic neoplasms

1. NONPARASITIC
• benign, focal, single or multiple
• Simple liver cyst
  asymptomatic with normal LFTs
• Polycystic disease
  associated with renal polycystic disease
  usually does not have abnormal LFTs

SS
• asymptomatic
• if large, can palpate mass
• may cause discomfort if huge
• normal LFTs

US
• well defined, smooth-walled, anechoic mass with posterior enhancement
• vary in size from < 1 cm to > 20 cm
• can have thin septations and still be considered benign
• can be multiple or solitary
• polycystic disease has cysts of multiple sizes found within liver parenchyma

2. PARASITIC–ECHINOCOCCAL (HYDATID)
• common in 3rd world or where people eat a lot of wild game or sheep
• cyst stage of infection by parasite tapeworm
Echinococcus granulosis
• travels from colon through portal system to liver
• generally do not aspirate as this can precipitate anaphylactic shock

SS
• pain, nausea, RUQ pressure, obstructive jaundice, ↑ WBC count

US
• well circumscribed cystic mass with smaller cysts surrounding it giving it a multilocular appearance
• variance in appearance may include:
  honeycomb: multiple simple cysts, calcified walls
  waterlily: daughter cysts collapse and appear to float within a larger cyst
  mother/daughter: endocyst cysts (internal to mother cyst) cause whole mass to appear as complex, multiloculated cystic mass with debris
• kidney and pancreas should be evaluated for associated cysts

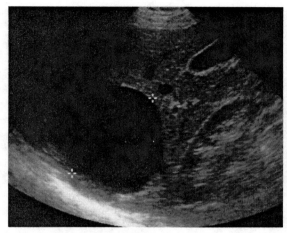

Large (8 cm) hepatic simple cyst

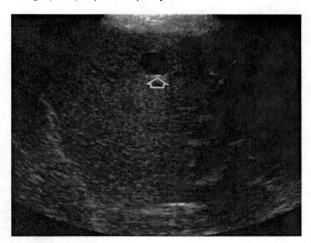

Small simple cyst

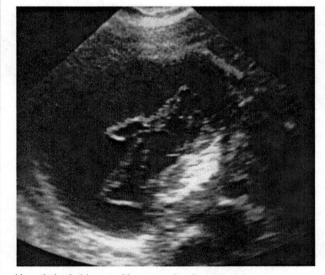

Hepatic hydatid cyst with ruptured collapsed endocyst

(*continued*)

US APPEARANCE OF HEPATIC CYSTS (*Continued*)

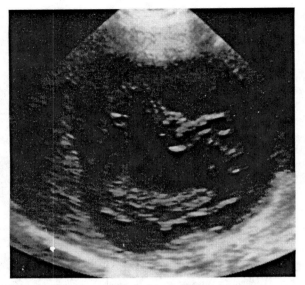

Hepatic hydatid cyst with ruptured collapsed endocyst

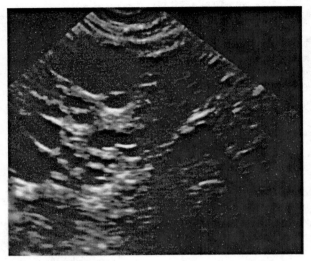

Polycystic liver disease

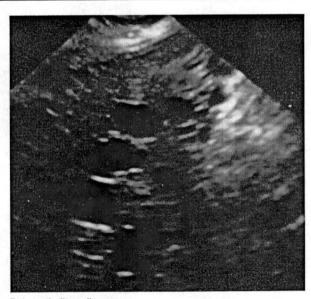

Polycystic liver disease

FOCAL ANOMALY	US APPEARANCE

FOCAL NODULAR HYPERPLASIA (FNH)

- not a true neoplasm but a malformation of liver cells
- benign process
- contain hepatocytes, Kupffer cells, and bile ducts
- uptake of tc^{99m} sulfur colloid in FNH has been reported in 60% of cases and may be of use in diagnosing these cases
- no tendency to rupture
- occurs in both sexes

US

- variable nonspecific appearance
- homogenous solid mass
- mildly more echogenic or isoechoic to liver
- may have a central scar

Diff. Dx.:

- any solid liver mass:
  liver cell adenoma (although it is usually more hypoechoic and inhomogenous)
  primary or secondary liver tumor
- hemangioma

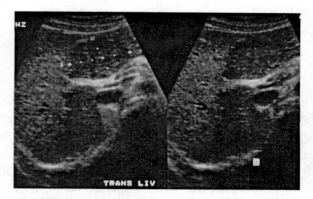

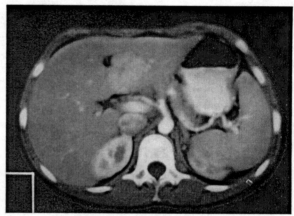

CT: early enhancement of lesion; note subtle hypodensity centrally, which represents central scar

FOCAL ANOMALY	US APPEARANCE

HEMANGIOMA—CAVERNOUS
- large sinusoidal spaces full of slowly moving RBCs
- most common benign tumor of liver
- small percentage may bleed
- most commonly subcapsular in right lobe

SS
- none, usually found incidentally in otherwise healthy people
- normal LFT, cold on liver nuclear medicine scan

US
- well circumscribed echogenic focal masses with acoustic enhancement
- sometimes do not show classical features

Doppler:
- small frequency shift that demonstrates little or no detectable flow

Diff. Dx.:
- primary or secondary malignancy of liver
- focal nodular hyperplasia
- adenoma

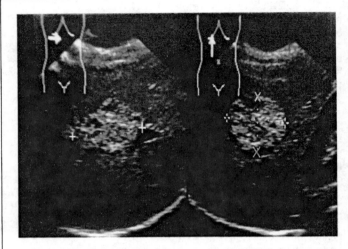

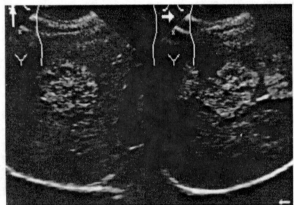

FOCAL ANOMALY	US APPEARANCE

HEMATOMA

- acquired traumatic lesion
- liver is 3rd most common organ injured after spleen and kidney
- frequently associated with other organs injured
- need for surgery depends on size of laceration

US
- CT used more frequently in diagnosis
- mixed echogenicity, which depends on age of hematoma
- irregular walls
- some through transmission
- peritoneal fluid (blood)
- Subcapsular hematomas
  hypo/hyperechoic possibly septated lenticular or curvilinear mass
- Internal hepatic hematomas
  < 24 hours—hypoechoic
  > 24 hours—complex, hyperechoic

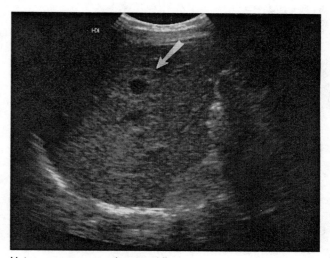

Heterogeneous mass in central liver

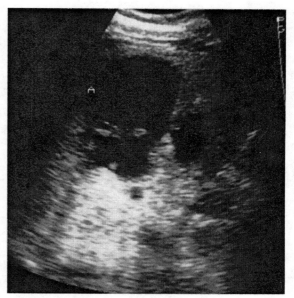

Liver hematoma

FOCAL ANOMALY	US APPEARANCE

LIVER CELL ADENOMA (LCA)/ADENOMA

- rare benign tumor
- most commonly seen in those who use oral contraceptive pills or steroids
- rapidly growing tumor
- tendency to rupture and hemorrhage
- 8% incidence of adenomas in glycogen storage disease (most commonly seen in type 1)

SS
- rarely palpable abdominal mass
- normal LFTs

US
- well defined solid mass
- can be hypo-, iso-, or hyperechoic
- may have fluid/fluid levels secondary to hemorrhage
- peritoneal fluid if ruptures

<u>Diff. Dx.:</u>
- FNH (more hyperechoic and homogeneous)

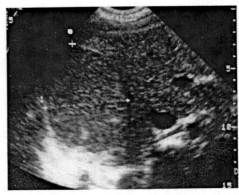

Transverse liver: LCA between calipers

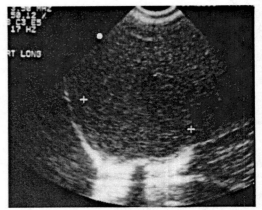

Sagittal liver: LCA between calipers

FOCAL ANOMALY	US APPEARANCE

MALIGNANCY OF LIVER

1. ANGIOSARCOMA (HEMANGIOSARCOMA)
- rare, highly malignant
- associated with distinct carcinogens such as arsenic, Thorotrast (old type of x-ray contrast), polyvinyl chloride

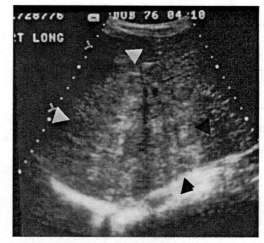

Hepatocellular carcinoma (arrows)

2. CHOLANGIOCARCINOMA
- 10% of primary liver cancers
- see section in Chapter 2—Bile Ducts

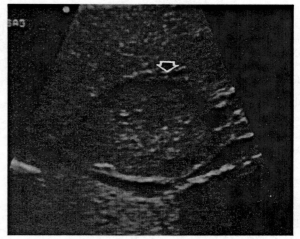

Round cell desmoplastic tumor of childhood

3. HEPATOCELLULAR CARCINOMA (Hepatoma, HCC)
- 90% of primary liver malignancy
- prevalence is increased by presence of chronic hepatocellular disease (cirrhosis due to ETOH abuse, hepatitis)
- more common in men
- elevation of α-fetoprotein in 2/3 of cases

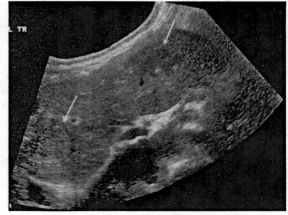

Transverse scan of liver in patient with HCC and cirrhosis; isoechoic lesion in right lobe and hypoechoic lesion in left lobe (from Siemens, with permission)

(continued)

143

FOCAL ANOMALY (*Continued*)	US APPEARANCE

4. HEPATOBLASTOMA
- primary pediatric liver tumor
- unless successfully resected, is usually fatal

5. METASTATIC DISEASE
- metastatic spread to liver is 20 times more common than primary malignancy
- most common primaries metastasizing to liver include lung, colon, pancreas, breast, stomach
  GI—spreads through portal system
  GB, stomach—direct spread

SS
- RUQ pain, hepatomegaly, weight loss, jaundice, and biliary stasis
- ascites, portal hypertension, splenomegaly

US
- variable and nonspecific
- small or large, diffuse or circumscribed
- "bull's eye" lesion: hypoechoic halo around tumor, which represents compressed liver tissue, tumor fibrosis
- focal lesion either echogenic (colon, pancreatic cancer) or hypoechoic
- mass effect: deviation of vessels to surround mass
- invasion of portal vein leading to portal vein thrombosis and hepatic veins leading to thrombus and Budd-Chiari syndrome

Doppler:
- neovascularization (AV communications) creates high-velocity shifts compared to normal liver tissue
- high systolic and diastolic signals from periphery of tumor that result from angiogenesis (RBC flow acceleration across AV fistulae and low-impedance neovessels lacking muscularis)
- vessel that does not deviate as it passes through mass suggests focal fatty infiltration rather than neoplasm

Pitfalls:
- absence of high-velocity signals does not exclude malignancy
- benign tumors with large AV shunts can mimic these Doppler signals

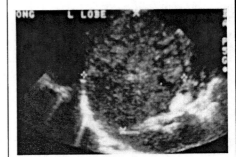

Hepatoblastoma (between calipers) in 17-month-old child

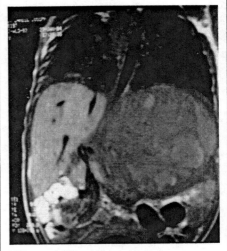

MRI correlation of hepatoblastoma

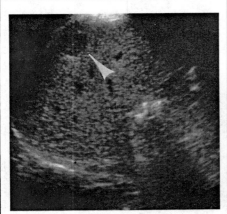

Metastatic liver disease: hypoechoic lesions from testicular primary (arrow)

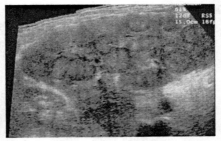

Longitudinal liver with multiple metastases (from Siemens, with permission)

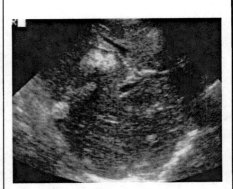

Metastatic liver disease: echogenic lesions from bowel primary

COMMON DIFFERENTIALS WITH FOCAL SONOGRAPHIC FINDINGS

ECHO PATTERN	DIFFERENTIAL	
SOLITARY SOLID MASS—GRANULOMA	• primary hepatoma • metastasis • adenoma, FNH, hemangioma • abscess or hematoma	
ANECHOIC LIVER LESIONS	• Caroli's disease • simple cysts • polycystic liver disease • hepatic vein or portal vein in cross section • biliary cystadenoma or carcinoma	• parasitic cyst (echinococcus) • hematoma • abscess • cystic metastases
HYPOECHOIC LESIONS	• abscess • cyst with cholesterol crystals • cystic tumor (cholangiocarcinoma, cystadenoma, hamartoma) • focal nodular hyperplasia	• hematoma • infarct • metastases
HYPERECHOIC LESIONS	• adenoma, focal nodular hyperplasia • abscess • cirrhosis (diffuse process) • focal fatty infiltration • foreign body	• granulomatous disease • hemangioma • hepatoma • liver cell adenoma, FNH • metastases (ovarian, pancreatic, GI or GU primaries)
COMPLEX SOLID MASS	• abscess • cavernous hemangioma • focal nodular hyperplasia • hepatocellular carcinoma • hydatid cyst (multiloculated with collapsed daughter/endocyst cysts) • metastasis (ovarian) • neoplams with liquefaction necrosis (hypoechoic) and infarcted nonliquefied areas (hyperechoic)	
ECHOGENIC FOCI WITHIN LIVER	• chronic abscess (amebic, polygenic) • gas in biliary tree • gas in portal veins • granulomatous disease (tuberculosis, histoplasmosis) • hydatid disease • neoplasm	

3) VASCULAR ANOMALIES OF LIVER

VASCULAR ANOMALY | US APPEARANCE

BUDD-CHIARI SYNDROME
- rare disorder caused by obstruction of hepatic veins
- obstruction can lie anywhere from the hepatic venules to the IVC
- rare in children
- causes:
  idiopathic 50%–75%
  secondary sources 25%–50%: thrombosis of hepatic veins, toxins, bone marrow transplantation, chemotherapy, lupus erythematosus, coagulation disorders, congenital malformations of hepatic vein, hepatic masses, oral contraceptives, pregnancy, trauma

SS
- nonspecific such as vague upper abdominal pain, ascites
- mildly abnormal LFTs
- hepatomegaly

US
- decreased echogenicity of liver
- enlarged hypoechoic caudate lobe
- IVC and/or hepatic vein thrombus
- reduced or nonvisualization of veins
- ascites

Pitfall:
- caudate lobe vein should not be mistaken for patent middle hepatic vein

Doppler:
- any reversal or lack of hepatic vein flow
- hepatic vein collaterals
- narrowing of the IVC causing accelerated and turbulent flow

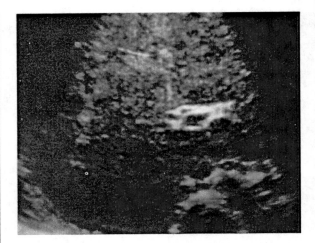

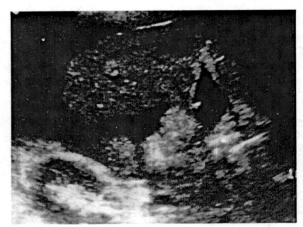

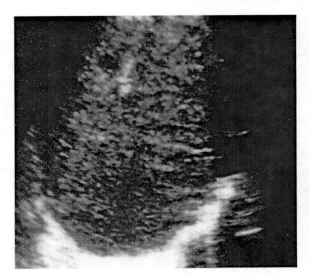

VASCULAR ANOMALY (*Continued*)	US APPEARANCE

PORTAL HYPERTENSION/OBSTRUCTION

- increase in the venous pressure of the portal system
- result of many diseases, but most commonly caused by cirrhosis
- occurs at 3 sites:
  1. Prehepatic: obstruction of splanchnic vein (e.g., portal)
  2. Intrahepatic: liver diseases (e.g., cirrhosis, hepatitis)
  3. Posthepatic: obstruction of hepatic veins, heart failure, constrictive pericarditis, thrombosis: (malignancy/HCC, chronic pancreatitis, hepatitis, trauma, shunts, hypercoagulable states/pregnancy), tumor compression

SS
- 4 major consequences: ascites, splenomegaly, portal systemic venous shunts, hepatic encephalopathy

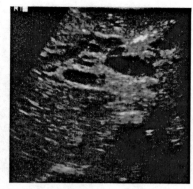

Multiple anechoic vascular collaterals seen on transverse scan through porta hepatis

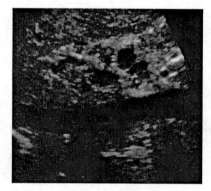

Multiple collaterals seen on sagittal scan through IVC

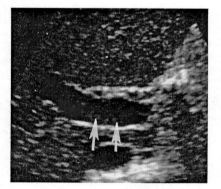

Portal vein thrombus: echogenic material noted in portal vein

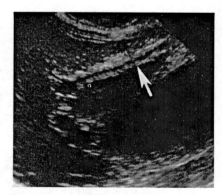

Patent umbilical vein (arrow)

US	PORTAL HYPERTENSION	PORTAL VEIN OBSTRUCTION
GRAY SCALE	• formation of collateral venous channels • portal vein and hepatic artery enlargement • splenomegaly	• lack of distention of splenic vein and SMV during respiration • enlarged vein filled with echogenic (acute) or hypoechoic (chronic) thrombus • chronic thrombosis can result in recanalization of portal vein also known as <u>cavernous transformation</u> • dilation of venous system proximal to point of obstruction
DOPPLER	• continuous low-velocity flow in portal vein (although normal velocity is variable and affected by age, cardiac diseases, hydration, nutrition state) • reversal (hepatofugal) of flow can be seen with increased portal pressures	• no blood flow at porta hepatis • high-frequency arterial signals in porta hepatis and intrahepatic branches • with portal vein occlusion, IVC and hepatic veins lose typical waveform and convert to a waveform more typical of portal vein (low-velocity continuous venous signal close to baseline)

TYPES OF PORTAL HYPERTENSION			
	PREHEPATIC PRESINUSOIDAL	**INTRAHEPATIC**	**SUPRAHEPATIC OR POSTHEPATIC**
CAUSE	• obstruction of splenic, mesenteric, or portal vein by thromboses	• cirrhosis: damaged hepatocytes cause sinusoids to become scarred and obstructed • abnormal portal venous flow occurs through any regenerated nodules • metabolic diseases, cirrhosis, hepatitis, ETOH or primary biliary cirrhosis	• obstruction of hepatic veins • Budd-Chiari syndrome
FACTORS	• vessel wall trauma • stagnant blood flow • abnormal clotting factors • tumor invasion • compression	• distorted hepatic parenchyma causes impedance to normal vascular flow	• coagulation abnormalities • congenital malformations of hepatic vein • congenital membranes of IVC
FINDINGS	CAVERNOUS TRANSFORMATION OR CAVERNOMA • collection of dilated paraportal veins and cystic vein channel blood into liver • appears as numerous small tortuous vessels at porta hepatis that represent recanalization secondary to portal venous obstruction • hepatopetal flow • portal hypertension often still persists despite these collateral channels	• intrahepatic blood flow decreases and portosystemic collaterals open • decrease or reversal of portal blood flow • hepatic blood supply maintained by increased flow in hepatic artery	• enlarged and congested liver • ascites, pleural effusions • splenomegaly • portasystemic collaterals • absence or reversal of flow in hepatic veins • areas of high velocity near stenoses of hepatic veins • arterial blood may be shunted into portal vein • portal venous flow may reverse

VASCULAR ANOMALY	US APPEARANCE

TRANSJUGULAR INTRAHEPATIC PORTOCAVAL SHUNTS (TIPS)

- used to relieve symptomatic portal hypertension in patients with chronic obstructive liver disease
- inserted under fluoroscopy percutaneously into a hepatic vein via the internal jugular vein
- the diameter of the stent can be altered to achieve the desired reduction in portal venous pressure
- shunt can be used to perform corrective angioplasty, thrombolysis, shunt dilatation, or varicocele embolization

US

- stent appears as parallel echogenic lines visualized within liver from right coronal, intercostal approach
- measure the angle-corrected velocity at the proximal, mid, and distal intrahepatic portions of stent and the main portal vein adjacent to the stent
- shunt stenosis should be considered with:
  decreasing velocity on interval scanning within the stent
  portal vein velocity > 40 cm/sec
  peak velocity < 50–60 cm/sec within stent
  and/or reversed flow in the proximal portion of the hepatic vein draining the stent

Diff. Dx.: for absence of flow in shunt:
- technical limitations
- reflective metal mesh wall of stent reduces sonographic visualization of flow
- completely thrombosed stent will not have any flow

Helpful Hint: to determine patent shunt when flow cannot be visualized in shunt:
- good flow in splenic and main portal vein toward the shunt with velocities higher than preshunt values

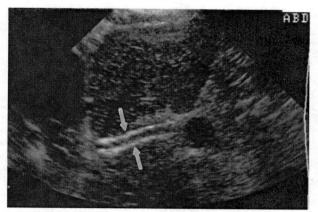

Longitudinal scan through liver showing TIPS (between arrows) in position

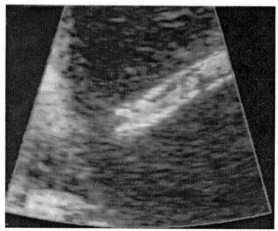

Power color flow through patent TIPS

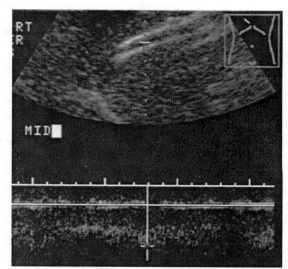

Pulsed Doppler signal within stent indicating an acceptable velocity of 77 cm/sec

F) TECHNICAL FACTORS

TRANSDUCER	• 3.0 MHz or 3.5 MHz • 5.0 MHz for very thin patient
TECHNIQUE	• deeply held inspiration
SCAN PLANES	• depending on liver shape and patient respiration, different degrees of subcostal and inferior angles should be used • intercostal scanning may be required • longitudinal and transverse views

TECHNICAL DIFFICULTIES HELPFUL HINTS	SMALL OR HIGH LYING LIVER	INTERCOSTAL VIEW • multiple intercostal scans taken using multiple intercostal windows can be used to visualize liver adequately RIGHT COSTAL MARGIN VIEW • angling up under the costal margin toward the patient's right shoulder

MINIMUM PROTOCOL	ROUTINE • aorta, IVC in liver region • main fissures and ligaments • hepatic veins and branches of portal vein • liver size in parasagittal scan plane from diaphragm to tip of liver • liver texture (echogenicity can be compared to right kidney) • documentation of any masses or abnormalities (e.g., location, size, echogenicity, whether they displace vessels, biliary tree)
	TRANSPLANTATION • accepted method of treatment for hepatic failure, cirrhosis, Budd-Chiari syndrome, biliary atresia, and tumor US ROLE Pretransplant • liver parenchyma and vasculature abnormalities must be ruled out • evaluation of anatomy, size, patency of IVC, hepatic and portal veins • other significant abdominal pathology must be ruled out Posttransplant • anastomotic sites as they are at an increased risk for stenosis, thrombosis, or occlusions: IVC—suprahepatic IVC—infrahepatic hepatic artery to aorta portal vein common bile duct • evaluation of hepatic parenchyma and size • evaluation of biliary system • volume of all extrahepatic fluid collections • common complications besides vascular and biliary include rejection and complications of immunosuppression 1. Hepatic artery thrombosis • most common and serious posttransplant problem • complications from this include infarction of liver parenchyma, biliary necrosis, bilomas, bile duct stenosis, sepsis, abscess • US is producing good sensitivity and specificity but presently gold standard for diagnosis is angiography

150

CHAPTER 8 - NECK AND HEAD
SALIVARY, THYROID, AND PARATHYROID GLANDS
A) NORMAL ANATOMY AND SONOGRAPHIC APPEARANCE OF SALIVARY GLANDS

DEFINITION	• 3 pairs of glands that secrete major portion of saliva

STRUCTURE

1. PAROTID GLAND
• composed of tubuloacinar glands
• largest salivary gland
• under and in front of ears
• between skin and masseter muscle
• occupies parotid fossa

2. PAROTID (STENSEN'S) DUCT
• pierces buccinator muscle to open into the mouth opposite the upper 2nd molar tooth

3. SUBMANDIBULAR GLAND
• 2nd largest of major salivary glands
• acinar glands
• beneath base of tongue in posterior part of mouth floor mainly in submandibular triangle
• between the platysma and mylohyoid muscle

4. SUBMANDIBULAR (WHARTON'S) DUCT
• runs superficially under mucosa of either side of midline of floor of mouth
• enter mouth just behind central incisor

5. SUBLINGUAL GLANDS
• smallest salivary gland
• acinar glands
• anterior to submandibular glands
• most deeply situated in sublingual sulcus

6. SUBLINGUAL DUCTS
a) Bartholin
• largest; 1 or 2 branches join submandibular duct
b) Rivinus
• smallest; some join submandibular duct, others open separately into floor of mouth

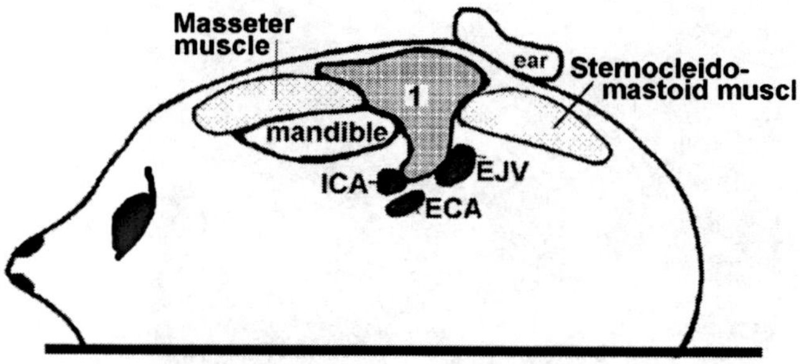

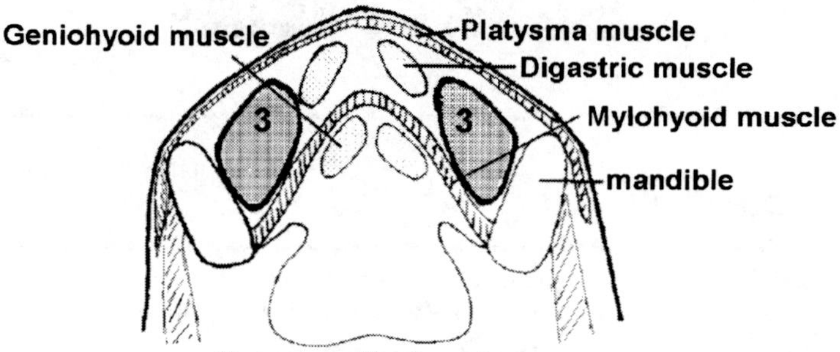

Submandibular view

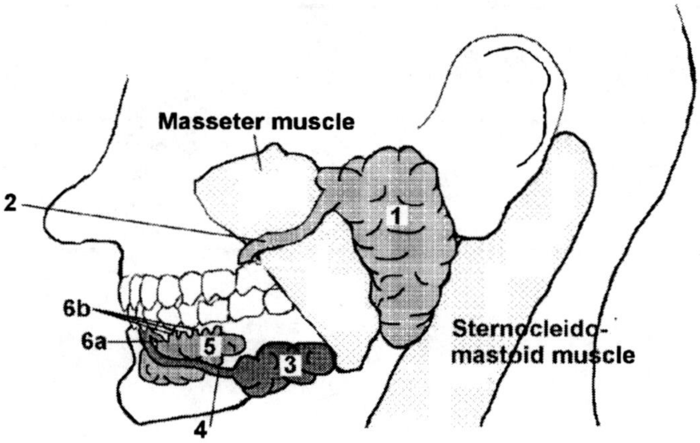

(continued)

US APPEARANCE

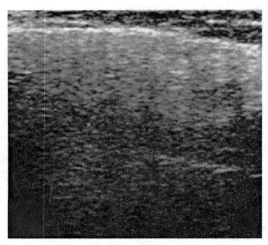

Sagittal scan through normal parotid gland

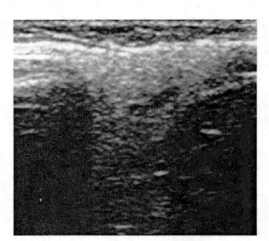

Coronal scan through normal parotid gland

B) VASCULATURE OF SALIVARY GLANDS

ARTERIAL	submandibular—branches of facial artery sublingual—branches of lingual artery
VEINS	follow arteries
LYMPHATICS	drain to submandibular nodes

C) PHYSIOLOGY OF SALIVARY GLANDS

PURPOSE AND FUNCTION	• moisten mucous membranes of mouth • secrete enzymes involved in initial stages of digestion of food • saliva is continuously secreted by glands in or near mouth • aids in the initial digestion of food

D) ANOMALIES OF SALIVARY GLANDS

ANOMALY	US APPEARANCE

CYSTS AND TUMORS
<u>1. CYSTS</u>
• types include true, dermoid, ductal, mucous retention, and mucoceles
 	
<u>2. TUMORS</u>
• incidence:
   65%–80% of salivary tumors are found in the parotid (15% are malignant)
   10% in the submandibular gland (40% are malignant)
   9% in the minor salivary glands (65% are malignant)
   1% in the sublingual glands (90% are malignant)
• the majority of salivary gland tumors are of epithelial origin
	• Benign neoplasms: less echogenic than normal parenchyma
	• Malignant neoplasms: inhomogeneous lesions with irregular and ill-defined borders
	• unilateral gland enlargement

BENIGN TUMORS	MALIGNANT TUMORS
<u>Pleomorphic Adenoma (Mixed Tumor)</u> • most common salivary tumor • benign tumor comprising 60% of all parotid tumors • composed of epithelial cells mixed in with mucoid, myxoid, and chondroid tissue <u>Warthin's Tumor (Adenolymphoma)</u> • 2nd most common benign salivary gland tumor	<u>Mucoid Epidermoid</u> • most common malignant tumor • found mainly in the parotid gland <u>Adenoid Cystic Carcinoma</u> • rare in parotids • most common malignant neoplasm in other salivary glands

ANOMALY	US APPEARANCE
ENLARGEMENT—SIALOSIS, ASYMPTOMATIC PAROTID ENLARGEMENT • nonneoplastic, noninflammatory chronic, or recurrent enlargement of salivary glands • associated with: malnutrition, alcoholic cirrhosis, diabetes • a common disturbance of parotid gland in adults	• nonspecific glandular enlargement
INFLAMMATION WITH SIALADENITIS/INFECTION • may be of viral, bacterial, or autoimmune origin • most common autoimmune disease is Sjögren's syndrome, which can lead to glandular destruction • most common viral infection is mumps mainly involving parotid • predisposing factors to infections are: obstruction of duct, debilitation, dehydration, irradiation, drug suppression of salivary secretions, immunosuppression	• nonspecific glandular enlargement • inhomogenous parenchyma • US can be used to check for abscess formation
SIALOLITHIASIS WITH SIALADENITIS/INFECTION • submandibular 80% • parotid 19% • sublingual 1% • only about 20% are shown on conventional x-rays • salivary calculi (sialoliths) are made primarily of calcium carbonate and calcium phosphate • form because of several factors (pH of saliva, mucous content of glands, obstruction of orifices by impacted food debris or edema) • secondary in frequency to mumps as a disease of salivary glands • occurs twice as often in men • dilatation of ducts is often associated with stones and/or strictures • peak occurrence between ages 30–50 SS • pain, swelling of glands • pus draining into mouth	• enlarged hypoechoic glands • echogenic focus with acoustic shadow • can have multiple calculi within gland and/or duct • increased blood flow (hypervascularity) on color Doppler and amplitude power mapping

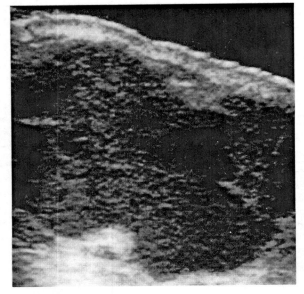

Pleomorphic adenoma

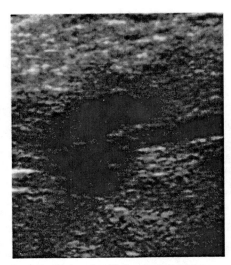

Submandibular gland inflammatory changes

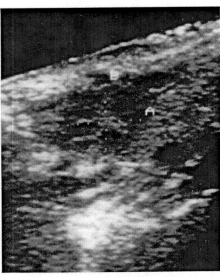

Submandibular gland: abscess

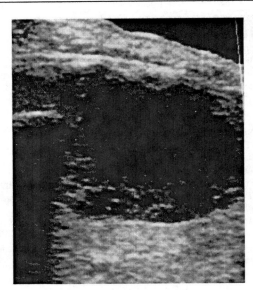

Submandibular malignant lymphoma

E) TECHNICAL FACTORS FOR SALIVARY GLANDS

TRANSDUCER	• high resolution 7–10 MHz • short focus
SCAN PLANES	Parotid Glands • scanned initially in axial plane, then coronal views Submandibular • coronal views are useful • scan patient in supine position with the neck hyperextended
HELPFUL HINTS	• glands are easily accessible to palpitation and therefore locate glands initially by feeling for them

A) NORMAL ANATOMY AND SONOGRAPHIC APPEARANCE OF THYROID AND PARATHYROID GLANDS

DEFINITION	THYROID • small butterfly-shaped endocrine gland in anterior part of throat PARATHYROIDS • 2 pairs, total 4 • small endocrine glands located adjacent to thyroid • secrete parathyroid hormone (PTH), which regulates calcium and phosphorus metabolism

STRUCTURE AND REGIONAL ANATOMY

1. THYROID GLAND
• bound by a fibrous capsule whose posterior layer encloses the 4 parathyroid glands
a) Right lobe
b) Left lobe
c) Isthmus
• superficial tissue that connects right and left lobes across the anterior tracheal wall
• between margins of sternohyoid and sternothyroid muscles
d) Pyramidal lobe
• variation of normal
• an extra lobe that extends superiorly from isthmus anterior to cricoid cartilage

2. PARATHYROID GLAND—superior (right and left)

3. PARATHYROID GLAND—inferior (right and left)

4. INTERNAL JUGULAR VEIN (IJV)
• located adjacent to CCA, at lateral aspect of thyroid

5. COMMON CAROTID ARTERY
a) External carotid artery

6. LONGUS COLLI MUSCLE
• posterior to each lobe of thyroid
• wedge-shaped hypoechoic structure (transverse plane) and long, narrow structure (longitudinal plane)
• normally cannot be distinguished from normal parathyroid or minor neurovascular bundle on longitudinal scan planes

7. SCALENUS MUSCLE
a) Anterior
• situated deeply at side of neck behind sternomastoid
b) Medial
• largest of scalenus muscles

8. STRAP MUSCLES
a) Sternohyoid muscle
b) Sternothyroid muscle
• thin hypoechoic bands adjacent to anterior surface of thyroid

9. STERNOCLEIDOMASTOID MUSCLE (SCM muscle)
• large muscle located anterior and laterally in neck
• extending from mastoid to sternum

10. OMOHYOID MUSCLE
• passes from the scapula to the hyoid bone

11. TRACHEA
• creates an echogenic curvilinear interface centrally

12. ESOPHAGUS
• bull's eye appearance posteromedial to left lobe of thyroid
• usually obscured by air in trachea

13. CRICOID CARTILAGE
• most inferior cartilage of larynx

14. HYOID BONE
• U-shaped bone lying at base of tongue
• muscles ascend and descend to it, but none cross it

15. THYROID CARTILAGE
• principal cartilage of larynx

16. PLATYSMA MUSCLE
• extends from fascia of both sides of neck to jaw and muscles around mouth

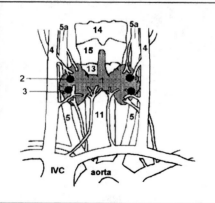

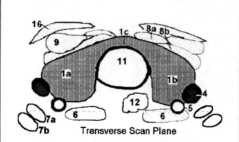

Transverse Scan Plane

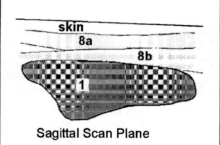

Sagittal Scan Plane

NORMAL ANATOMY

	THYROID	PARATHYROID
SIZE (EACH LOBE)	5 × 5 × 2 cm Length: 4–6 cm Width: 2–3 cm (each lobe) Thickness: 1–2 cm Isthmus: 1.25 × 1.25 cm	5 × 3 × 1 mm Length: 4–6 mm Width: 2–4 mm Thickness: 0.5–2 mm abnormal if > 6 mm

SHAPE	• whole gland is butterfly shaped
	• each lobe is pear shaped
	• lobes can by asymmetrical with right often larger than left
	• Lobes:
	  Medially—concave
	  Laterally—convex
		• oval, button shaped
		• become oblong when enlarged

LOCATION	• located in the lower front and sides of neck from C5 to T1 • superficial glands below larynx • lobes lie on either side of trachea	• located within the thyroid capsule or external to the posterior surface of each thyroid lobe • may occur anywhere within neck and even superior mediastinum
NEUROVASCULAR BUNDLES (NVB)	**a)** Major = CCA + IJV + vagus nerve • posterolateral to thyroid **b)** Minor = recurrent laryngeal nerve + inferior thyroid vessels • near parathyroid • appears as transverse structure between longus colli and lateral aspect of thyroid • to differentiate from parathyroid: in long axis parathyroid is oval and minor NVB is circular	

SONOGRAPHIC APPEARANCE

THYROID

TEXTURE ECHOGENICITY	• uniform, homogeneous, medium-level echogenicity • hyperechoic to surrounding neck muscles • visualization of fibrous septae, vascular calcifications, dilated follicles can normally be visualized and not indicate significant pathology

LANDMARKS

ISTHMUS Posterior: • trachea	**RIGHT LOBE** Lateral: right CCA right IJV Medial: trachea	**WHOLE GLAND** Anterior: muscle groups of neck including: SCM, sternothyroid, sternohyoid Posterior: longus colli muscle neurovascular bundle carotid sheath	**LEFT LOBE** Lateral: left common carotid artery left internal jugular vein Medial/posterior esophagus Medial: trachea

PARATHYROID

TEXTURE ECHOGENICITY	• hypoechoic or isoechoic to thyroid • homogeneously solid • surrounded by a fibrous sheath that appears as a dense echogenic band • normal parathyroids are not usually visible sonographically

LANDMARKS	**SUPERIOR GLANDS** • located close to upper posterior aspect of midportion of thyroid	**INFERIOR GLANDS** • anywhere from lower pole thyroid to thymus • anterior to longus colli muscle • medial to NVB	**ECTOPIC ADENOMAS** • retrotracheal/ tracheoesophageal groove • superior mediastinal • intrathyroid • carotid sheath

SONOGRAPHIC APPEARANCE

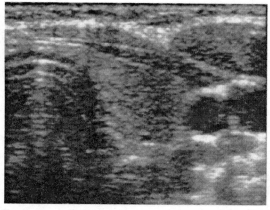

Transverse left lobe

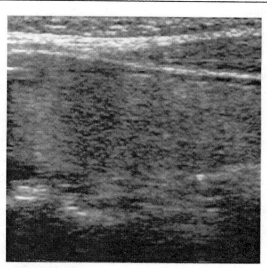

Sagittal left lobe

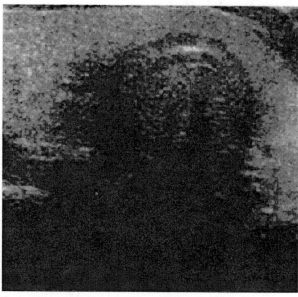

Transverse scan plane imaging bilateral thyroid gland
(Courtesy of Siemens SieScape)

B) VASCULATURE OF THYROID AND PARATHYROID GLANDS

ARTERIAL	External Carotid Artery → Superior Thyroid Artery **(1a)**
	Subclavian Artery → Thyrocervical Branches → Inferior Thyroid Artery **(1b)**
VENOUS	Superior **(2a)** + Middle Thyroid Veins **(2b)** → Internal Jugular Veins
	Inferior Thyroid Veins **(2c)** → Brachiocephalic Veins
LYMPHATICS	empty into deep cervical chains, posterior to SCM muscles

C) PHYSIOLOGY OF THYROID AND PARATHYROID GLANDS

THYROID GLANDS	

FUNCTION	1. Distribution of iodide into the body
	2. Coupling with iodide and other enzymes to produce
	   T_4—thyroxine
	   T_3—triiodothyronine
	   whose principal effects of thyroid hormones are:
	   a) regulation of metabolism (carbohydrate, lipid catabolism, protein synthesis)
	   b) regulation of growth and development
	   c) regulation of activity of nervous system
	3. Store and release hormones steadily over a long period of time
	4. Produce calcitonin
	• lower blood levels of calcium by accelerating calcium absorption by bones

HORMONE CYCLE	• respond to thyroid-stimulating hormone (TSH) secreted by pituitary gland • TSH is produced in response to release of thyroid-releasing hormone (TRH) by hypothalamus
PARATHYROID HORMONE	
PURPOSE	• secrete parathormone (PTH), which is involved in calcium and phosphorus metabolism, vitamin D activation 1. decrease blood phosphate level 2. increase blood calcium level
FUNCTION	• not controlled by pituitary gland, but controlled by a negative feedback control system of calcium levels in blood In GI tract: • increases rate of calcium, magnesium, and phosphate absorption into blood In bone: • causes release of calcium into bloodstream by increasing the number of osteoclasts (bone-destroying cells) In kidneys: • increases removal of calcium and magnesium from filtrate and returns them to blood • accelerates transportation of phosphate from blood into urine for elimination

D) LAB TESTS FOR PARATHYROID AND THYROID GLANDS

PARATHYROID GLANDS

TEST	ELEVATED	DECREASED
ALKALINE PHOSPHATASE	• hyperparathyroidism	
CALCIUM • serum calcium and phosphorus levels are reflective of parathyroid function	• hyperparathyroidism • malignant tumors (multiple myeloma, lymphoma, carcinoma of breast, lung, kidney, bone metastases) • hyperthyroidism • excessive calcium intake • parathyroid adenoma	• therapeutic hemapheresis • massive blood transfusion • vitamin D deficiencies • hypoparathyroidism (due to removal of parathyroids usually) • acute pancreatitis
PARATHYROID HORMONE • secreted by parathyroid glands • decrease in calcium stimulates PTH release	• hyperparathyroidism due to solitary adenoma, or secondary hypoplasia (most commonly as a result of renal disease)	• hypoparathyroidism (most commonly secondary to postoperative thyroid surgery, and can also be idiopathic, congenital (DiGeorge syndrome, which is also associated with absence of thymus)

THYROID GLANDS

TEST	PRINCIPLE	COMMENTS
RADIOACTIVE IODINE UPTAKE (RAIU) ^{131}I uptake	• determines thyroid function	• hyperthyroidism does not always cause high iodine uptake NORMAL OR HIGH • Graves' disease • toxic multinodular goiter • hypopituitary disease LOW • subacute thyroiditis • hyperthyroiditis • thyrotoxicosis • metastatic thyroid carcinoma • struma ovarii (ectopic thyroid tissue in ovarian teratoma)
TSH LEVEL	• secreted by anterior pituitary on stimulation by TRH from the hypothalamus • it stimulates the release of T_3 and T_4 by the thyroid	• most sensitive test for primary hyperthyroidism HIGH • hyperthyroidism, thyroid cancer LOW • hypothyroidism, thyroiditis
T_4 (THYROXINE)	• secreted by the thyroid gland in response to TSH • only a small amount circulates freely in blood	TOTAL T_4 • detects 90% of hyperthyroid cases • affected by thyroxine-binding globulin (TBG) FREE T_4 • fraction of total T_4 • independent of TBG levels
T_3 (TRIIODOTHYRONINE)	• the more potent thyroid hormone • 50% is derived from T_4 • secretion occurs in response to TSH secretion	• used to detect hyperthyroidism • low value does not always indicate hypothyroidism

E) ANOMALIES OF PARATHYROID AND THYROID GLANDS

PARATHYROID ANOMALIES	US APPEARANCE
HYPERPARATHYROIDISM (PRIMARY) • excessive PTH that causes hypercalcemia: bone resorption and calcium mobilization from the skeleton (can cause bone to be highly susceptible to fracture) increases renal tubular reabsorption and retention of calcium enhances GI calcium absorption • secondary hyperparathyroidism is associated with renal failure, vitamin D deficiency • primary hyperparathyroidism is caused by: 1. PARATHYROID ADENOMA (75%–80%) • most common cause of enlargement of parathyroid gland • occurs in both sexes, any age but peak incidence in middle decades of life • usually involves only one of the glands US • sharply marginated, discrete solid, oval masses • can be round, usually oblong and homogeneously solid • less echogenic than thyroid gland • can have cystic changes, calcification and be multilobulated • usually < 1.5 cm in length • 10%–15% are situated in sonographically inaccessible locations 2. PARATHYROID CARCINOMA (< 5%) • very rare • usually larger than adenomas US • frequently have lobulated contour • heterogeneous internal architecture • cystic components • usually indistinguishable sonographically from large benign adenomas 3. PRIMARY HYPERPLASIA OR PARATHYROID (10%–15%) • can be diffuse or nodular • usually involves all of the parathyroid glands SS • elevated serum calcium • may include renal stones or nephrocalcinosis same sonographic appearance as other adenomas • can be inconsistently and asymmetrically enlarged **HYPOPARATHYROIDISM** • functional disorder with few distinctive anatomic changes; therefore, not visualized sonographically • can be caused by the inadvertent removal of the glands, congenital absence of the glands, autoimmune disease, or rare syndromes SS • tetany (stiffness, cramps, spasms, convulsions) due to muscle instability brought on by reduced available calcium	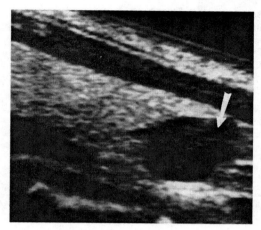 Adenoma (arrow) 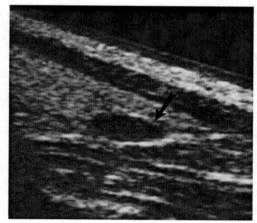 Adenoma (arrow)

THYROID ANOMALIES	US APPEARANCE

ADENOMAS AND CYSTS

1. ADENOMAS
- 90% of thyroid neoplasms are adenomas
- nearly all present as solitary, discrete masses
- not premalignant
- FOLLICULAR ADENOMA
  most common benign thyroid tumor
  encapsulated true neoplastic nodules
  can undergo hemorrhage and necrosis

US
- low level homogeneous echotexture
- may contain some irregularity, internal septations, debris, or calcification
- can have "halo" or hepoechoic rim in 60%–80% of cases

2. CYSTS
- true simple cyst is very rare
- both benign and malignant lesions can have cystic components, therefore sonographic determination of a cystic lesion will need further clinical follow-up

US
Simple: same as elsewhere in body (echo free with through transmission and well defined walls)
Other: most have thickened walls secondary to internal degeneration (degenerating adenoma)

- THYROGLOSSAL DUCT CYST
  congenital anomaly found in midline of neck anterior to trachea
  usually form fusiform-shaped cysts smaller than 3 cm
  may communicate with skin, producing draining sinuses or drain into base of tongue

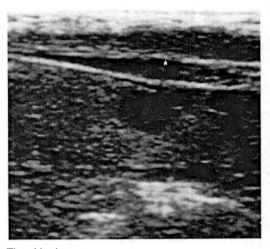

Thyroid adenoma

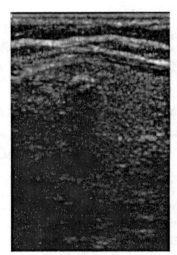

Adenomas can "burn" out and show as small calcified lesions

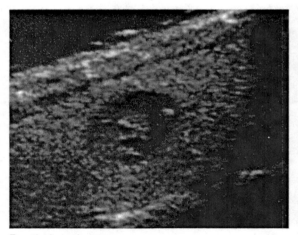

Functioning adenoma

THYROID ANOMALIES	US APPEARANCE

CANCER
• differentiated into 4 types microscopically:

1. ANAPLASTIC (UNDIFFERENTIATED)
• < 5% of thyroid cancers
• more common in age group 70–80
• rapidly growing fatal tumor

2. FOLLICULALR ADENOCARCINOMA
• 2nd most common thyroid malignancy (5%–15%)
• occurs in older age group, women more commonly than men
• malignant counterpart of the benign follicular adenoma

3. MEDULLARY CARCINOMA
• makes up 5%–10% of thyroid malignancies
• frequently familial
• more aggressive than follicular and papillary tumors with poorer prognosis
• may demonstrate echogenic foci with shadowing, which represent fibrosis and calcification around amyloid deposits

4. PAPILLARY CARCINOMA
• most common thyroid carcinoma (75%–85%)
• occurs often in young females
• slow-growing tumor

SS
• lump in neck, hard mass on palpation, history of enlarging goiter, hoarseness, difficulty in swallowing, pressure symptoms, pain, satellite lymphadenopathy

US
• primarily solid but can appear complex
• may have smooth or irregular borders
• size varies from 2–10 cm
• usually singular and hypoechoic
• cystic degeneration can occur
• small fine punctate microcalcifications are a predictor of carcinoma

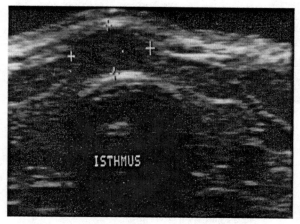

Papillary carcinoma (calipers) within isthmus of thyroid

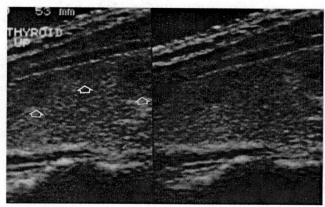

Follicular carcinoma (arrows)

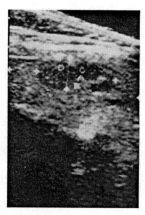

Follicular carcinoma
(calipers)

THYROID ANOMALIES	US APPEARANCE

GOITERS

- any unusual enlargement of the thyroid gland
- occurs with lack or excess of iodine, chronic alcoholism, Graves' disease, Hashimoto's disease

1. SIMPLE/DIFFUSE (ENDEMIC)

- diffuse enlargement of one or both lobes of gland
- occurs if gland does not receive enough iodine to produce suffucient thyroxine for body's needs
- usually caused by dietary insufficiency of iodine
- not associated usually with either hyperfunction or hypofunction
- endemic goiter refers to the high incidence in particular areas of world (i.e., Alps, Andes, central Africa)
- nonendemic or sporadic simple goiter is much less common

2. MULTINODULAR GOITER

- derived from chronic simple goiter
- may be nontoxic or may induce thyrotoxicosis
- rarely associated with hypothyroidism

SS

- enlargement of gland with multiple nodules of varying size
- can lead to cosmetic disfigurement, dysphasia, inspiratory stridor
- hemorrhage into goiter may cause sudden painful enlargement

US

- varies widely
- initially may enlarge and have normal or heterogeneous echogenicity without discrete nodules
- later stages may develop:
  multiple focal solid nodules within normal tissue
  diffusely nodular with no normal tissue
  areas of punctate calcifications
- glandular asymmetry

Diff. Dx.:

- neoplastic involvement of thyroid

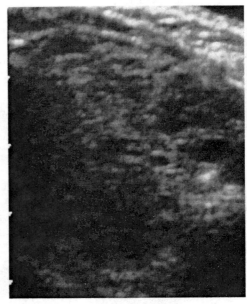

Transverse scan of right lobe goiter

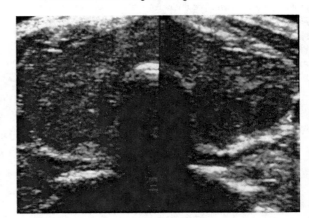

Transverse split image of diffuse goiter involving both lobes

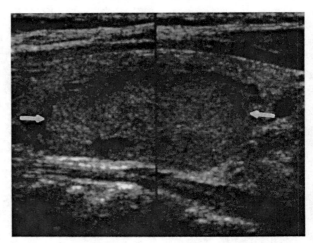

Sagittal scan of thyroid with large nodule (between arrows)

HYPERTHYROIDISM	HYPOTHYROIDISM
• hypermetabolic state of thyroid with elevated serum T_3 and T_4 levels	• low levels of T_4
• caused by: hyperfunction (hyperthyroidism) leakage of hormone in nonhyperactive gland (thyrotoxicosis)	• caused by: postoperative thyroidectomy diseases that can destroy the thyroid or the production of thyroid hormone deficiency of TSH stimulation of a normal thyroid gland deficiency of TRH from hypothalamus peripheral resistance to the action of thyroid hormone (rare)
• disorders that can cause this include:	• clinical manifestation depends on age of occurrence
1. GRAVES' DISEASE—hyperfunction	**1. CRETINISM**
• most common diffuse abnormality of thyroid gland • autoimmune disorder in which antibodies are produced against TSH receptors • occurs in younger ages • exophthalmic goiter • exophthalmos (protruding eyeballs)	• onset in utero or infancy • results in physical and mental retardation • seldom apparent at birth
2. METASTATIC THYROID CANCER	**2. MYXEDEMA**
3. SUBACUTE OR ACUTE THYROIDITIS	• onset in older children and adults
4. CHORIOCARCINOMA, HYDATIDIFORM MOLE	SS
5. OVERDOSE OF THYROID HORMONE	• slowing of mental and physical activities • nonspecific symptoms, i.e., lethargy, depression, constipation, thick puffy skin, cold intolerance, impaired memory, slowing of speech, slow heart rate, low body temperature, muscular weakness
SS • abnormally high metabolic rate (increased skin temperature, pulse rate, blood pressure, tremor, muscular weakness, weight loss, restlessness, anxiety)	US • depends on etiology • postoperative: absence of thyroid gland
US • enlargement of gland that otherwise appears normal • thickening of isthmus > 1.25 cm	
Doppler: • "thyroid inferno": multiple tiny areas of flow in entire gland	

THYROID ANOMALIES	US APPEARANCE

THYROID ANOMALIES

THYROIDITIS
- many forms
- inflammatory enlargement of gland

1. HASHIMOTO'S DISEASE
- most common cause of goitrous hypothyroidism
- autoimmune disorder: chronic inflammatory disease of thyroid
- more common in women and incidence increases with age

SS
- goitrous enlargement of gland
- ↑ serum TSH levels, ↓ T3, T4 levels

US
- diffuse, possibly asymmetric moderate enlargement of gland
- diffusely abnormal echo pattern, inhomogeneous
- decreased in overall echogenicity of gland
- occasionally seen with discrete nodules

2. SUBACUTE THYROIDITIS
- viral disorder with possible hyperthyroidism
- any sonographic changes in thyroid resolve in weeks
- women more commonly affected than men

SS
- ear pain, dysphagia
- thyroid is slightly enlarged, firm, and tender
- can cause hyperthyroidism

US
- causes diffuse coarsening of parenchymal echotexture
- diffuse decreased echogenicity of gland
- glandular enlargement
- discrete nodules may be present
- calcifications can be present
- often difficult to distinguish from multinodular goiter

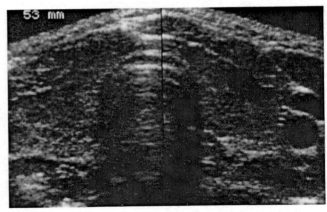

Transverse split image of both lobes of thyroid in Hashimoto's disease

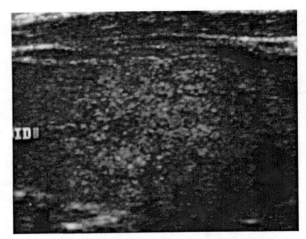

Sagittal scan of inhomogeneous thyroid with thyroiditis

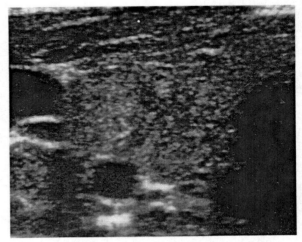

Transverse scan of inhomogeneous thyroid with thyroiditis

THYROID NODULES

- there is a significant overlap with appearance of benign and malignancy nodules and at present differentiating benign from malignant lesions is not possible sonographically
- fine needle aspiration (FNA) is a more accurate method to distinguish benign from malignant nodules
- calcifications are found in 13% of all nodules

	BENIGN		MALIGNANT
US FEATURES	• multiple nodules (2%–4% risk of malignancy) • cystic components • course, large or peripheral (eggshell-like) calcifications • hyperechoic texture • well defined margin • thin, complete halo		• solitary nodule (15%–25% risk of malignancy) • irregular and poorly circumscribed • hypoechoic to adjacent normal thyroid parenchyma (although benign hypoechoic nodules are commonly seen) • varies from solid to purely cystic • thick, incomplete halo • fine, punctate internal calcifications
CONDITIONS	FOCAL	DIFFUSE	• primary malignant thyroid disease
	adenomas hemorrhagic cysts simple cysts	goiter thyroiditis post-neck irradiation of gland	

RADIONUCLIDE SCANS

FUNCTION	• radionuclide imaging that can evaluate function, morphology, size, and location of thyroid gland

COLD NODULE—Nonfunctioning nodule • nodule that takes up little or none of the radionuclide	HOT NODULE—Hyperfunctioning nodule • nodule that takes up a lot of radionuclide
• solitary cold, 15%–25% are malignant • cold nodule in multinodular gland, < 1% are malignant (although sonographic detection of additional nodules is not a reliable sign for excluding malignancy) Diff. Dx.: • cysts (usually degenerating adenoma) • carcinomas, lymphomas, metastases • focal thyroiditis	• malignancy is extremely rare • almost always a benign adenoma

F) TECHNICAL FACTORS FOR THYROID AND PARATHYROID GLANDS

	THYROID	**PARATHYROID**
TRANSDUCER	7.5–10 MHz linear array • water bath or stand-off pad if required to visualize very superficial structures	7.5–10 MHz linear array
TECHNIQUE	• patient scanned in supine position with head flat and neck hyperextended (pad under shoulders) and supported by cushion • scanned in sagittal, transverse, and oblique scan planes	• patient scanned in same position as for thyroid • locate and scan thyroid in transverse, sagittal, and oblique scan planes • evaluate superior to thyroid • evaluate inferior to thyroid to clavicles • patient swallowing will elevate thyroid and some of parathyroid lesions caudal to thyroid
SCAN PLANES	Transverse: • superior, middle and inferior right gland, left gland • isthmus Longitudinal: • lateral, middle and medial right and left gland	• best visualized on sagittal views
MINIMUM PROTOCOL	• document size and shape of gland • assess texture (use split screen images to compare lobes) • examination extended to carotid artery and jugular vein to visualize any parathyroid masses or nodes	• use standard thyroid imaging protocol • scan below inferior aspect of thyroid • look for discreet hypoechoic masses adjacent to thyroid • document size, shape, and echogenicity of any nodules

TECHNICAL DIFFICULTIES AND HELPFUL HINTS	• lower poles of thyroid gland can be visualized by having the patient swallow
	• to fully measure length of thyroid gland, a 5-MHz transducer that has a wider footprint might be needed
		False-positive results:
		• other neck structures can simulate parathyroid adenomas
		  perithyroid veins
		  esophagus
		  longus colli muscles
		  thyroid nodules
		  cervical lymph nodes
		False-negative results:
		• some reasons why visualization of adenomas does not occur
		  minimally enlarged adenomas
		  enlarged thyroid displaces and obscures them
		  ectopic adenomas

OTHER PROCEDURES	FINE NEEDLE ASPIRATION (FNA) • most effective way for diagnosing malignancy in thyroid nodule • palpable nodules can undergo biopsy without sonographic guidance • FNA under sonographic guidance enables selective sampling of solid elements of mass • accuracy of FNA is about 95% FNA PROCEDURE • small echogenic foci within thyroid nodule is the tip of a 25-gauge needle during aspiration of cells • use of high-resolution small parts 10-MHz transducer is noted	PERCUTANEOUS BIOPSY • done under US guidance • frequent preoperative confirmation of parathyroid pathology • biopsy failures are usually due to inadequate recovery of tissue for analysis • cytologic, histologic, and radioimmunoassay for PTH can be done

CHAPTER 9 - PANCREAS

A) NORMAL ANATOMY AND SONOGRAPHIC APPEARANCE

DEFINITION	• lobulated organ extending obliquely and transversely across the mid to upper abdomen

DUCTAL SYSTEM	PANCREAS

1. MAIN (PRINCIPAL) PANCREATIC DUCT (WIRSUNG'S DUCT)
• extends length of pancreas
• originates in small ducts of lobules in tail
• lies transverse in pancreas, nearer the posterior surface and anterior to splenic vein
• increases in size toward neck, but normally ≤ 2 mm
• joins the CBD in entering descending duodenum at the ampulla of Vater
 	
2. AMPULLA OF VATER (SPHINCTER OF ODDI/ HEPATOPANCREATIC AMPULLA)
• formed by union of CBD and main pancreatic duct
• opens into major duodenal papilla
 	
3. MAJOR DUODENAL PAPILLA
 	
4. ACCESSORY PANCREATIC DUCT (DUCT OF SANTORINI)
• small and sometimes absent
• additional duct from upper pancreatic head
• opens into minor duodenal papilla 2 cm above level of ampulla of Vater separately from Wirsung's duct
 	
5. MINOR DUODENAL PAPILLA
• also known as accessory duct papilla or Santorini papilla
• no capsule
	6. HEAD
	a) Uncinate process
	• medial projection from left lower aspect of head
	
	7. NECK
	• junction and head and body
	
	8. BODY
	• three surfaces
	  anterosuperior: concave, covered with peritoneum
	  posterior: not covered with peritoneum
	  anteroinferior: covered with peritoneum
	
	9. TAIL
	• contained within 2 layers of splenorenal ligament

REGIONAL ANATOMY OF PANCREAS

HEAD	UNCINATE PROCESS	NECK	BODY	TAIL
• lies in curve of duodenum • right of SMV • anterior to IVC • caudad to portal vein	• encircles SMV, but not always SMA • anterior to aorta, posterior to superior mesenteric vessels • variable in size	• lies in transpyloric plane posterior to pylorus • anterior to confluence of SMV and splenic vein • often lies posterior to SMV and SMA	• most anterior aspect of pancreas • anterior to SMA, splenic vein	• commonly lies cephalad to body directly anterior to upper pole of left kidney • tip lies in splenic hilus • left adrenal lies posterior to splenic vein and pancreatic tail

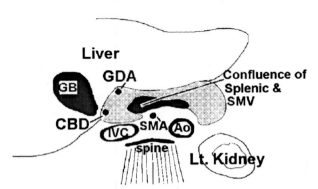

Transverse through midline at level of pancreas

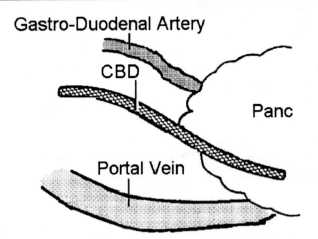

Longitudinal through portal hepatis showing relationship of portal vein, GDA and CBD to head of pancreas

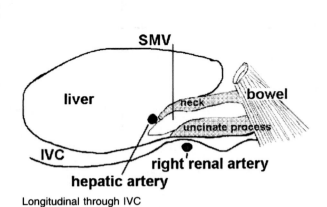

Longitudinal through IVC

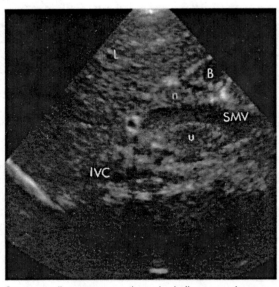

Corresponding sonogram through similar scan plane

REGIONAL ANATOMY OF PANCREAS

Longitudinal through aorta

Corresponding sonogram through similar scan plane

NORMAL ANATOMY

SHAPE	• lobulated sideways J-shaped gland tapering from head to tail
CONGENITAL ANOMALIES	• both of these conditions are usually diagnosed by ERCP, occasionally on CT and not seen sonographically 1. ANNULAR PANCREAS • rare anomaly • formed by failure of normal regression of left ventral bud • head of pancreas encircles duodenum causing duodenal or biliary obstruction 2. PANCREAS DIVISUM • failure of the normal fusion of the 2 separate pancreatic buds • associated with higher incidence of pancreatitis
SIZE	• 15–20 cm long • no AP measurement should exceed 3 cm • tail measurements are taken at 90° to long axis

	HEAD	BODY	TAIL
ADULT	2.5 cm	2.0 cm	2.0 cm
CHILD	< 2.0 cm	< 1.0 cm	< 1.6 cm
MAIN DUCT	2–3 mm	2 mm	1.5 mm

LOCATION	• upper abdomen in anterior pararenal space in the retroperitoneum • extends from the hilum of the spleen to the duodenum • posterior and slightly inferior to stomach • variable lie, but usually in an oblique rather than transverse plane with the head at a more inferior level than the tail

SONOGRAPHIC APPEARANCE

SONOGRAPHIC ANATOMY

LANDMARKS	TRANSVERSE SCAN PLANE	SAGITTAL SCAN PLANE
PORTAL SPLENIC CONFLUENCE	• splenic vein joins with SMV posterior to neck to form portal vein	• circular sonolucent structure anterior to IVC and superior to head of pancreas
COMMON BILE DUCT	• sonolucent structure posterior aspect of head of pancreas	• tubular sonoluceny coursing posteriorly to pancreatic head
GASTRODUODENAL ARTERY	• sonolucent structure anterior border of head of pancreas	• sonolucency coursing anterior-medially to CBD over pancreatic head
SPLENIC VEIN	• courses posterior and parallel to body and tail of pancreas	• circular sonolucency posterior to cephalad portion of pancreas
SPLENIC ARTERY	• tortuous vessel in anterior aspect of body	• rounded sonolucent structures along anterior border
SUPERIOR MESENTERIC VEIN	• left of pancreatic head	• anterior to uncinate process
SUPERIOR MESENTERIC ARTERY	• sonolucent circular structure posterior to pancreatic body, anterior to aorta	• posterior-inferior to pancreatic body and splenic vein
ANTRUM OF STOMACH	• superior to body of pancreas • when full appears as oval cystic structure • when contracted appears with lucent walls with echodense lumen	• bull's eye appearance anterior and caudal to head and body

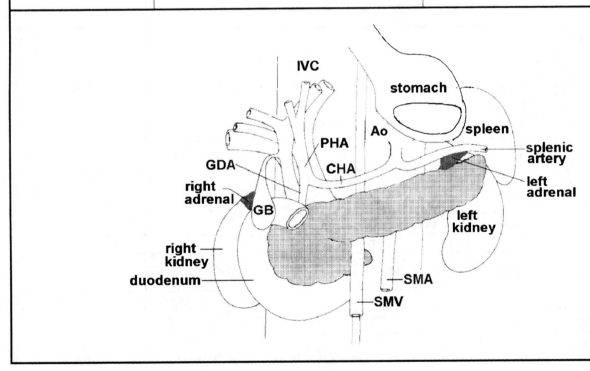

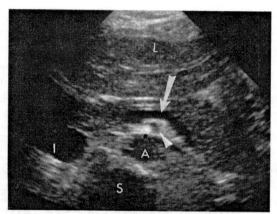

Transverse pancreas: liver (L), IVC (I), aorta (A), spine (S), SMA (arrowhead), splenic vein (arrow)

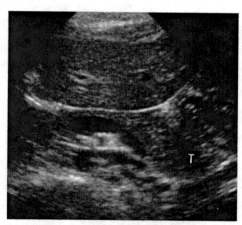

Transoblique scan plane that enables better visualization of tail of pancreas (T)

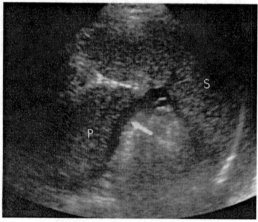

Coronal left: splenic vein (arrow) from hilum of spleen (S) coursing along posterior aspect of tail of pancreas (P)

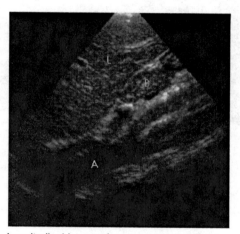

Longitudinal image of pancreas through body (B), aorta (A), liver (L)

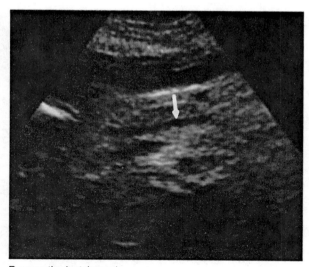

Pancreatic duct (arrow)

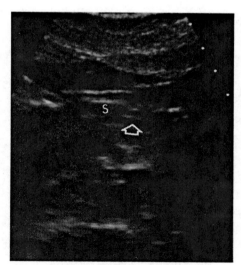

Pitfall: hypoechoic wall (arrow) of stomach lying adjacent to pancreas can appear as pancreatic duct

SONOGRAPHIC ECHOGENICITY	
TEXTURE	• fine homogeneous echos • no true capsule, which limits its definition sonographically

ECHOGENICITY	• variable
	• medium-level echos
	• isoechoic or more echogenic than liver
	   Children < liver
	   Adults ≥ liver
	
	Normal Variations:
	• echogenicity depends on fat content; therefore, will be more echogenic and coarse in elderly and obese
	   ↑ fat = ↑ echogenicity
	• can have focal areas of decreased echogenicity or fatty sparing, especially in obese people
	
	Pitfall:
	• fluid-filled stomach anterior to pancreas may make the pancreas appear more echogenic due to through

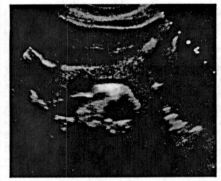

Young adult: 18 year old

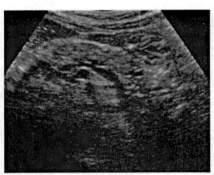

Adult: increasing amount of echogenicity in 55 year old

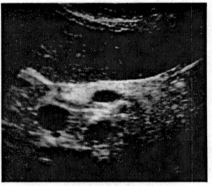

Geriatric (fatty) pancreas: 85 year old

NORMAL AGING OF PANCREAS: INCREASING ECHOGENICITY

B) VASCULATURE

ARTERIAL SUPPLY → **INTO PANCREAS** → VENOUS RETURN
Gastric Duodenal Artery + Superior Mesenteric Artery → HEAD AND NECK → Portal Vein + Superior Mesenteric Vein Splenic Artery + Superior Mesenteric Artery → BODY AND TAIL → Splenic Vein + Inferior Mesenteric Vein

C) PHYSIOLOGY

FUNCTION	
ENDOCRINE	EXOCRINE
PANCREATIC ISLETS (OF LANGERHANS) • 1% of cells that are embedded into main mass • form endocrine portion that secretes hormones, glucagon, insulin, and somatostatin • pancreatic hormones: **Insulin** • lowers blood glucose levels **Glucagon** • increases blood glucose levels by stimulating the breakdown of glycogen and the release of glucose stored in liver **Somatostatin** • suppresses insulin/glucagon release	**ACINAR CELLS** • main mass (99% of cells) • glandular secretory acinar cells secrete pancreatic juice, which is a clear, colorless liquid consisting mostly of water, some salts, sodium bicarbonate, and enzymes • cells are arranged in saclike clusters (acini) and connected by ducts that converge into the main duct of Wirsung then the ampulla of Vater where the juice mixes with bile and empties into duodenum • regulated by nervous and hormonal mechanisms • pancreatic enzymes: **Amylase** • digests carbohydrates **Lipase** • digests fats **Trypsin, Chymotrypsin, Carboxypolypeptidase** • digests proteins

CONDITIONS AFFECTING BLOOD GLUCOSE

SERUM LEVEL	CONDITIONS THAT CAUSE IT

HYPERGLYCEMIA
• elevation of glucose in the blood
• excess excretion of glucose in urine
	1. hyperthyroidism, elevated estrogen levels, acromegaly, hyperaldosteronism
	2. diabetes mellitus
	   disorder of carbohydrate metabolism
	   divided into two major types:
	      Type 1 Insulin-Dependent Diabetes (IDDM)
	         occurs abruptly and presents in childhood or teens
	         absolute deficiency of insulin due to a marked decline in the number of insulin-producing beta cells
	      Type 2 Non−insulin-Dependent Diabetes (NIDDM)
	         also known as mature-onset diabetes
	         more common (90% of all cases)
	         occurs in people overweight and over 40 years of age
	         can be controlled by diet alone

HYPOGLYCEMIA • decrease of normal glucose levels in blood	1. alcoholism, severe liver or kidney disease 2. insulin overdose 3. fasting hypoglycemia 4. tumor (e.g., insulinoma)

PANCREATIC ISLETS (OF LANGERHANS)

ALPHA CELLS
control release of glucagon

BETA CELLS
control release of insulin

DELTA CELLS
secrete somatostatin and growth hormone inhibiting factor

insulin levels rise when blood glucose rises

-act on liver to manufacture glucose (glycogenolysis and gluconeogenesis)
-release glucose into blood

-decrease serum glucose level by
1. accelerating transport of glucose from blood into cells
2. accelerating conversion of glucose into glycogen
3. decreasing glucose manufacturing in liver

increase in serum glucose

decrease in serum glucose level

D) LAB TESTS

PRINCIPLE	INTERPRETATION	
BLOOD STUDIES	INCREASED VALUE	DECREASED VALUE
ALKALINE PHOSPHATASE • obstruction of bile ducts	• carcinoma of head of pancreas • common duct stone	
BILIRUBIN • obstruction of bile ducts limits bilirubin's path into duodenum resulting in elevated levels	• carcinoma of head of pancreas • common duct stone	
AMYLASE • enzyme produced by pancreas and essential in the digestion of starches • can seep into tissues surrounding pancreatic ducts when the ductal system is blocked by edema, stricture, stone, or tumor	• within 24 hours, lasting 1–3 days, then starts to decrease acute pancreatitis • Other cause of elevated results: pancreatic pseudocysts renal failure intestinal obstruction mumps	• chronic pancreatitis • cirrhosis • hepatitis
LIPASE • acinar cells of pancreas are major source of lipase to body • test done when damage to pancreas is suspected	• acute, chronic pancreatitis • pancreatic cancer • pancreatic pseudocysts	• viral hepatitis

GLUCOSE TESTING
• measures the amount of glucose (sugar) in the blood
• detects disorder of glucose metabolism
1. <u>Blood Glucose</u>
   FBS = Fasting blood sugar gives the best indication of glucose metabolism
2. <u>Glucose Tolerance</u>
• measures body's ability to process sugar
   Oral Glucose Tolerance Test
   Intravenous Glucose Tolerance Test
   Cortisone Glucose Tolerance Test
3. <u>2-hr PP = 2-Hour Postprandial Blood Sugar</u>
• reflects body's response to a carbohydrate challenge
• normally blood sugar levels return to fasting levels in 2 hours
	• diabetes mellitus
	• chronic liver disease
	• chronic pancreatitis
		• tumor (islet of Langerhans) islet cell adenoma
		• hypoglycemia

URINE STUDIES		
AMYLASE • generally parallels levels found in blood • lag time differs between blood and urinary levels, as urinary levels return to normal more slowly than blood levels	• remain elevated for 7–10 days: acute pancreatitis chronic pancreatitis	

E) ANOMALIES

ANOMALY	US APPEARANCE
ADENOCARCINOMA • often present for awhile before they produce symptoms • increased incidence in males (also greater in those > 50 years of age), diabetics, persons with hereditary chronic pancreatitis • most common site is head (60%), which can cause obstruction of CBD • spreads mainly to liver (via portal vein) and lungs, but can involve other sites including bone SS • abdominal and back pain, weight loss, nausea, palpable mass (Courvoisier's GB) • ↑ alkaline phosphatase, ↑ bilirubin • jaundice (secondary to obstruction of biliary tree) • ascites US • hypoechoic mass with irregular borders mostly found in head of pancreas • secondary changes include enlarged pancreatic duct distal to carcinoma, Courvoisier's (distended) GB with obstruction of CBD, SMV and SMA displacement, compressed IVC	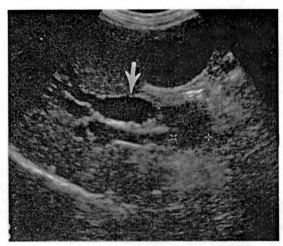 Sagittal scan plane through midline demonstrating large hypoechoic mass (between calipers) in the head of the pancreas. Note dilated CBD (arrow).

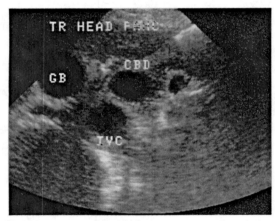

Transverse scan of head of pancreas: mass found at level of ampulla of Vater causing enlarged CBD

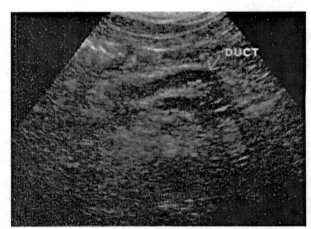

Transverse pancreas: dilated pancreatic duct from carcinoma in head of pancreas

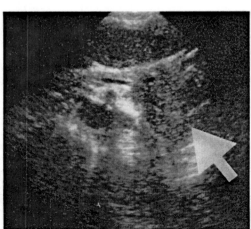

Transverse: adenocarcinoma in tail of pancreas (arrow)

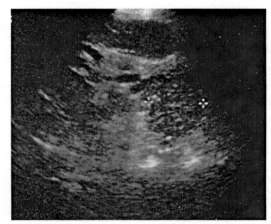

Transverse: calipers measuring mass in tail of pancreas

ANOMALY	US APPEARANCE

CYSTIC TUMORS OF PANCREAS

- 5% of all pancreatic neoplasms

1. MUCINOUS CYSTIC TUMORS (MACROCYSTIC)

- malignant
- uni- or multilocular with large cyst, usually > 5 cm
- increased incidence in females
- seen primarily in pancreatic body and tail

US

- large cystic areas with excellent through transmission
- well circumscribed

Diff Dx.:

- pseudocyst

2. SEROUS CYSTIC TUMOR (MICROCYSTIC)

- benign
- cystic tumor composed of multiple tiny cysts which are < 2 cm in size
- 60% found in body and tail

US

- seen commonly in body and tail
- variable appearance:
  a) complex mass that may appear solid ± small fluid collection within it
  b) occasionally large cysts
  c) central scar with thick calcifications

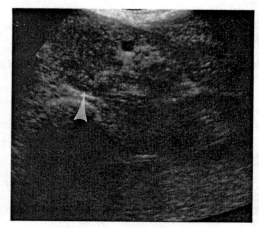

Mucinous mass in head of pancreas

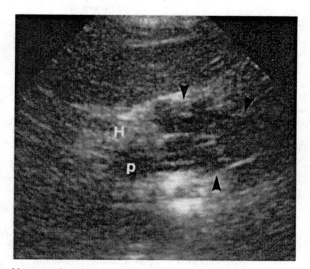

Macrocystic adenocarcinoma demonstrated as cystic lesions in body and tail (between arrows)

ANOMALY	US APPEARANCE

CYSTS

1. TRUE
- lined with epithelium
- can occur in 10% of patients with APKD disease and 30% of patients with von Hippel-Lindau syndrome and occasional cystic fibrosis
- can occasionally occur on their own secondary to anomalous development of pancreatic duct

US
- smooth walls, anechoic, good through transmission

Diff. Dx.:
- tortuous splenic artery

2. PSEUDOCYSTS
- most common cystic pancreatic lesions
- encapsulated collections of leaked pancreatic juices secondary to acinar and ductal disruption
- result from trauma (post-traumatic) to gland or secondary to acute or chronic pancreatitis (postinflammatory)
- body walls off leakage, which may remain contained within gland or may break through to collect within the abdomen or thorax

SS
- persistent abdominal pain

US
- sharply defined, echogenic, thick smooth walls
- sonolucent masses with or without acoustic enhancement
- may contain internal echos and septations
- usually uniloculated but can be multiloculated
- generally take the contour of space they occupy

Diff. Dx.:
- distinguish between fluid-filled bowel and stomach
- neoplastic cystic lesions (which are usually more multiloculated)

Pitfall:
Cystic fibrosis:
- hereditary disease seen in children and young adults that causes abnormal mucous secretion by exocrine glands
- this can sometimes appear on US as a pancreas with increased size and echogenicity and tiny multiple cysts, which are actually dilated ducts

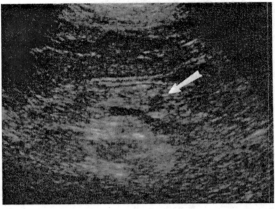

Simple cyst (arrow)

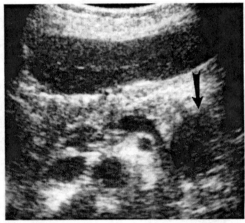

Pseudocyst (arrow)

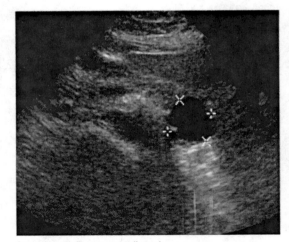

Pseudocyst (between calipers)

ANOMALY	US APPEARANCE

ISLET CELL TUMOR
• endocrine tumor
• rare in comparison with tumors of the exocrine pancreas
• most commonly found in tail and body as that is where there is an increased concentration of Langerhan islets
• usually small, 1–2 cm in diameter
• may be single or multiple, benign or malignant
• well encapsulated
 	
1. <u>NONFUNCTIONAL</u>
• silent, until large usually with evidence of metastases at time of diagnosis
• 80% are malignant
 	
2. <u>FUNCTIONAL</u>
• detected earlier due to signs and symptoms produced by tumor's secretions
• Gastrinoma
   increased gastrin causes peptic ulcerations
   60% are malignant
 	
SS
• serum gastrin level increases
• peptic ulcers
• gastric hypersecretion
• Insulinoma (beta cell tumors)
   most common islet cell tumor
   5%–10% malignant
 	
SS
• hypoglycemia
• elevated insulin levels as it produces insulin
• CNS symptoms (confusion, stupor)
 	
US
• hypoechoic, solid homogeneous
• well circumscribed small 1–2-cm mass
• due to small size, may be difficult to locate
	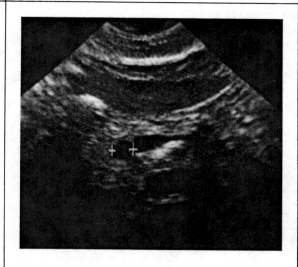

ANOMALY	US APPEARANCE

PANCREATITIS

- causes:
  - in adults 80% caused by ETOH abuse and biliary tract disease can also be caused by drugs, trauma, extension of adjacent inflamed tissues, mass lesions, iatrogenic
  - in children by blunt abdominal trauma, also infectious diseases, cystic fibrosis
  - rare forms include hereditary pancreatitis caused from ductal malformation, which is an autosomal dominant disorder
  - 10%–20% of causes are idiopathic
- two forms, acute and chronic

1. ACUTE

- destructive effect of pancreatic enzymes released from acinar cells, which breaks down tissue and can cause hemorrhage, thrombosis, and inflammation

MILD

- reversible

SS

- epigastric abdominal pain radiating to back
- ↑ levels of pancreatic enzymes

MODERATE (EDEMATOUS PROCESS)

- reversible
- diffuse spread to anterior and posterior pararenal compartments of the retroperitoneum
- used to be referred to as a phlegmon process

US

- depends on age of process
- focal to diffuse enlargement of pancreas
- decreased echogenicity due to a generalized edema (early)
- ill defined borders
- peripancreatic fluid, pseudocyst may be present (depends on time course)

SEVERE (ACUTE HEMORRHAGIC/NECROTIZING)

- least common but most severe form of pancreatitis
- enzyme destruction of pancreas (autodigestion) leads to abscess, pseudocysts, areas of fresh blood, fat necrosis

SS

- abdominal pain, nausea, vomiting
- patient very ill, shock, ileus
- decreased hematocrit

US

- mixed appearance due to areas of edema or focal areas of necrosis
- pancreatic duct may be enlarged secondary to underlying chronic pancreatitis
- peripancreatic fluid, pseudocyst may be present (depends on time course)
- pancreatic abscess may arise from neighboring infection from bacteria, which reaches pancreas via lymphatic channels

2. CHRONIC

- continued destruction of pancreatic tissue
- usually associated with ETOH abuse and biliary tract disease
- rare forms include nonalcoholic tropical pancreatitis and familial hereditary pancreatitis

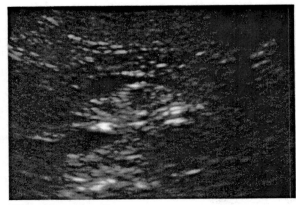

Mild acute pancreatitis

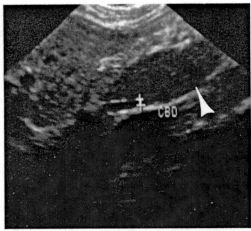

Focal pancreatitis (arrow) in head

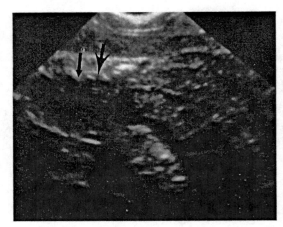

Focal pancreatitis in head (arrows)

ANOMALY	US APPEARANCE

PANCREATITIS (*Continued*)

SS
- may have vague symptoms
- constant midepigastric pain radiating to back
- mild jaundice, nausea, vomiting—attacks may be precipitated by alcohol, overeating, or drug use

US
- normal to small pancreas (atrophic) with a lumpy, irregular contour
- increased echogenicity (focal or diffuse)
- inhomogeneous, coarse (irreversible fibrotic scarring)
- ducts can be enlarged and contain calcifications (ducts can be ≥ 2 mm usually < 6 mm)
- pancreatic pseudocyst
- dilated CBD (secondary to fibrosis)

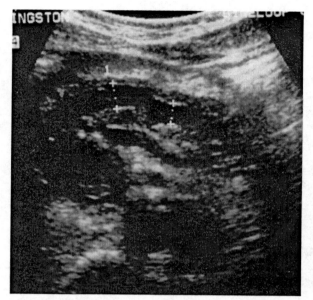

Chronic pancreatitis: atrophic pancreas with enlarged duct (between calipers)

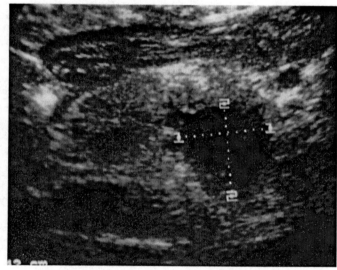

Transverse pancreas with chronic pancreatitis and pseudocyst (calipers)

COMMON DIFFERENTIAL DIAGNOSIS IN REGION OF PANCREAS	
APPEARANCE	ANOMALY
CYSTIC LESION	abscess fluid collection aneurysm/pseudoaneurysm polycystic disease cystic fibrosis pseudocyst cystic pancreatic tumors true cyst
HYPOECHOIC MASS	carcinoma; islet cell tumor metastases focal pancreatitis thrombosed aneurysms lymphoma
FOCAL SHADOWING AND CALCIFICATION	calcification from chronic pancreatitis calculi in pancreatic duct splenic artery calcification
ENLARGED DUCT (> 2 mm)	chronic pancreatitis pancreatic carcinoma (if > 5 mm carcinoma is the more likely diagnosis)

F) TECHNICAL FACTORS

TRANSDUCER	• 3.0–3.5 MHz
PATIENT PREPARATION	• nothing to eat or drink for 8–12 hours to reduce bowel gas anterior to pancreas and to ensure biliary tract dilatation • perform prior to any barium studies Exception: • using stomach as a sonographic window by filling it with 2–4 cups of noncarbonated drink • works best with patient in erect position • glucagon can be used to decrease peristalsis so water stays in stomach longer
TECHNIQUE	• patient initially supine then change into left decubitus • erect or upright position can displace stomach downward, using left lobe of liver for window
MINIMUM PROTOCOL	• pancreatic head, body, and tail in transverse and longitudinal scan planes for size, shape, and texture • assess pancreatic and bile ducts • document any masses or calcifications • document any peripancreatic nodes or fluid collections
HELPFUL HINTS	• use left lobe of liver as a window • full inspiration • when scanning sit high with transducer and angle inferiorly Body: • once you locate it, rotate the transducer varying degrees to visualize the longitudinal plane Tail: • try with the patient prone, using the left kidney as a window • tail lies anterior to superior pole of left kidney

CHAPTER 10 - PERITONEUM AND CAVITY, MESENTERIES, RETROPERITONEUM, DIAPHRAGM, AND ABDOMINAL WALL

A) NORMAL ANATOMY AND SONOGRAPHIC APPEARANCE

PERITONEUM	
DEFINITION	• largest serous membrane of the body; lines the abdominal cavity
STRUCTURE	• has a parietal and visceral layer • consists of layer of simple epithelium (mesothelium) + underlying supporting layer of connective tissue
FUNCTION	1. attach organs to each other and to the posterior abdominal wall 2. minimize friction between organs 3. resist infection (in response to injury or infection will attempt to localize and wall it off)

1. PARIETAL PERITONEUM
• lines wall of abdominal and pelvic cavities and forms the mesenteries and omenta

2. VISCERAL PERITONEUM
• peritoneum that covers some organs and constitutes their serosa

3. PERITONEAL CAVITY

4. FOLDS (LIGAMENTS, OMENTA, MESENTERIES) OF PERITONEUM

Intraperitoneal organ (small bowel)

Retroperitoneal organ (kidney)

PERITONEAL CAVITY

- space between parietal and visceral peritoneum; contains serous fluid
- divided into several pouches or compartments that are created by the peritoneal folds
- Females: uterine tubes open into it
- Males: completely closed sac

1. SUBPHRENIC SPACE
- inferior to diaphragm
- divided into right and left spaces by falciform ligament

a) Right subphrenic space
- separated from right subhepatic space by right coronary ligament
  - i) Anterior—anterior to liver
  - ii) Posterior—lies amid right lobe of liver, right kidney, and right colic flexure

b) Left subphrenic space
- inferior to diaphragm, anterior and posterior to spleen
  - i) Anterior—perigastric
  - ii) Posterior—perisplenic

2. SUBHEPATIC SPACE
- inferior to liver
- divided into anterior and posterior spaces by stomach and lesser omentum

a) Anterior subhepatic space
- not clearly delineated by ligaments, but in region of GB fossa

b) Posterior subhepatic/hepatorenal space (MORRISON'S POUCH)
- formed by right subhepatic recess + hepatorenal recess
- anterior to right kidney, posterior and inferior to liver
- common location for free fluid as it is the most dependent portion of the abdominal cavity
- communicates with the lesser sac via the epiploic foramen, right subphrenic space, and right paracolic gutter

3. LESSER SAC (lesser omental bursa)
- enclosed portion of peritoneal space behind liver and stomach
- diverticulum from main cavity between pancreas and stomach
- Boundaries
  - anterior: caudate lobe, lesser and greater omentum, stomach
  - posterior: great omentum, mesocolon, left adrenal and kidney, pancreas, and great vessels
  - superior: liver
  - inferior: transverse colon
  - right: opens into greater sac; accessed by epiploic foramen, an opening at right side
  - left: phrenicolic ligament, hilum of spleen, gastrosplenic ligament

a) Superior recess of lesser sac
- between caudate lobe of liver and diaphragm

b) Lienal recess
- between spleen and stomach

4. FORAMEN OF WINSLOW (EPIPLOIC/OMENTAL FORAMEN)
- Boundaries:
  - anterior: edge of lesser omentum (portal triad—CBD, hepatic artery + portal vein)
  - posterior: IVC
  - cephalad: caudate lobe of liver
  - caudad: duodenum
- communication between greater and lesser sac
- fluid/infection can track through this opening although it is very small; however, most fluid within the lesser sac is from direct causes
- common site for pancreatic pseudocysts

5. PARACOLIC GUTTERS
- longitudinal channels alongside ascending (right) and descending (left) colon
- pathway of communication between supra and infra mesocolic spaces where free abdominal fluid can flow

a) Right paracolic gutter
- deepest; therefore, naturally the first pathway for free fluid
- communicates freely with Morrison's pouch and the right subphrenic space

b) Left paracolic gutter
- fluid in this area is confined by the phrenocolic ligament and cannot enter the left subphrenic space

c) Right infracolic gutter
- below and behind transverse colon and mesocolon and right of mesentery
- appendix often located here

d) Left infracolic gutter
- below and behind transverse colon and mesocolon and left of mesentery
- in free communication with pelvis

6. PELVIC CUL-DE-SACS
a) Anterior cul-de-sac (vesicouterine pouch)

b) Posterior cul-de-sac
- females: rectouterine pouch or pouch of Douglas
- males: rectovesicle pouch

c) Space of Retzius (prevesical/retropubic space)
- space between bladder and pubis filled with extraperitoneal adipose tissue

186

PERITONEAL CAVITY

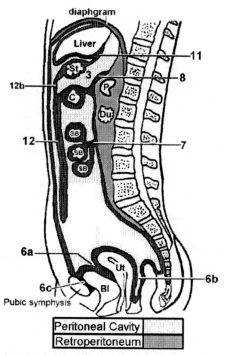

Longitudinal section of abdomen

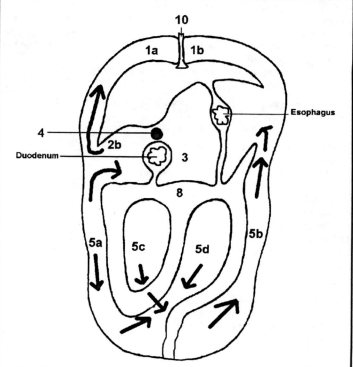

Flow of ascites

Key for Diagrams

PERITONEAL CAVITY
1. Subphrenic space: (A) Right (B) Left
2. Subhepatic space: (A) Anterior (B) Posterior
3. Lesser sac: (A) Superior (B) Lienal
4. Foramen of Winslow
5. Paracolic gutters: (A) Right (B) Left (C) Right Infra (D) Left Infra
6. Pelvic cul-de-sac: (A) Anterior (B) Posterior (C) Space of Retzuis

MESENTERIES
7. Mesentery proper
8. Transverse mesocolon
9. Sigmoid mesocolon
10. Falciform ligament
11. Lesser omentum
12. Greater omentum: (A) Gastrolienal ligament (B) Gastrocolic ligament (C) Splenorenal ligament
13. Coronary ligaments: (A) Anterior (B) Posterior (C) Bare area
14. Triangular ligaments: (A) Right (B) Left

MESENTERIES

- folds of peritoneum that unite the abdominal wall with intestines
- carry blood vessels, nerves, and lymphatics to organs and can direct disease and infection
- normal mesenteric fat and blood vessels can be visualized sonographically
- peritoneal folds encircling parts of the bowels and the abdominal wall

Omenta and Ligaments:
- term used to describe more complex peritoneal folds

7. MESENTERY PROPER (SMALL BOWEL)
- double sheet of peritoneum suspending jejunum and ileum from posterior body wall
- fans out to encircle the small bowel loops

8. TRANSVERSE MESOCOLON
- dorsal mesentery of transverse colon
- divides the abdominal cavity into supra and infra mesocolic compartments, which communicate via the paracolic gutters
- connects large bowel to the anterior aspect of the pancreas and posterior body wall
- continuous with
a) Splenorenal ligament
b) Phrenicolic ligament—from left colic flexure to diaphragm, helps to support spleen

9. SIGMOID MESOCOLON

10. FALCIFORM LIGAMENT
- extends from umbilicus to diaphragm
- attaches liver to anterior abdominal wall
- ligament teres (remnant of fetal umbilical vein) runs in its inferior free edge
- divides:
  subphrenic space into right and left compartments
  medial and lateral left lobe of liver

11. LESSER OMENTUM
- peritoneal fold passing from porta hepatis at inferior surface of liver to lesser curvature of stomach and duodenum
- continuous with:
a) Gastrohepatic ligament
b) Hepatoduodenal ligament
- arises as 2 folds from the lesser curvature of the stomach and duodenum to the ligamentum venosum from liver
- portal triad runs in its right free margin

12. GREATER OMENTUM
- 4-layer fold from the greater curvature of stomach that hangs down like an apron over the front of the intestines then reflects anteriorly to transverse colon, wraps around it, and attaches to parietal peritoneum of posterior wall
- contains large quantities of adipose tissue
- in disease states may contain enlarged lymph nodes or tumor and is known as an omental band or omental cake
a) Gastrolienal/splenic ligament
- left lateral extension of anterior layer of greater omentum
- continues from stomach to spleen
b) Gastrocolic ligament
- omentum between the colon to stomach
c) Splenorenal ligament (SLR)
- posterior reflection of dorsal mesentery/peritoneum of spleen and does NOT extend to kidney but passes inferiorly to overlie left kidney
- important pathway for spread of disease between the peritoneal (spleen) and extraperitoneal spaces (pancreas, left kidney, adrenal)

13. CORONARY LIGAMENTS OF LIVER
- a portion of peritoneum that forms border of bare area
a) Anterior layer
- continuous with right side of falciform ligament where peritoneum is reflected from the diaphragm to right lobe of liver
b) Posterior layer
- from the back of right lobe to right adrenal and kidney
c) Bare area of liver
- area of liver not covered by peritoneum, which lies mostly between the layers of the coronary ligaments

14. TRIANGULAR LIGAMENTS
- a portion of peritoneum that forms border of bare area where posterior coronary ligaments meet
a) Right triangular ligament
b) Left triangular ligament

KEY: Bl, bladder; C, colon; Du, duodenum; IVC, inferior vena cava; LK, left kidney; P, pancreas; RK, right kidney; SB, small bowel; Sp, spine; St, stomach; Ut, uterus

MESENTERIES

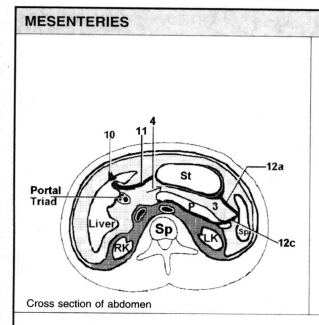

Cross section of abdomen

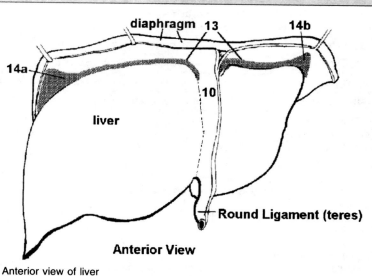

Anterior view of liver

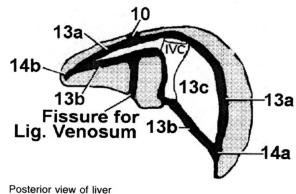

Posterior view of liver

Key for Diagrams Above

PERITONEAL CAVITY
1. Subphrenic space: (A) Right (B) Left
2. Subhepatic space: (A) Anterior (B) Posterior
3. Lesser sac: (A) Superior (B) Lienal
4. Foramen of Winslow
5. Paracolic gutters: (A) Right (B) Left (C) Right Infra (D) Left Infra
6. Pelvic cul-de-sac: (A) Anterior (B) Posterior (C) Space of Retzuis

MESENTERIES
7. Mesentery proper
8. Transverse mesocolon
9. Sigmoid mesocolon
10. Falciform ligament
11. Lesser omentum
12. Greater omentum: (A) Gastrolienal ligament (B) Gastrocolic ligament (C) Splenorenal ligament
13. Coronary ligaments: (A) Anterior (B) Posterior (C) Bare area
14. Triangular ligaments: (A) Right (B) Left

RETROPERITONEUM

- area posterior to the parietal peritoneal membrane
- retroperitoneal organs are ones that adhere to the posterior abdominal wall and are not suspended by a mesentery

LOCATION	• between the posterior parietal peritoneum and the posterior abdominal wall
LENGTH	• extends from diaphragm to pelvis
LATERAL BOUNDARIES	• extends to extraperitoneal fat planes within transversalis fascia
MEDIAL BOUNDARIES	• space encloses the great vessels

STRUCTURE

RETROPERITONEUM:
- subdivided into 2 major spaces

1. PERIRENAL SPACE
- extends from diaphragm to iliac crest
- defined anteriorly and posteriorly by Gerota's fascia
- contains:
  kidneys, ureters
  adrenal glands
  aorta, IVC
  retroperitoneal nodes and fat
- pathology includes hematomas, urinomas, lymphoceles
- the center contains the aorta and IVC, which are surrounded by connective tissue that isolates them from the other spaces and prevents fluid crossing across midline

2. PARARENAL SPACES
a) Anterior pararenal space
- defined anteriorly by the posterior parietal peritoneum and posteriorly by Gerota's (anterior renal) fascia
- extends laterally to the lateroconal renal fascia
- contains:
  pancreas
  "C" loop of duodenum
  ascending and descending colon
- communicates across midline

b) POSTERIOR PARARENAL SPACE
- defined anteriorly by Gerota's fascia and posteriorly by the transversalis fascia
- contains:
  blood vessels and lymphatics
  posterior abdominal wall
  iliopsoas and quadratus lumborum muscle
- communicates with the anterior pararenal space and the iliac fossa
- collection in this area clearly delineated lateral to the psoas muscle and displaces kidneys anterior and laterally

OTHER STRUCTURES
3. EXTERNAL OBLIQUE MUSCLE
4. INTERNAL OBLIQUE MUSCLE
5. TRANSVERSE ABDOMINUS MUSCLE
6. PARIETAL PERITONEUM
7. TRANSVERSALIS FASCIA
8. ANTERIOR AND POSTERIOR RENAL (GEROTA'S) FASCIA
9. INTRAPERITONEAL CAVITY

RETROPERITONEUM
- Consists of:
  prevesical space (Retzius)
  rectovesical space
  presacral space
  pararectal space

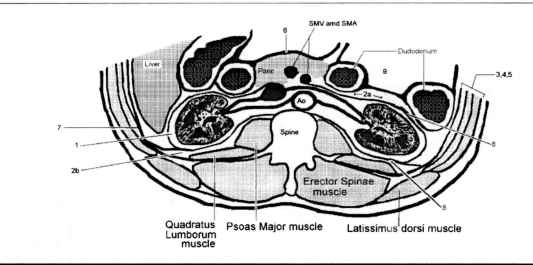

REGIONAL ANATOMY OF RETROPERITONEUM

SPACE	ANTERIOR	POSTERIOR	COMMUNICATES WITH:	CONTAINS:
ANTERIOR PARARENAL	• posterior parietal peritoneum	• anterior renal (Gerota's) fascia	• inferiorly with posterior pararenal space • across midline	• pancreas • ascending colon • descending colon • duodenum
PERIRENAL/ PERINEPHRIC	• renal (Gerota's) fascia	• renal (Gerota's) fascia	• inferiorly with posterior pararenal space • closed superiorly, laterally and across midline	• adrenals and kidneys • ureters • great vessels (in a connective tissue sheath, which seals off midline)
POSTERIOR PARARENAL	• posterior renal fascia	• transversalis fascia	• inferiorly perirenal and anterior pararenal space	• fat • lymph vessels • blood vessels

DIAPHRAGM

DEFINITION	• dome-shaped structure separating the abdominal cavity from the thorax
FUNCTION	• active muscle of respiration

STRUCTURE
• musculofibrous sheet

1. CRURA
• fibromuscular bundles that attach to lumbar vertebra
• anchor the diaphragm
a) Right
• attaches to L3 vertebra
b) Left
• attaches to L1 vertebra

2. SUBPHRENIC SPACE
• space between diaphragm and spleen or diaphragm and liver
• common site for abscess formation or fluid accumulation

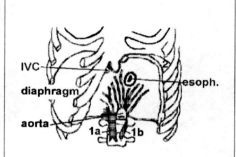

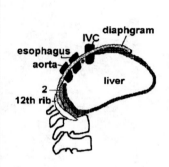

MEASURING DIAPHRAGM MOVEMENT
• with patient supine, find the diaphragm/liver interface with a longitudinal scan plane
• with full expiration, place a cursor on the edge of the diaphragm
• have patient take a large breath in
• place another cursor on the edge of the diaphragm at maximum inspiration
• normal diaphragm movement requires that the diaphragm moves inferiorly on inspiration and superiorly on expiration

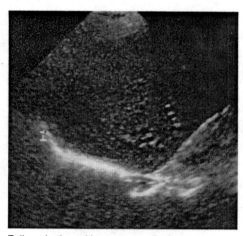

Full expiration with cursor on diaphragm

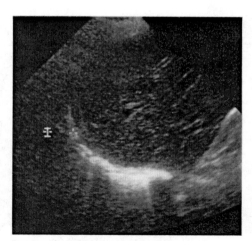

Full inspiration with second cursor on new position of diaphragm indicating movement of diaphragm with respiration

US APPEARANCE OF DIAPHRAGM

MUSCLES	thin hypoechoic band	
LIVER–DIAPHRAGM INTERFACE	thin echogenic liver mirror-image artifact of diaphragm–liver interface appears as another thin echogenic line cephalad to the lung–diaphragm interface	
LUNG–DIAPHRAGM INTERFACE	prominent, thick echogenic band	
	TRANSVERSE SCAN PLANE	**LONGITUDINAL SCAN PLANE**
DIAPHRAGMATIC "SLIPS"	• normal prominent muscular insertions that can be mistaken for focal liver or peritoneal lesions • small rounded hypoechoic masses	• appear elongated and enlarge on inspiration
CRURA **RIGHT CRUS**	• posterior to IVC • extends between IVC and aorta • anterior medial to right kidney and adrenal gland	• solid hypoechoic longitudinally oriented structure • posterior and parallel to IVC • anterior and parallel to aorta • ends superiorly near esophagogastric junction
LEFT CRUS	• hypoechoic structure • runs anterior and lateral to aorta • in close proximity to left adrenal, splenic vasculature and esophagogastric junction	• not visualized sonographically

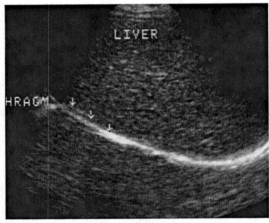

Sagittal right lobe liver and diaphragm interface

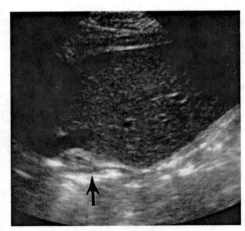

Diaphragm crura (arrow)

ABDOMINAL WALL

1. ANTERIOR ABDOMINAL MUSCLES
a) External oblique
b) Internal oblique
c) Transversus abdominus
d) Rectus abdominis
e) Serratus anterior

2. PECTORALIS
a) Major
b) Minor

3. EXTERNAL INGUINAL RING

4. LINEA ALBA

5. RECTUS SHEATH

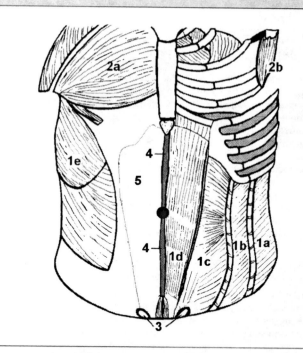

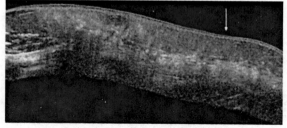

Longitudinal scan of left abdominal wall (Courtesy of Siemens SieScape)

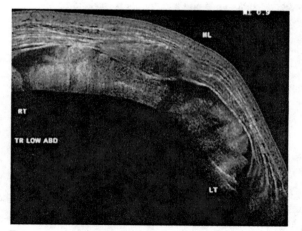

Transverse scan through abdominal wall (Courtesy of Siemens SieScape)

B) ANOMALIES

ANOMALY	US APPEARANCE

ABDOMINAL WALL PATHOLOGY
 	
1. HEMATOMAS
• Bladder flap hematoma
  potential space between bladder and uterus is filled with collection of blood caused by bleeding from a transverse cesarean section sonographically appear as complex masses with poorly defined borders
• Subfascial hematoma
  posterior to rectus muscle, most commonly seen in prevesical space
• Superficial hematoma
  located anterior to rectus muscle
• Rectus sheath
  common superficial abdominal wall hematoma that is within the anterior abdominal musculature
  can be post-traumatic or secondary to anticoagulant treatment
 	
SS
• fever, ↓ hematocrit
• if infected can have ↑ WBCs and more pain
 	
2. HERNIAS
• peritoneal structures may protrude through weakened abdominal wall muscles resulting in a hernia
• common locations are umbilical, epigastric, inguinal, femoral, and at the separation of recti abdominis muscle
• incarcerated hernia is one that cannot be pushed back into the abdominal cavity (reduced)
 	
US
• abdominal wall defect: interruption of abdominal wall musculature
• peritoneal structures seen anterior to abdominal wall musculature
• can note peristalsing bowel and typical bowel shadowing artifact within mass
 	
3. NEOPLASMS
• Desmoid tumor
  benign fibrous neoplasm of aponeurotic structures
  more frequent in women
• Lipoma
  benign fatty tumor with echogenic texture
• Metastases
  related usually to extension from nearby primary carcinoma
  most commonly from melanoma
	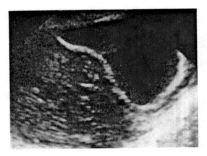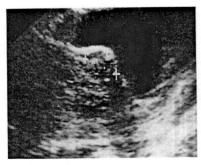
	Sagittal scan of uterus with small complex mass (calipers), which is a small bladder flap hematoma at anterior aspect of uterus
	
	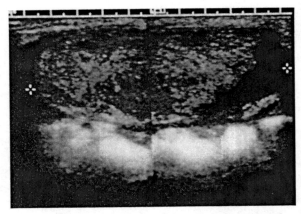
	RLQ rectus sheath hematoma. A 5 × 12 × 15 cm complex anterior abdominal wall fluid mass seen following RLQ trauma in a 67-year-old man. (Courtesy Catherine Carr-Hoefer, RT[R], RDMS RDCS, Good Samaritan Hospital, Corvallis, OR)

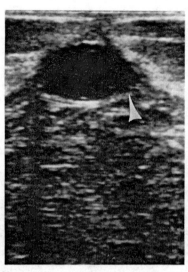

Nonspecific postsurgical fluid collection: differential would include hematoma, abscess, seroma

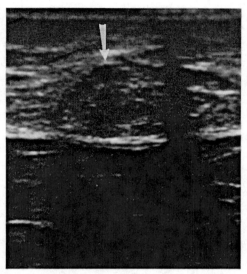

Anterior abdominal hernia (arrow) right of midline

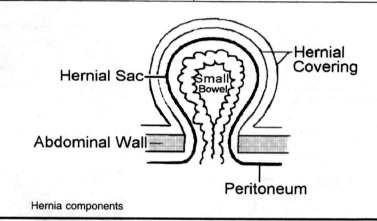

Hernia components

ANOMALY	US APPEARANCE

ABSCESS
• a localized collection of pus
• common regions for location of abscess include the RUQ and the pelvis
• can occur in any part of the body as the result of:
  1. perforated bowel
  2. secondary to malignancy
  3. complication of surgery, trauma, pancreatitis or in immunocompromised patients
 	
Treatment:
• aspiration and drainage under US guidance
• antibiotics
 	
SS
• fever of unknown origin, pain, chills, tenderness
• ↑ WBCs, ↑ sed rate, ↓ platelets
• nuclear medicine—gallium scans indicate "hot spot"
• Peritonitis
  inflammation of the peritoneum usually as a result of infection
  can result in abscess formation
  may be generalized or localized process
 	
US
• difficulties finding abscess include:
  lack of specificity
  presence of incisions, drains, ostomies
  obscured by bowel gas
• appearance is mixed:
  classic appearance is of an elliptical sonolucent mass with thick and irregular margins
  predominantly fluid filled, may appear solid or with debris levels
  tend to displace structures
  possible loculations
  with gas appears with echogenic foci with acoustic shadowing
• US can guide drainage and subsequent follow-up of these masses
 	
Diff. Dx.:
• neoplastic disease, hematoma, seroma, urinoma, cyst, biloma, pseudocyst, bowel
	• Suspected locations for abscess are:
	  splenic and hepatic recesses and borders
	  liver/right kidney
	  pericolic gutters
	  lesser omentum
	  transverse mesocolon
	  Morrison's pouch
	  gastrocolic, phrenicosplenic, extrahepatic falciform, broad ligaments
	  pouch of Douglas
	
	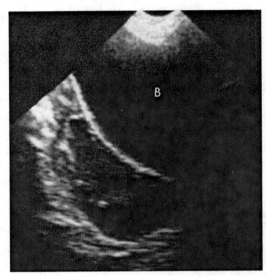
	Pelvis abscess posterior to bladder (B) and adjacent to rectum

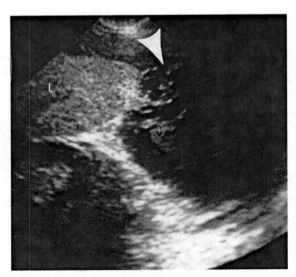

Loculated fluid (arrow) beneath liver (L): differential includes infectious process, neoplasm

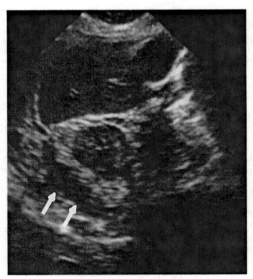

Abscess within the posterior pararenal space in the retroperitoneum (arrows)

ANOMALY	US APPEARANCE

ASCITES

- abnormal collection of serous fluid in peritoneal cavity
- gravity causes it to accumulate in the pelvis first
- if loculated, care must be used to differentiate it from intraperitoneal cystic neoplasm
- can also be blood, pus, urine

Pathology Associated with Ascites

congestive heart failure	pyogenic peritonitis
infection	tuberculosis
kidney or liver failure	portal venous obstruction
malignancy	obstruction of lymph nodes
ruptured aneurysm	acute cholecystitis
ectopic gestation	postoperative complications

1. EXUDATIVE—MALIGNANT ASCITES

- focal or diffuse thickening of peritoneum, which can be solid or cystic in nature
- fine or coarse internal echos, loculations
- matting and clumping of bowel or bowel fixed to posterior abdominal wall

2. TRANSUDATIVE—SEROUS

- anechoic, simple
- bowel moves freely within fluid
- usually benign

US

- small amounts of ascites usually lie in the most dependent portion of the pelvic cul-de-sac, lower end of mesenteric root at the ileocecal junction, sigmoid mesocolon, right paracolic gutter
- fluid accumulates in the following order in these regions:
  1. pelvis cul-de-sac
  2. right paracolic gutter
  3. Morrison's pouch
  4. right subphrenic space

Other sonographic findings include:

- displacement of liver, spleen, bowel (massive ascites)
- GB wall thickening
- patent umbilical vein (in portal hypertension)
- visualization of extrahepatic portion of falciform ligament

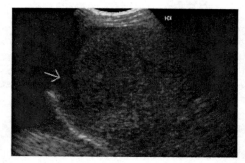

Subhepatic fluid (arrow)

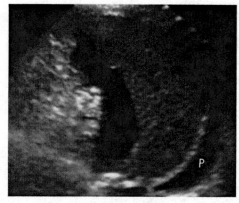

Bowel loops (B) freely floating in ascites

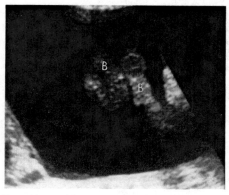

Pleural effusion (P) with subsplenic fluid

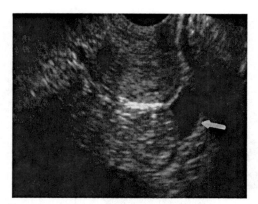

Posterior cul-de-sac/pelvic fluid (arrow) as seen on a transvaginal longitudinal scan of the cervix. First area of fluid collection is in the pelvis.

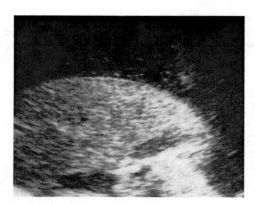

Malignant ascites adjacent to liver

ANOMALY	US APPEARANCE

CYSTIC COLLECTIONS AND CYSTS

- congenital, traumatic, inflammatory, or neoplastic cysts can arise in mesentery
- range from small to quite large

1. BILOMAS
- localized collections of bile within peritoneal cavity
- formed by bile leakage after surgery or trauma (usually postcholecystectomy)

US
- sharply defined anechoic mass with acoustic enhancement
- can be loculated
- continuous with liver or biliary system
- can perform nuclear medicine biliary scan to confirm diagnosis

2. HEMATOMAS/HEMORRHAGE
- many causes, including trauma, bleeding disorders, leaking aneurysm, vasculitis
- may be well localized
- early hemorrhage presents as sonolucent areas become more echogenic as thrombus organizes and clot forms

3. LYMPHOCELES
- lymph-filled space without a distinct epithelial lining caused by disruption of a lymphatic channel usually after surgery
- can be retroperitoneal or intraperitoneal, uni- or bilateral
- accumulate slowly over a period of months to years
- will recur after simple drainage

US
- elliptical shape with sharp margins
- usually unilocular and small
- increased through transmission
- uncomplicated lymphoceles have no internal echos but can have thin septations
- can cause mass effect

4. MESENTERIC/OMENTAL CYSTS
- obscure etiology, congenital or acquired
- may be septated and/or contain debris
- omental cysts usually follow contour of bowel
- mesenteric cysts often occur in root of mesentery

US
- unilocular cystic lesions that may be septated

5. PSEUDOCYSTS
- see Chapter 9—Pancreas

6. URINOMAS
- encapsulated collection of urine outside the urinary tract
- may result from closed renal trauma, surgical intervention, spontaneously secondary to an obstruction
- usually occur about the kidney or upper ureter in the perinephric space

US
- anechoic fluid-filled collection with posterior acoustic enhancement

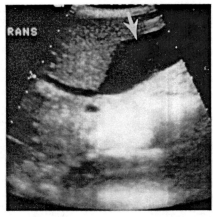

Biloma (arrow)

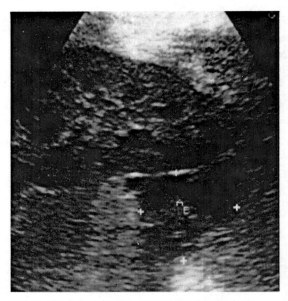

Nonspecific fluid collection around renal transplant (calipers): differential includes lymphocele, urinoma, hematoma, seroma, abscess

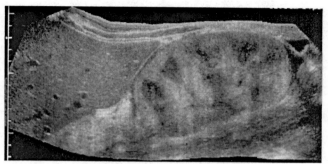

Fluid collection distal to renal transplant (Courtesy of Siemens SieScape)

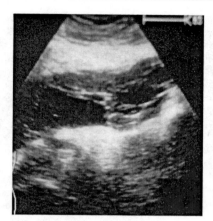

Lymphocele in left lower abdomen

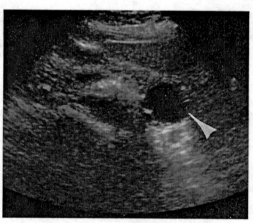

Pseudocyst (arrow) in region of tail of pancreas

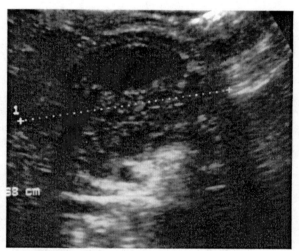

Pseudocyst (calipers)

ANOMALY	US APPEARANCE

MESENTERITIS

- diffuse or focal mesenteric
  edema/infection/inflammation
- associated with
  acute pancreatitis
  appendicitis
  diverticulitis
  superior mesenteric vein thrombosis
  Crohn's disease
  trauma

US
- thickened mesenteric folds of variable echogenicity

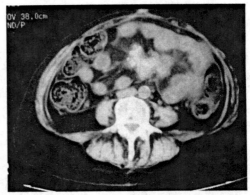

CT findings of nonspecific mesenteritis: soft tissue mass with calcifications in root of mesentery, anterior to abdominal aorta

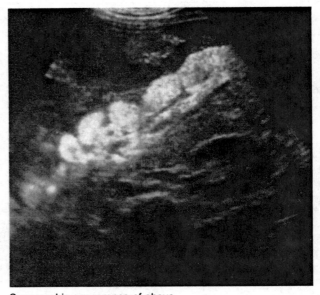

Sonographic appearance of above

200

ANOMALY

PERITONEAL NEOPLASMS	RETROPERITONEAL NEOPLASMS
• mesenteric and omental neoplasms are rare • benign or malignant • grow to large proportions • types include:	• most primary retroperitoneal tumors arise from kidney and adrenal gland • can be quite large and undergo hemorrhage and necrosis • biopsy or excision is required to differentiate type of mass

PERITONEAL NEOPLASMS

1. CARCINOMATOSIS (SECONDARY)
metastatic spread of disease (pseudomyxoma peritonei—see next section)

2. DESMOID TUMORS
• locally aggressive fibrous tumors
• nonmetastasizing
• commonly occur in anterior abdominal wall

US
• hypoechoic mass with areas of acoustic shadowing

3. LYMPHOMA
• most common primary mesenteric malignancy

US
"sandwich" sign—trapped mesenteric vessels are surrounded by hypoechoic masses

4. MESOTHELIOMA
• rare neoplasm arising from mesothelium
• most often occurs in middle-aged men as the result of exposure to asbestos
• causes thickening of omentum

US
"omental mantle or cake"—sheet-like superficial mass (anterior surface follows contour of abdominal wall + posterior surface which is adjacent to bowel loops)
• ascites

5. PSEUDOMYXOMA PERITONEI
• peritoneal seeding of mucinous peritoneal implants and gelatinous ascites
• caused by secondaries from mucin-producing adenocarcinoma of the ovary, pancreas, appendix, colon, and rectum

US
• cystic and/or solid masses of varying echogenicity throughout the peritoneal cavity

RETROPERITONEAL NEOPLASMS

1. NEUROGENIC TUMORS
• originate from nerve tissue
• occur mostly in paravertebral region

2. SARCOMAS
• generally large with bull's eye appearance (thick hypoechoic rim that represents viable tumor with echogenic dense core representing necrosis)
• arise from underlying muscle, bone, connective tissue
  leiomyosarcomas (smooth muscle)
    undergo necrosis and cystic degeneration
  liposarcoma (fat)
    complex echogenic, irregularly thickened wall
  malignant fibrous histiocytoma (connective/fibrous tissue)
    invasive and infiltrate into muscle and adjoining tissue
  rhabdomyosarcoma (muscle)
    same as fibrous histiocytoma

3. TERATOMAS
• originate from all 3 germ layers
• occur mostly in upper pole of left kidney region
• arise within upper retroperitoneum and pelvis
• most are benign

US
• variable echopattern; complex, homogeneous
• irregularly thickened wall

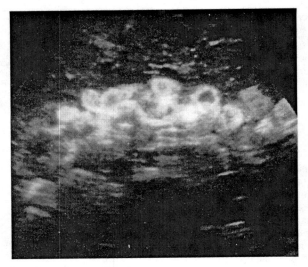

Pseudomyxoma peritonei

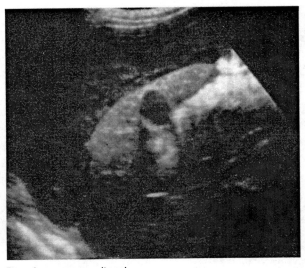

Pseudomyxoma peritonei

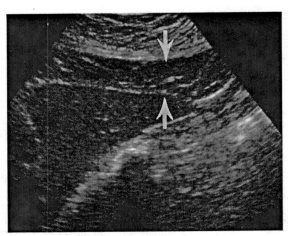

Longitudinal midline image of liver: normal layers of fat between arrows not to be mistaken for pathology

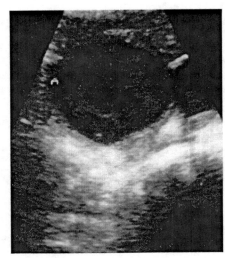

Mesothelioma

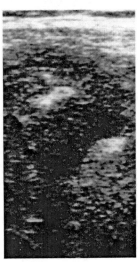

Metastasis to peritoneum: nonspecific mass

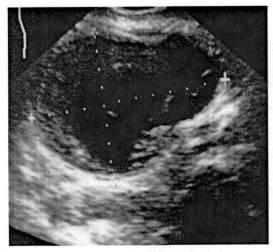

Nonspecific neoplastic mass within the anterior peritoneum

ANOMALY	US APPEARANCE

PLEURAL EFFUSION

- fluid in the thoracic cavity between the visceral and parietal pleura
- nonspecific reaction to an underlying pulmonary or systemic disease
- abdominal causes:
  cirrhosis
  trauma
  malignancy

US

- echo-free, wedge-shaped area posteromedial to diaphragm
- can contain echos (blood, infectious process)

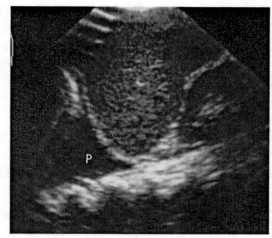

Sagittal scan showing fluid in lung (P)

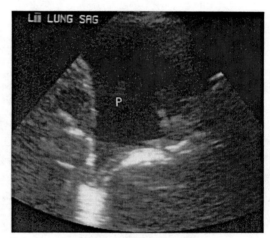

Scanning through the patient's back with patient sitting, as in thoracentesis procedure, shows large amount of pleural fluid (P)

ANOMALY	US APPEARANCE

RETROPERITONEAL FIBROSIS

- dense proliferation of fibrotic tissue located in perirenal space between renal hila to dome of bladder
- centrally located
- may envelop aorta, IVC, ureters, and lymphatics and can cause obstruction
- more frequent in males, and more common from 50–60 years of age
- obscure etiology

SS
- can present with symptoms secondary to hydronephrosis

US
- large bulky mass with ill defined, irregular margins
- anechoic to hypoechoic
- surrounding or envelopes great vessels and does NOT displace them

Diff. Dx.:
- retroperitoneal nodes
- lymphoma
- retroperitoneal sarcoma or hematoma
- aortic aneurysm with thrombus

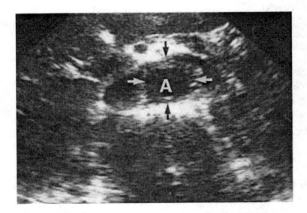

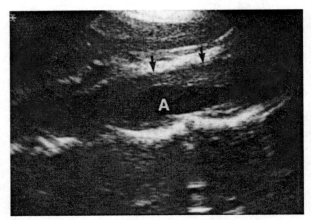

Retroperitoneal fibrosis appears as rim of tissue anterior to aorta with loss of tissue plane between mass and aorta

204

ANOMALY	US APPEARANCE

URACHAL CYSTS/PATENT URACHUS
- failure of urachal canal to close
- in the embryo the urachus is a hollow tube continuous with the allantois and bladder
- usually fibroses at birth to become the middle umbilical ligament of the bladder connecting the apex of the bladder to the umbilicus in the space of Retzius
- adenocarcinoma may arise within
- can remain patent resulting in an:
- Umbilical urinary fistula
  complete patent urachus from bladder to umbilicus
- Urachal cyst
  midportion of urachus is patent with both cephalic and caudal ends closed
- Urachal sinus
  partially patent urachus
  cephalic portion of urachus is patent and opens into umbilicus
- Vesicourachal diverticulum
  partially patent urachus
  internal portion is patent and opens into bladder with cephalic portion blind

SS
- cyst typically asymptomatic unless infected

US
Cyst
- anechoic tubular structure in lower anterior midabdominal wall (space of Retzius)
- may extend from umbilicus to bladder
- can be missed in reverberation artifact anteriorly
- no Doppler flow or changes of appearance with breathing

Urachal fistula

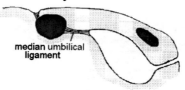

Urachal Cyst

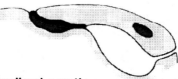

Urachal sinus

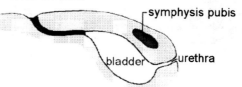

Longitudinal section through pelvis

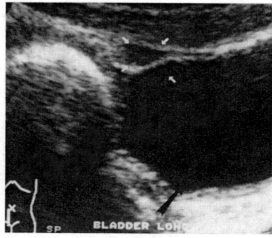

Longitudinal scan demonstrating anechoic mass anterior and superior to bladder consistent with urachal cyst

IDENTIFYING FLUID COLLECTION LOCATIONS

PLEURAL VERSUS SUBDIAPHRAGMATIC

PLEURAL	SUBDIAPHRAGMATIC/SUBPHRENIC
• pleural effusion if fluid is posterior to IVC • transverse scan plane—fluid posterior to diaphragm • longitudinal scan plane—fluid superior to diaphragm	• subphrenic fluid can mimic a pleural effusion • diaphragm must be identified using a parasagittal scan plane • because of coronary ligament attachments, collections in right posterior subphrenic space cannot extend between bare area of liver and diaphragm • a higher frequency transducer should be used to find superficial small fluid collection superior and anterior to liver

SUBCAPSULAR VERSUS INTRAPERITONEAL

SUBCAPSULAR	INTRAPERITONEAL
• subcapsular fluid will be: unilateral conform to shape of organ (unless it is a large collection, which can cause some indentation of the organ tissue)	• will change in location relative to organs during respiration

RETROPERITONEAL VERSUS INTRAPERITONEAL

RETROPERITONEAL	INTRAPERITONEAL
• retroperitoneal fluid can displace retroperitoneal structures anteriorly • large right-sided retroperitoneal mass rotates intrahepatic portal vessels to left Retroperitoneal structures: • kidneys, adrenals, body and head of pancreas, most of duodenum, great vessels, descending and ascending colon, ureters, bladder	Intraperitoneal structures: • sigmoid and transverse colon, small bowel, stomach, liver, spleen, lesser sac, tail of pancreas • most common site of intraperitoneal pelvic fluid is posterior cul-de-sac (pouch of Douglas)

EXTRAPERITONEAL VERSUS INTRAPERITONEAL

EXTRAPERITONEAL	INTRAPERITONEAL
• delineation of an undisrupted peritoneal line • if in space of Retzius, will displace bladder laterally or posteriorly • is generally lenticular in shape with an acute angle (e.g., fluid in rectus sheet or prevesical space)	• intraperitoneal fluid will indent dome of bladder inferiorly

C) TECHNICAL FACTORS

TRANSDUCER	3.5–5 MHz sector probe
TECHNIQUE	• patient usually scanned in supine position
TECHNICAL DIFFICULTIES AND HELPFUL HINTS	• decubitus or erect positions will help determine whether a fluid collection is free or loculated
DIAPHRAGM	
TECHNIQUE	• patient in supine or sitting position • quiet respiration
HELPFUL HINTS	• coughing may be used to evaluate diaphragm motion

CHAPTER 11 - PROSTATE GLAND AND SEMINAL VESICLES

A) ANATOMY AND SONOGRAPHIC APPEARANCE OF PROSTATE GLAND AND SEMINAL VESICLES

PROSTATE GLAND	
DEFINITION	• tubuloalveolar gland composed mainly of fibromuscular tissue that surrounds neck of male bladder and urethra
STRUCTURE	• composed of posterior glandular portion and a nonglandular anterior portion • the urethra and ejaculatory ducts pass through these zones • anatomically divided into several zones, which is important to understand because cancers within each zone have different clinical implications

ZONAL ANATOMY

1. PERIPHERAL ZONE (PZ)
• posterior lateral, apical gland
• surrounds distal urethral segment
• separated from TZ and CZ by surgical capsule
• apex of gland is a weak spot due to thin or absent capsular coverage
• 70% of gland
• 70% of malignancy

2. CENTRAL ZONE (CZ)
• pyramidal-shaped structure at base of prostate
• extends from base to where it narrows at the verumontanum
• 25% of gland
a) Invaginated extraprostatic space (IES)
• inward extension of extraprostatic space composed of loose connective tissue
• site where seminal vesicles and/or ejaculatory ducts enter the CZ
• this spot is devoid of prostatic capsule and is a potential route of spread of tumor to outside space
• 5%–10% of malignancy
b) Verumontanum
• area where the ejaculatory ducts join the urethra
• an elevation of the floor of the prostatic portion of the urethra

3. TRANSITIONAL ZONE (TZ)
• on both sides of preprostatic/proximal urethra
• 5% of gland in absence of benign prostatic hyperplasia (BPH), which originates in this zone
• 10%–20% of malignancy

4. PERIURETHRAL GLANDS
• 1% of glandular tissue
• embedded in longitudinal smooth muscle or proximal urethra

5. PROSTATIC URETHRA
• preprostatic and prostatic portion form a 35° angle at the verumontanum
• prostatic urethra is surrounded by striated muscles

6. ANTERIOR FIBROMUSCULAR STROMA (AFS)
• nonglandular region formed by smooth muscle and connective tissue

7. SURGICAL CAPSULE
• line dividing PZ and CZ from TZ
• line of surgical demarcation when performing TURP

8. SEMINAL VESICLES

9. EJACULATORY DUCTS

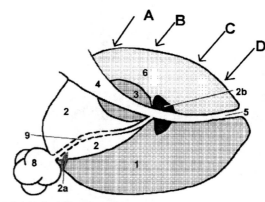

Sagittal midline prostate

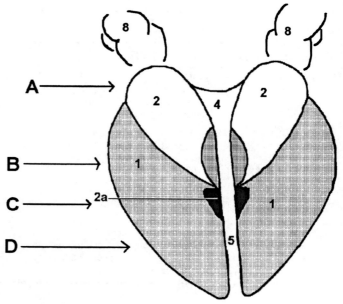

Coronal prostate
(*see next page for corresponding diagrams of coronal slices through prostate*)

207

PROSTATE GLAND

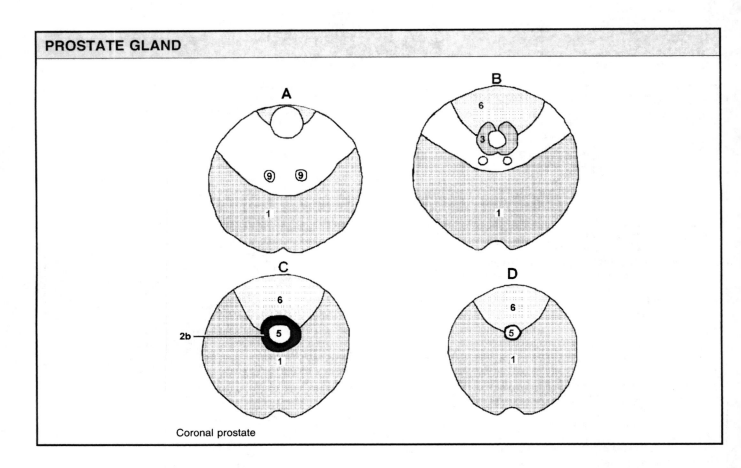

Coronal prostate

NORMAL ANATOMY OF PROSTATE GLAND

SIZE AND WEIGHT	VOLUME $= (W \times H \times L) \times 0.523$ • if spherical shape $= 4/3 \, \pi \, r^3$ • if cylindrical shape $= \pi \, r^2 \times$ height	
	WEIGHT 1 cc of prostate tissue $= 1$ g as specific gravity of prostatic tissue is approximately 1 Normal weight: $= 20$ g in younger men < 40 g in older men (heavier glands are considered to be enlarged in older men)	SIZE (W) Transverse $= 4$ cm (L) Length $= 3–3.5$ cm (H) AP diameter $= 2–2.5$ cm
LOCATION	• directly beneath bladder • between symphysis pubis and rectum • encircles neck of bladder and urethra • retroperitoneal	

REGIONAL ANATOMY OF PROSTATE GLAND

ANTERIOR (BASE OF PROSTATE)	• pubis symphysis • symphysis pubis, abdominal wall, previsicle space of Retzius • urethra enters near anterior border
INFERIOR (APEX OF PROSTATE)	• perineum • urogenital diaphragm
INTERIOR	• surrounds portion of urethra
POSTERIOR	• rectum • ejaculatory ducts enter posterosuperiorly
SUPERIOR (BASE)	• bladder

1. URETER
2. BLADDER
3. SEMINAL VESICLE
4. EJACULATORY DUCT
5. PROSTATE
6. RECTUM
7. UROGENITAL DIAPHRAGM
8. BULBOURETHRAL GLAND
9. URETHRA
10. PENIS
11. SCROTUM
12. EPIDIDYMIS
13. DUCTUS DEFERENS
14. TESTIS
15. SYMPHYSIS PUBIS

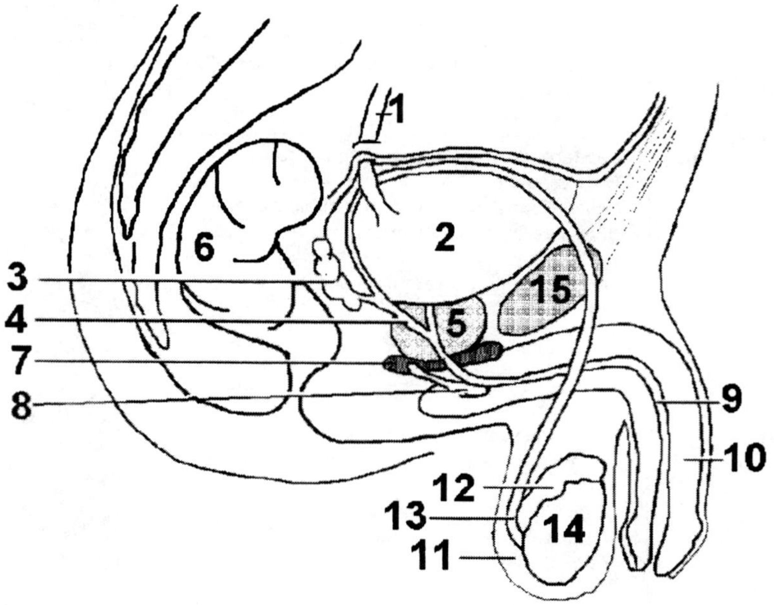

SONOGRAPHIC ECHOGENICITY AND APPEARANCE OF PROSTATE GLAND

- homogeneous low-level echos
- margins are defined by bright linear echos representing the fibrous capsule
- in transverse plane, the gland is symmetric with the PZ being slightly more echogenic
- in normal gland, 4 zones can rarely be seen; therefore for sonographic purposes, it is often more useful to separate the prostate into:
  peripheral zone
  inner gland = transitional + central zone + periurethral glandular area

PERIPHERAL ZONE (PZ)	• homogeneous texture • middle-range echos	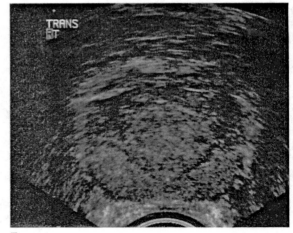 Transverse
CENTRAL ZONE (CZ)	• more echogenic than PZ • corpora amylacea with or without calcifications causes diffuse hyperechoic foci within CZ • "beak": hypoechoic band formed by entrance of seminal vesicles and vas deferens into CZ tissue (IES) and extends to the verumontanum	
TRANSITION ZONE (TZ)	• appearance varies depending on degree of BPH present • "Eiffel Tower"-shaped hyperechoic pattern produced by deposits of corpora amylacea within glands of proximal urethra and verumontanum (marks the caudal portion of the TZ and CZ)	
SURGICAL CAPSULE	• hypoechoic, although may calcify and become hyperechoic	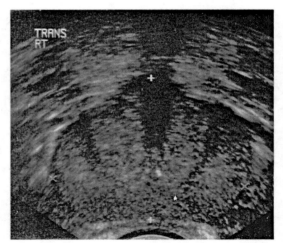 Transverse
CORPORA AMYLACEA	• echogenic foci • can develop at level of surgical cap creating boundary between inner gland and peripheral zone • when filling the periurethral glands may form linear hyperechoic configuration appearing as "Eiffel Tower" sign	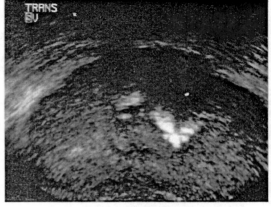 Transverse: bright echos represent corpora amylacea, which may or may not be calcified

SONOGRAPHIC ECHOGENICITY AND APPEARANCE OF PROSTATE GLAND

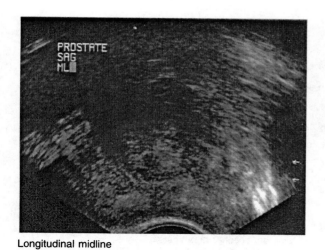

Longitudinal midline

Longitudinal right

TRANSABDOMINAL US OF PROSTATE

TRANSVERSE	LONGITUDINAL
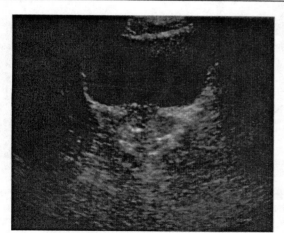	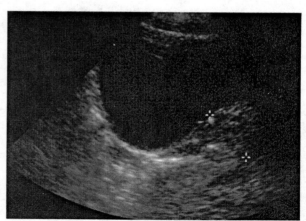
Prostate seen as a rounded or ovoid structure and differentiation of internal structures is not usually possible	A slightly hypoechoic defect (a portion of the periurethral tissues) may occasionally be seen at the bladder neck

SEMINAL VESICLES

DEFINITION	• saclike structures in male, lying behind the bladder close to prostate
STRUCTURE AND SHAPE	• paired, mostly symmetrical ovoid structures containing cystlike spaces
SIZE	Thickness = 1 cm thick–3 cm (bulky) Length = 3–4 cm long • size and shape vary, depending on age and sexual activity
LOCATION	• superior to and at the most posterior portion of prostate gland • posterior to base of bladder • lateral to ampulla of ductus deferens • join the vas deferens to form the ejaculatory ducts
PHYSIOLOGY AND FUNCTION	• depend on hormones for their development and growth and ability to produce secretions • secrete an alkaline, viscous fluid into the ejaculatory duct • this fluid constitutes about 60% of semen volume and contributes to sperm viability
SONOGRAPHIC APPEARANCE	• bilateral hypoechoic, multiseptated structures surrounding rectum • slightly less echogenic than prostate, often without distinct borders • could appear multicystic depending on the amount of retained sperm • normal vesicles are virtually always imaged • symmetric midgray or medium to low-level echo textures, superior to prostate

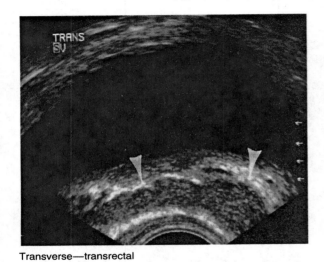

Transverse—transrectal

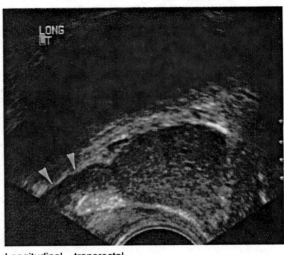

Longitudinal—transrectal

B) PHYSIOLOGY OF PROSTATE GLAND

FUNCTION

• produce fluid for transportation of sperm
• this secretion contributes to sperm motility and makes up about 1/3 of semen volume
• storehouse for many tiny glands that form 15–30 secretory ducts that empty into urethra
• during orgasm prostate's muscles contract and force this fluid into urethra along with sperm from testes and fluid from seminal vesicles
• regulated by androgens (testosterone) produced by testes but controlled by luteinizing hormone from pituitary gland

C) LAB TESTS

PRINCIPLE	INTERPRETATION
	ELEVATED
ACID PHOSPHATASE (ACP/SAP) • found in prostate gland and semen in high concentration • prostate epithelium normally produces large amounts of acid phosphatase	• carcinoma that has spread beyond prostate capsule
ALKALINE PHOSPHATASE • produced by osteoblasts; therefore, level will rise whenever there is an increase in osteoblastic activity	• not specific to prostate cancer but associated with bony metastases
PROSTATE SPECIFIC ANTIGEN (PSA) • enzyme whose purpose is to break down coagulated semen • made almost exclusively in prostate • normally secreted and disposed of through tiny ducts in prostate, but in prostate cancer the ductal system does not drain into urethra, and PSA builds up and leaks out of prostate and shows up in bloodstream **Serum PSA Test** • tumor marker and a second-line screening parameter for prostate cancer PREDICTED PSA VALUES: 2 methods 1) = 0.2×BPH* (wt) *dimensions of BPH part of gland only 2) = 0.14×(W×H×L)	• BPH • infection • carcinoma • the higher the PSA, the larger the tumor burden and the higher the risk of spread beyond the prostate

NORMAL VALUES			
AGE SPECIFIC	< 50 years of age	< 2.5 ng/mL	
	> 50 years of age	normal values increase 1.0 ng/mL for each successive decade after age 50	
	• lacks specificity for malignancy and 2/3 of men with an elevated PSA do not have cancer • an increase in PSA of 20% between 2 years, even if total PSA is normal, can be an indication for TRUSP biopsy		
PSA DENSITY (PSAD)	• calculates the corrected serum PSA level relative to the size of the prostate • helps to distinguish BPH from prostatic cancer in patients with PSAs in the intermediate area • inaccurate volumes may potentially undermine the value of PSAD in early prostate cancer $\dfrac{\text{PSA (ng/mL)}}{\text{Prostate volume (cc)}}$ Normal level < 0.12 ng/mL/cc		
SCREENING	• best system for early detection is a multimodality detection effort with a combination of PSA, direct recal exam (DRE) adn transrectal ultrasound (TRUS) • TRUS should not be used in isolation for prostate cancer screening		

D) ANOMALIES

ANOMALIES OF PROSTATE GLAND

ANOMALY	US APPEARANCE

BENIGN PROSTATE HYPERPLASIA (BPH)

- prostate enlarges with age, beginning with innermost cells (TZ)
- growing prostate narrows the urethra, which impedes urine flow
- small number (7%) who develop BPH at an earlier age probably have inherited a gene that predisposes them to it
- caused by aging, hormones, genetics
- Treatments include:
  TURP: prostate core is removed in fragments by means of electrosurgical cautery and a scope through the urethra
  Prostatectomy (open laser)
  Transurethral incision of prostate
  Balloon dilation
  Transurethral microwave thermal therapy

SS
- size of gland does not always correlate with symptoms
- frequent urination and sense of urgency and constant feeling of fullness in bladder

US
- AP dimension is enlarged initially
- enlargement of the inner gland, which remains relatively hypoechoic to PZ
- echopattern varies from hypo- to hyperechogenic depending on the predominance of fibromuscular tissue or degree and type of glandular hyperplasia
- cystic areas and calcifications can be seen
- hyperplasia can create hypoechoic nodules that mimic carcinoma
- hyperplasia in TZ may displace urethra posteriorly
- asymmetry of gland can be an indication of carcinoma
- secondary changes of bladder include hypertrophy, trabeculation, diverticuli
- large, fairly discrete nodules in periurethral region of prostate
1. Homogeneous stromal (fibromuscular) hyperplasia
   hypoechoic (similar to myometrium in uterus)
2. Glandular hyperplasia
   hypoechoic or hyperechoic depending on gland size and cystic changes
3. Mixed
   stromal and glandular hyperplasia

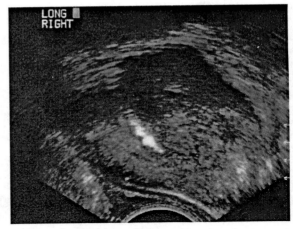

Transrectal scan right sagittal

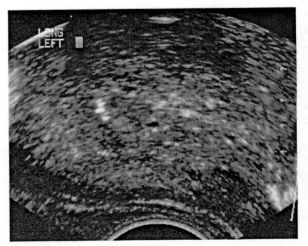

Transrectal scan left sagittal

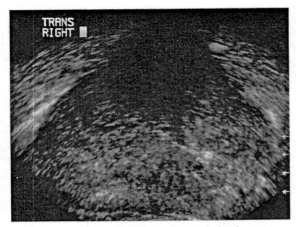

Transverse prostate with enlarged central gland

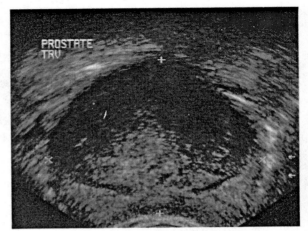

Transrectal scan transverse showing enlarged central portion of gland compatible with BPH (gland measured with calipers)

ANOMALY	US APPEARANCE
CANCER—ADENOCARCINOMA • common cancer in men • prevalence increases rapidly with age • tendency to metastasize to bone SS • BPH-like symptoms, blood in urine or semen, back pain, pelvis, hips or thighs, less rigid erections or impotence, decrease in amount of fluid ejaculated US • areas of hypervascularity in PZ associated with isohypoechoic definable lesions • varied appearance with small masses appear primarily as hypoechoic nodule and larger masses that can appear more hyperechoic • many are isoechoic and may only appear as a bulge in the capsule, areas of attenuation or asymmetry of gland • can be multifocal • indistinct or bulging margin of tumor suggests infiltrative tumor and larger than it appears Doppler: • can potentially differentiate benign from malignant flow patterns in and around mass • small tumors (< 1 cm)—Doppler may not yield signals • large tumors—neovascularization; increased diastolic blood flow	Location: • 70% arise in PZ usually at the posterior part of gland • 20% arise in TZ • 10% arise in CZ • surgical capsule acts as a barrier to inner gland spread 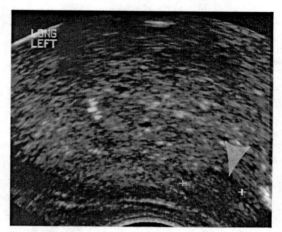 Transrectal sagittal scan demonstrated 1 cm hypoechoic nodule in peripheral zone representing a small prostatic carcinoma (arrow)

CYSTS
1. CONGENITAL
i) Prostatic utricle cysts
    due to dilation of prostatic utricle
    associated with unilateral renal agenesis
    small midline cyst
ii) Mullerian duct cysts
    arise from remnants of mullerian duct
    may extend lateral to midline and can be large
    tend to be central and superior to verumontanum
    classified as utricle cysts if continuous with verumontanum
    do not contain spermatozoa
iii) Seminal vesicle cysts
    can be associated with ipsilateral renal agenesis
 	
2. OBSTRUCTION
i) Ejaculatory duct cysts
    cystic dilation of ejaculatory duct
    contain spermatozoa
 	
3. WITHIN PROSTATE (ACQUIRED CYSTS)
• can be caused by benign hyperplasia, inflammation, trauma
• lateral in gland
 	
SS
• asymptomatic, can become infected if large
 	
US
• anechoic mass within or adjacent to prostate
	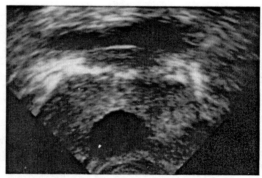
	
	Transrectal transverse scan demonstrated 1.5-cm simple cyst in the posterior aspect of the prostate consistent with a ejaculatory duct cyst
	
	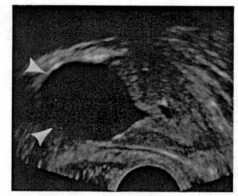
	
	Sagittal transrectal scan of mullerian duct cyst (arrows) superior to base of prostate

ANOMALY	US APPEARANCE

PROSTATITIS/PROSTATE ABSCESS

- inflamed, swollen, and tender prostate
- umbrella diagnosis that encompasses acute and chronic bacterial and nonbacterial prostatitis and prostatodynia
- common in men, rare in prepubertal boys

SS
- pain in joints, muscles, lower back, area behind scrotum
- aches, fever chills
- blood in urine, pain and burning urination
- painful ejaculation

US

1. ACUTE PROSTATITIS
- limited role of US, although can help in early diagnosis of abscess, which appears as a hypo-anechoic mass with or without internal echos
- hypoechoic gland or hypoechoic rim (edema) surround the periurethral tissues

2. CHRONIC PROSTATITIS
- focal masses of varying degrees of echogenicity within central or peripheral zones
- ejaculatory duct calcifications
- capsular thickening or irregularity

3. PROSTATODYNIA
- chronic prostatitis with no known etiologic factor
- enlargement of periprostatic veins and distended seminal vesicles

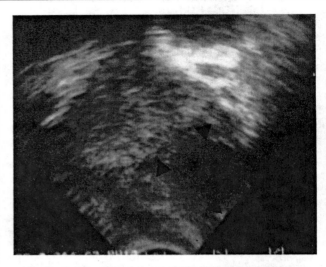

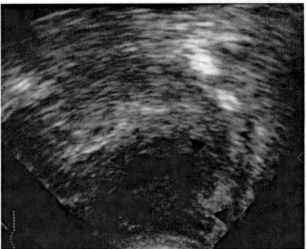

Both images are transverse transrectal scans showing a complex hypoechoic area (arrowheads) within the prostate indicating an abscess

ANOMALIES OF SEMINAL VESICLES

ANOMALY	US DESCRIPTION
• seminal vesicle pathology is very rare	
CONGENITAL ABSENCE • infertile man with agenesis of vas and azospermia • can be unilateral • rare finding	• absence of seminal vesicles • vas deferens can be seen
DILATION OF SEMINAL VESICLES • caused by obstruction (tumor) • can occur following TURP, but the ejaculatory duct is usually dilated as well	• anechoic tubular area within the seminal vesicle • with tumors there can be obliteration or displacement of the beak of seminal vesicle
SEMINAL VESICLE ABSCESSES • can be caused by seminal vesiculitis, recurrent epididymitis, congenital anomalies (ectopic ureteral insertion)	• asymmetric enlargement of one seminal vesicle • anechoic or hypoechoic partially fluid-filled lesion

SEMINAL VESICLE CYST
• rare
• usually congenital
• result from:
  incomplete absorption of mesonephric duct with ureter attached to side of seminal vesicle
  atresia of the ejaculatory duct creating a cyst
SS
• dysuria, pelvic pain, ejaculatory disturbances
	• thin-walled cystic structure within seminal vesicle
	• can be large
	• may be difficult to distinguish from tubular dilatation
	• may be seen occasionally on transabdominal USs
	
	<u>Diff. Dx.:</u>
	• Wolffian duct cysts, mullerian duct remnant cysts, prostatic cysts, diverticula of the ejaculatory duct, seminal vesicle dilatation duct to obstruction

SEMINAL VESICULITIS (INFLAMMATION) • usually a secondary inflammatory process due to prostatitis • unusual to have it without any inflammation of prostate SS • hemospermia	• US is limited diagnostic benefit • may be enlarged with decreased echogenicity
TUMOR • one of the most common neoplasms affecting the seminal vesicle is an adenocarcinoma of the prostate	• asymmetry in size, shape, echogenicity • mass in one seminal vesicle

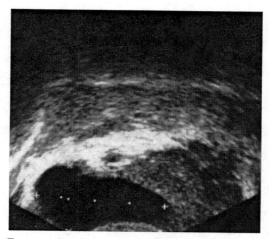

Transrectal sagittal scan of seminal vesicle cyst
(between calipers)

E) TECHNICAL FACTORS

TRANSRECTAL ULTRASOUND SCANNING (TRUS)	
INDICATIONS FOR TRUS	• evaluating size, shape, and weight of prostate • evaluate rectum and seminal vesicles • evaluate palpable lump, asymmetry, or area of induration on DRE • abnormal lab tests for PSA, acid phosphatase • screening, staging, and monitoring treatment response of prostate cancer • evaluate prostate infection • assist in TRUS biopsy guidance
PATIENT PREPARATION	• patients might require cleansing enema • patients placed in left lateral decubitus position with legs bent to chest • DRE is suggested to rule out any obstruction to probe placement

TRANSDUCER	• transrectal probes
	• use the highest frequency (5–10 MHz) available
	• variety of different types of biplane or dual probe transducers such as
	  1) phase array or mechanical sector scanners
	  2) flat faced
	  3) curved linear array
	  4) rotating (radial) endfire and multiplane probes
	• latex condom places over probe to ensure cleanliness
	• make sure patients do not have latex allergies
	• between usage probe should be soaked in antiseptic solution following manufacturer's recommendations
	• some probes require water path to decrease near-field artifact and allow better visualization of PZ close to the rectal wall

SCANNING TECHNIQUE	• a rectal examination before probe insertion can ensure no abnormalities that could create a problem with the scan • probe is lubricated and inserted into rectum and moved cephalad until prostate visualized • systematic approach using at least 2 orientations such as axial and longitudinal imaging • use near focus settings
SCAN PLANES	Coronal/axial: • probe is rotated clockwise and counterclockwise to evaluate the lateral aspect of the gland, and moved cephalad and caudad to evaluate the whole gland from superior to inferior aspect • preferred plane for assessment of lateral portions and symmetry of gland Sagittal: • probe is again rotated to image the outermost aspects of the gland • preferred plane to examine base and apex of gland
MINIMUM PROTOCOL	• thoroughly image prostate and seminal vesicles in coronal/axial and sagittal scan plans • include thorough examination of PZ • assess prostate for shape, contour, symmetry, and echogenicity • measure gland • assess seminal vesicles for size, shape, position, symmetry, and echogenicity • evaluate the perirectal area
BIOPSY	Indications: • presence of hypoechoic lesion in both longitudinal and transverse planes on TRUS, palpable nodule with DRE, elevated PSA values, or staging when a diagnosis of prostate cancer has been established Purpose: • main purpose is to obtain tissue for histologic diagnoses • several tissue samples are necessary to enable accurate evaluation Techniques: • needle-guidance system that clamps onto side of probe with an automatic biopsy gun is a commonly used device • electronic guidelines show the needle path and precise localization throughout the procedure is possible • site-specific biopsy should be performed on any identified lesion • 6 quadrant systematic biopsies from 6 standardized locations to sample whole gland Patient care: • may be performed in ambulatory setting with little preparation (enema) • patients taking anticoagulants or aspirin should stop taking them several days before biopsy • antibiotic should be prescribed just before and after biopsy • informed consent should be obtained

CHAPTER 12 - SCROTUM AND TESTES

A) NORMAL ANATOMY AND SONOGRAPHIC APPEARANCE

DEFINITION	Scrotum: • supporting structure for the testes • 2-compartment sac divided by a septum Testes: • paired male reproductive organs suspended within the scrotum by the spermatic cord

STRUCTURE

1. SCROTUM
• cutaneous, fibromuscular sac
• divided internally into two sacs by median raphe
• each contains a single testis
• consisting of following layers:
a) skin
b) dartos
   layer of muscle lying beneath skin that forms the median raphe
c) tunica vaginalis
   serous covering of testis, which is a double-layer extension of peritoneum
   separates scrotal layers from the tunica albuginea
   covers testes except at the back where the epididymis is attached
   i) Parietal (outer) layer of tunica vaginalis
      lines walls of scrotal sac
   ii) Visceral (inner) layer of tunica vaginalis
      covers testis, epididymis, lower portion of spermatic cord
   iii) Vaginalis sac
      potential space between two layers of tunica vaginalis, which normally contains a small amount of fluid

2. TESTES/TESTICLES (plural) TESTIS (single)
• paired oval glands
a) Tunica albuginea
   dense, fibrous capsule covering testis
   extends inward and divides each testis into 250–400 lobules
b) Lobules
   internal compartments formed by projections of tunica albuginea
   contain seminiferous tubules and interstitial cells
   bases are near surface and apices converge toward mediastinum testis
c) Seminiferous tubules
   each lobule contains 1–3 of these tightly coiled tubules
   produce sperm by spermatogenesis
d) Straight tubules
   spermatozoa are moved through seminiferous tubules to straight tubules that lead to rete testis
e) Rete testis
   seminiferous tubules converge to form rete testis
   located at testicular mediastinum
f) Mediastinum teste
   thickened portion of albuginea along posterior border of testis that projects into it creating a linear fibrous structure
   point where tubules converge and exit into rete testis and efferent ducts
g) Appendix testis
   paramesonephric duct in male degenerates except for this small portion at its cranial end

3. DUCTUS (VAS) DEFERENS/SEMINAL DUCT
• muscular cord designed to pump sperm into the prostatic segment of the urethra
• ascends along posterior border of testis and enters pelvic cavity by the inguinal canal where it travels over the side and posterior surface of bladder
• seminal vesicles connect to vas deferens to form ejaculatory ducts
• stores sperm for up to several months

4. SPERMATIC CORD
• supporting structure of testes
• contains blood vessels, nerves, lymph nodes, cremaster muscle
• attached to posterior border of testis
• travels through inguinal canal toward posterior surface of bladder where it joins the seminal vesicle duct to form the ejaculatory ducts

5. EPIDIDYMIS
• comma-shaped structure that curves along posterior border of testis
a) Head/globus major
   most superior aspect
   consists of first part of efferent ducts that transport sperm out of testes
b) Body/corpus
   contains ductus epididymis, which is a tightly coiled single tube that efferent ducts empty into
c) tail/globus minor
   distal part of epididymal ducts that exit and continue as ductus (vas) deferens in spermatic cord
d) Appendix epididymis
   mesonephric duct persists to form the ductus deferens, except for its most cranial portion, which becomes the appendix epididymis
   appears as a small stalk projecting from the head of epididymis
e) Efferent ductules pass from the rete to enter upper portion of the epidermis

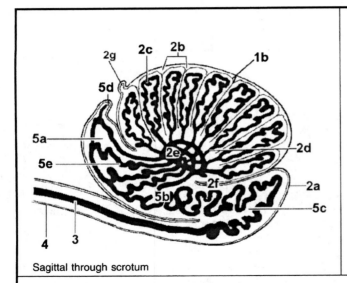

Sagittal through scrotum

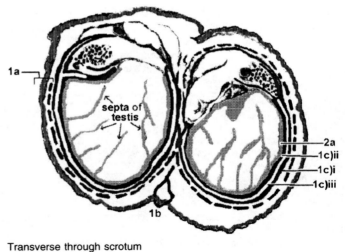

Transverse through scrotum

septa of testis

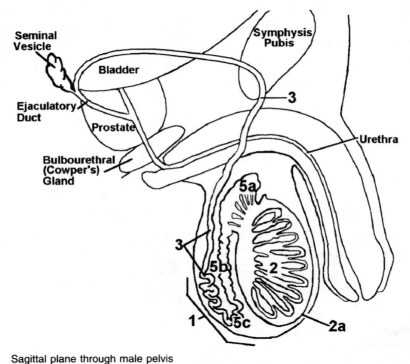

Seminal Vesicle

Bladder

Symphysis Pubis

Ejaculatory Duct

Prostate

Bulbourethral (Cowper's) Gland

Urethra

Sagittal plane through male pelvis

Key for Diagrams Above

1. SCROTUM
   a) skin
   b) dartos
   d) tunica vaginalis
      i parietal
      ii visceral
      iii vaginalis sac

2. TESTES
   a) Tunica albuginea
   b) Lobules
   c) Seminiferous tubules
   d) Straight tubules
   e) Rete testis
   f) Mediastinum teste
   g) Appendix testis

3. DUCTUS (VAS) DEFERENS
4. SPERMATIC CORD
5. EPIDIDYMIS
   a) Head
   b) Body
   c) Tail
   d) Appendix Epididymis
   e) Efferent Ductules

NORMAL ANATOMY

SIZE	TESTES	EPIDIDYMIS		
	Weight: 12.5–19 g Length: 3–5 cm Width: 2–4 cm Thickness: 3 cm	**HEAD**	**BODY**	**TAIL**
		10–12 mm diameter	< 4 mm diameter	< 4 mm
SHAPE	• symmetric, oval-shaped glands with smooth contour	• triangular with smooth edges	• elongated structure	• tapered end of body
LOCATION	• each testis lies protected in scrotum attached to spermatic cord • sit obliquely in scrotum upper pole more anterolateral lower pole more posteromedial	• rest directly on upper pole of testis lateral to superior pole of testis	• along posterior lateral aspect of testicle	• curved structure at inferior aspect of testicle

SONOGRAPHIC APPEARANCE

DOPPLER	SCROTUM	TESTES	EPIDIDYMIS
• largest vessels are visualized peripherally Testicular Artery • low peripheral resistance • broad systolic peaks and high diastolic flow Deferential Artery • high resistance • narrow systolic peaks and low diastolic flow	Wall/Scrotal Layers 2–8 mm thick • usually inseparable sonographically and appear as single echogenic stripe Tunica Vaginalis Sac • potential space that normally can contain a few cc of fluid	• homogenous with medium-level echos • smooth wall • each testis and epididymis should be compared for matching size and echogenicity Mediastinum Testis • highly echogenic linear structure peripherally located in posterior-superior aspect of testis (parallel to epididymis) Appendix Testes • small ovoid structure beneath head of epididymis	Head • isoechoic or slightly more echogenic than testis Body • isoechoic or slightly less echogenic than head and testes Tail • slightly thicker than body

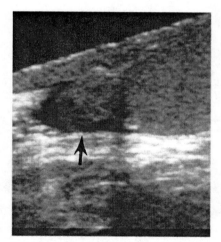

Epididymis: longitudinal (arrowhead)

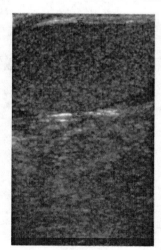

Testis: longitudinal

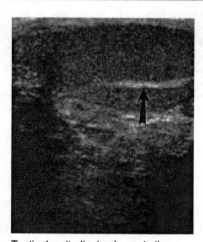

Testis: longitudinal-echogenic line = mediastinum testis (arrow)

(continued)

221

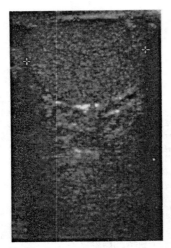

Testis: transverse

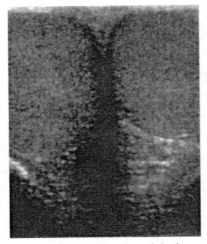

Transverse scan plane through both testes, comparing echogenicity

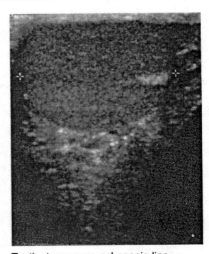

Testis: transverse-echogenic line = mediastinum testis

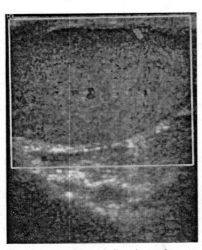

Normal color Doppler flow in testis

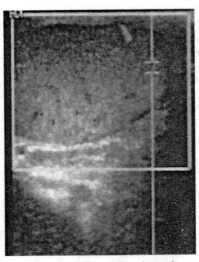

Normal Doppler flow pattern in testis

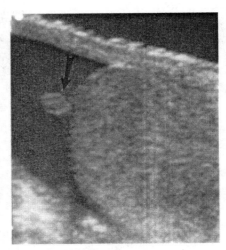

Appendix testis (arrow)

B) VASCULATURE

ARTERIAL			VENOUS
• Some anastomoses between these 3 major vessels			
AORTA ↓ **TESTICULAR ARTERY** ↓ travels in retroperitoneum ↓ enters inguinal canal in spermatic cord ↓ branch into CAPSULAR ARTERIES (run in layer beneath tunica albuginiea) ↓ surround testis as CENTRIPETAL ARTERIES (run into testicular parenchyma toward mediastinum)	INFERIOR EPIGASTRIC ARTERY ↓ **CREMASTERIC (EXTERNAL SPERMATIC) ARTERY** (spermatic cord) ↓	INFERIOR VESICLE ARTERY ↓ **DEFERENTIAL ARTERY** (spermatic cord) ↓ courses tail of epididymis ↓ divides into capillary network	INTRATESTICULAR VEINS exit through mediastinum ↓ VENOUS OUTFLOW ↓ PAMPINIFORM PLEXUS ↓ INTERNAL SPERMATIC VEIN ↓ LEFT INTERNAL SPERMATIC VEIN / RIGHT INTERNAL SPERMATIC VEIN LEFT INTERNAL SPERMATIC VEIN ↓ ; RIGHT INTERNAL SPERMATIC VEIN ↓ LEFT RENAL VEIN ; IVC ↓ IVC
SUPPLIES **TESTIS**	SUPPLIES SOFT TISSUES OF **SCROTUM AND EPIDIDYMIS**		DRAIN ↓ **IVC**
FLOW PATTERN • testes have low resistance to arterial flow • broad systolic peaks and high levels of diastolic flow throughout cardiac cycle RI average = 0.55–0.64	FLOW PATTERN • do not supply testicular tissue • high resistance pattern • narrower systolic peaks and diminished or absent diastolic flow		FLOW PATTERN • typical venous flow pattern

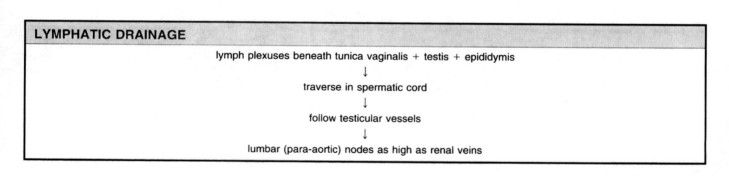

LYMPHATIC DRAINAGE

lymph plexuses beneath tunica vaginalis + testis + epididymis
↓
traverse in spermatic cord
↓
follow testicular vessels
↓
lumbar (para-aortic) nodes as high as renal veins

C) PHYSIOLOGY

	FUNCTION	OPERATION
SCROTUM	1. supporting structure for testes 2. regulates temperature of the testes	• holds testicles outside the body where the temperature is more optimum for sperm maturation • contraction of the cremaster muscles adjusts scrotum's position from the pelvic cavity • this ensures an environment of about 3°C below body temperature for sperm production and survival
EPIDIDYMIS	1. site of sperm maturation, which requires 18 hours to 10 days 2. site of sperm storage	• stores sperm until orgasm, then propels sperm from testicle to vas deferens within spermatic cord
TESTES	1. functions as an exocrine gland by producing spermatozoa (male germ cells) 2. functions as an endocrine gland by synthesizing and secreting testosterone (male sex hormone)	• interstitial cells among tubules include secretory cells of "Leydig," which produce and secrete testosterone into adjacent capillaries • excretion is influenced by pituitary gland • function of testosterone: stimulates development of glands and ducts at puberty secondary sex characteristics

D) LAB TESTS

	INTERPRETATION	
	ELEVATED	DECREASED
HUMAN CHORIONIC GONADOTROPIN • increased pituitary secretion of FSH or production of gonadotropin by tumors can raise levels in blood	seminoma embryonal tumors of testes	
TESTOSTERONE • principle androgen secreted by Leydig cells • induces puberty in male • maintains male secondary sex characteristics	testicular tumor adrenal hyperplasia benign or malignant adrenal tumor	orchectomy testicular or prostatic cancer cirrhosis of liver primary or secondary hypogonadism

E) ANOMALIES

ANOMALY	US APPEARANCE
CALCIFICATION 1. MICROCALCIFICATION IN TESTES • benign condition • may be secondary to vascular calcification, inflammation, and/or granulomas 2. SCROTAL CALCULI • extratesticular focus • arise then break away from tunica vaginalis • appear as echogenic foci between layers of tunica vaginalis US • echogenic free-floating calculus outside testicle • visualization aided by hydrocele Other causes: • resolved hematoma • neoplasm (teratoma, choriocarcinoma)	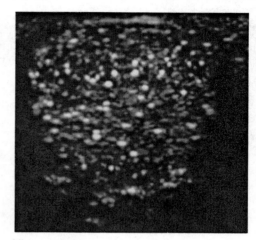 Microcalcifications within testes 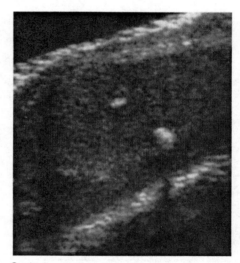 Sagittal scan through testis with 2 echogenic foci with shadow: old hematomas can leave residual calcification *(continued)*

ANOMALY (*Continued*)	US APPEARANCE

CRYPTORCHIDISM (UNDESCENDED TESTIS)

- normally testes descend into scrotal sac at 8 months' gestational age
- Ectopic location
  Child—usually found in inguinal canal
  Adult—small testis with normal echogenicity usually found in inguinal canal
- Potential concerns
  −increased chance of malignancy (seminoma) in undescended testicle
  −infertility

US

- malpositioned testes situated anywhere along the normal track of decline from retroperitoneum to scrotum
- most commonly found at or below level of inguinal canal
- appear more echogenic than muscle

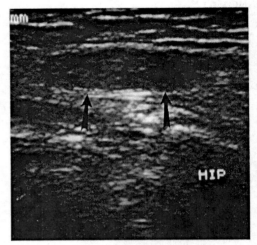

Undescended testis in the left inguinal canal (arrows)

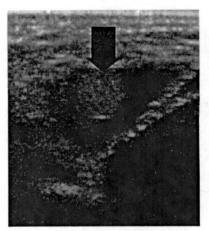

Transverse scan plane: testis in inguinal canal (arrow)

ANOMALY	US APPEARANCE

CYSTS
EXTRATESTICULAR
1. EPIDIDYMAL CYST
- benign serous-containing cysts
- similar in appearance to spermatocele
- single or multiple and usually in head but can occur throughout epididymis

US
- variable, but usually appear as a cyst of mass with a hyperechoic, calcified wall

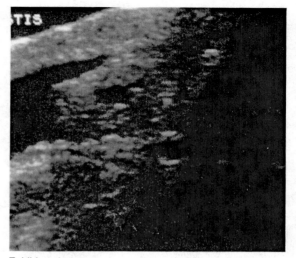

Epididymal cyst

2. SPERMATOCELE
- common, cystic mass of epididymis containing spermatozoa
- located in head epididymis, superior to testis
- if large can be septated and palpable
- can be uni- or bilateral, single or multiple
- may be loculated and contain low-level echos

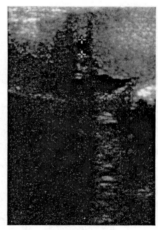

Epididymal cyst (caliper)

3. TUNICA ALBUGINEA CYSTS
- located within the tunica albuginea, usually anterior and lateral aspects of testis
- well defined, single or multiple, uni- or multilocular
- occur most often in 5th to 6th decade
- asymptomatic, but can present as small firm nodule at margin of testes in superficial location
- etiology unknown

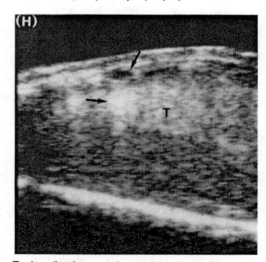

Tunica albuginea cyst in anterior surface of tunica albuginea (arrow)

(*continued*)

227

ANOMALY	US APPEARANCE

CYSTS (*Continued*)
INTRATESTICULAR
- less common than extratesticular cysts

<u>5. TESTICULAR CYST</u>
- rare, benign cyst more commonly found in elderly
- vary in size between 2–18 mm
- usually located near mediastinum testis

US
- well circumscribed anechoic mass with regular margins (simple)
- enhance (but necrotic tumors also enhance)
- cystic tumor must be excluded where septations, echos, solid components, or a thick wall is seen

<u>6. EPIDERMOID CYST</u>
- 1% of testicular neoplasms
- benign

SS
- none

US
- homogeneous, well circumscribed that may have wall thickening
- hypo- to hyperechoic
- main contain calcification

<u>Diff. Dx.:</u>
<u>DILATED RETE TESTIS</u>
- focal enlargement of rete testis due to obstruction at level of epididymis
- appears as a cluster of hypoechoic, small cystic spaces adjacent to mediastinum
<u>VARICOCELE</u>
- collection of tortuous dilated veins arising from pampiniform venous plexus
- vessel size increased with Valsalva or with patient standing
- 95% occur on left (right-sided varicocele should raise the possibility of underlying right-sided abdominal pathology)

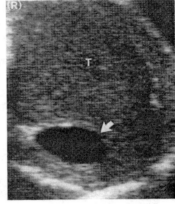

Single intratesticular cyst (arrow) in inferior aspect of testis (T)

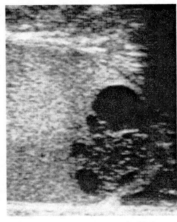

Benign intratesticular cystic changes within the mediastinum testis

ANOMALY	US APPEARANCE

HERNIA INTO SCROTAL SAC
- intestine or omentum herniates and extends into scrotum
- can be further distinguished into:
- Indirect (external)
- bowel passes through external inguinal ring into inguinal canal and then to scrotum from abdominal cavity
- Direct (internal)
- caused by weakness in floor of inguinal canal

SS
- persistent or intermittent scrotal mass
- may have abdominal pain, blood in stool

US
- mass that may contain air or fluid-filled loops of bowel within the scrotal sac
- look for peristalsis to confirm diagnosis
- bowel haustral can be sometimes seen
- if only omentum is present, an echogenic mass is seen

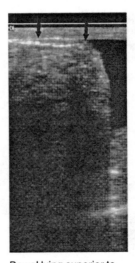

Bowel lying superior to testis in scrotal sac (arrows)

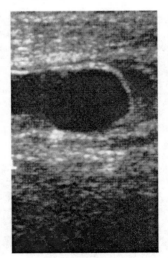

Fluid within inguinal canal

ANOMALY	US APPEARANCE

HYDROCELE, PYOCELE, HEMATOCELE

- abnormal collection of fluid (serous, blood, pus, or urine) in potential space between the 2 layers of tunica vaginalis

1. HYDROCELE: (SEROUS)
- painless swelling of scrotum
- congenital or acquired, often idiopathic or associated with epididymitis, torsion, trauma (25%–50%)
- usually occur in anterior aspect of scrotum and displace testis posteriorly

2. PYOCELE: (PUS)
- infectious process, debris within fluid

3. HEMATOCELE: (BLOOD)
- hemorrhage in sac of tunica vaginalis
- due to trauma, surgery, tumor, torsion, or hemophilia

SS
- enlargement of scrotum

US
- hydrocele
- anechoic fluid collection anterior and lateral to testis between layers of tunica vaginalis
- pyoceles and hematoceles
- can be septated with low- to medium-level echos

Helpful Hint:
- normal scrotum contains a few milliliters of fluid

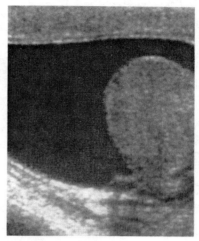

Hydrocele

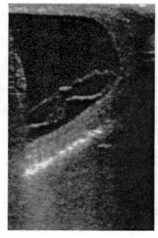

Septations within hydrocele

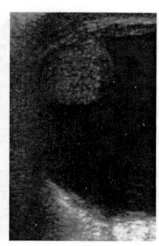

Hydrocele

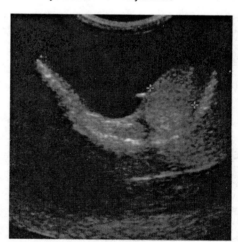

Hydrocele (testes between calipers)

ANOMALY	US APPEARANCE

INFECTION AND INFLAMMATION

1. ABSCESS
- complication of epididymo-orchitis, torsion, tumor, or diabetes
- can lead to pyocele

SS
- hypoechoic, mixed echogenicity, sonolucent, irregular border mass
- similar appearance to seminoma and if it does not resolve, further investigation is necessary

Doppler:
- hypervascularity (peripheral)
- decreased RI indices

2. EPIDIDYMITIS
- most common cause of acute scrotum
- caused by retrograde spread of bacterial infection from bladder or prostate and is associated with prostatitis
- common cause in young men are sexually transmitted organisms gonococci and chlamydia

US
ACUTE
- enlarged, hypoechoic epididymis
- mainly involves head
- entire epididymis involved in 50% of cases
- hypoechoic areas are secondary to edema

CHRONIC
- thickened echogenic epididymis
- may contain calcifications

3. EPIDIDYMO-ORCHITIS
- inflammation of the testis and epididymis
- 20% of epididymitis involves the testes
- testicular involvement can be focal or diffuse

US
- hypoechoic area extending from epididymal region

4. ORCHITIS
- inflammation of testis due to trauma, metastasis, mumps, or other infection
- isolated orchitis is rare as usually occurs as a secondary result of epididymitis
- can be focal and if persists, a neoplasm must be ruled out by serial US examinations or surgery
- orchitis will eventually resolve, where a neoplasm will not

SS
- acute scrotal, pain, with or without fever

US
1. ACUTE ORCHITIS
Diffuse—decreased echogenicity and increased size
Focal—focal areas of decreased echogenicity
Doppler:
Testicular hyperemia with:
  increased number and concentration of blood vessels in affected area
  increased venous flow in epididymis

2. CHRONIC ORCHITIS
- thickened tunica albuginea
- echogenic, thickened, irregular epididymis
- both may contain calcifications
- affected testis is smaller

3. GRANULOMATOUS ORCHITIS
- multiple focal hypoechoic lesions
Diff. Dx.:
- neoplastic process

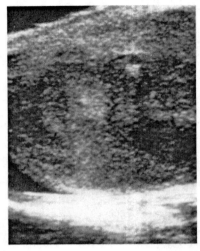

Abscess

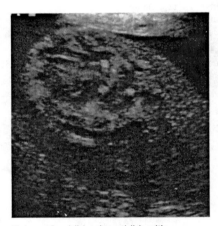

Enlarged epididymis: epididymitis

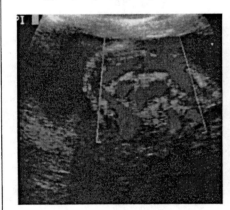

Epididymitis: increased blood flow

US APPEARANCE OF INFECTION AND INFLAMMATION

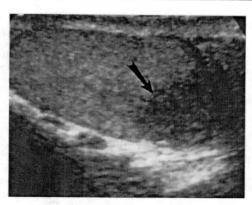

Focal orchitis: focal hypoechoic area of
inflammation (arrows) on longitudinal scan of testis

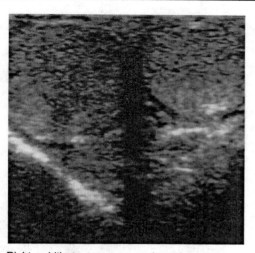

Right orchitis: transverse scan through scrotum
showing enlarged hypoechoic right testis

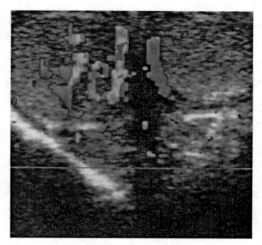

Right orchitis: transverse scan through both testes
showing increased blood flow on right

ANOMALY	US APPEARANCE

LYMPHOMA/LEUKEMIA

- 5% of testicular neoplasms
- leukemia is the most common metastatic tumor to testes
- leukemia can escape chemotherapeutic effect in the testicle due to a blood–gonad barrier
- most common testicular neoplasm in men over 60
- most common bilateral testicular tumor
- associated with disseminated lymphoma (non-Hodgkin's)
- poor survival (5%–20% 5-year survival)

SS
- painless testicular mass

US
- enlargement of testis with uniform decreased echogenicity
- can appear either as
  focal unilateral or bilateral hypoechoic masses
- diffuse inhomogeneous enlargement with hypervascularity

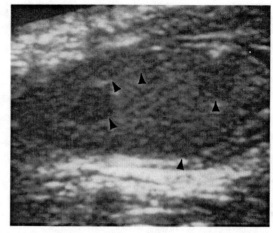

Longitudinal scan through testis showing multiple focal
hypoechoic masses (arrows) within testis representing
neoplastic involvement

ANOMALY	US APPEARANCE

SPERMATIC CORD AND TESTICLE TORSION

1. ACUTE INFARCTION
- spermatic cord and testicle twist
- limits vascular flow and drainage, which compromises blood supply (ischemia)
- occurs in individuals with abnormal suspension of testicle within scrotum
- surgical treatment within 4–6 hours is necessary as testicular viability can be lost quickly
- peak incidence in neonatal period and at puberty

SS
- sudden onset of extreme pain

US
- appearance depends on duration of symptoms
- after a period of ischemia:
  testis: enlarges with decreased echogenicity
  scrotum: thickened wall, edematous, hypervascular

Doppler:
- testicular ischemia: complete or near complete absence of detectable flow in symptomatic testicle

Diff. Dx.:
- global infarction of testis and epididymis due to an inflammatory process

Pitfall:
- some diminished flow may be seen in early or partial torsion
- spontaneous resolution of torsion may show normal or increased blood flow to testis
- ischemia can be also caused by trauma
- settings are not sensitive enough to detect normal blood flow (especially in pediatric cases, where normal blood flow is very low)

2. CHRONIC INFARCTION ("MISSED TORSION")
- history of acute pain in past

US
- heterogeneous appearance of testes with peripheral rim of normal-appearing testicular tissue

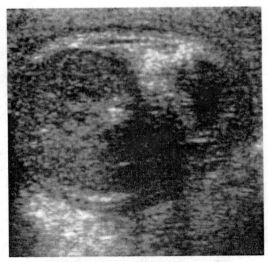

Transverse scan through testes demonstrated inhomogeneous echotexture

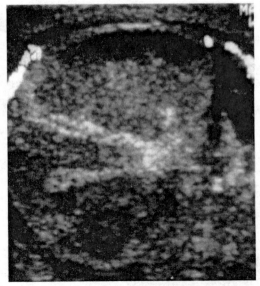

Testicular torsion: note only peripheral blood flow is present

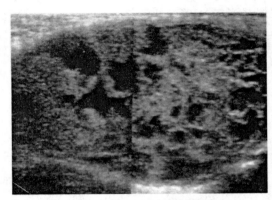

Complete infarction with necrosis of testicular parenchyma

ANOMALY	US APPEARANCE

TRAUMA/HEMATOMA

1. EFFUSION
- blood in scrotal wall

2. INTRATESTICULAR HEMATOMAS
- irregular hypoechoic area in region of hemorrhage, which undergoes cystic changes as hematoma resolves

3. TESTICULAR FRACTURE/RUPTURE
- contour abnormality of tunica albuginea
- hemorrhage or infarction appearing as focal areas of altered texture
- hematocele

US
- complex nonspecific predominantly hypoechoic pattern whose appearance depends on age of hematoma/infarction
- correlate findings with clinical history and if in doubt rescan to document any changes in sonographic appearance over time
  change in appearance = trauma
  no change = neoplasm

Rupture:
- can see discrete fracture plane
- irregular testicular contour
- altered echogenicity consistent with infarct/hematoma
- hematocele in 33% of cases
- requires immediate surgery

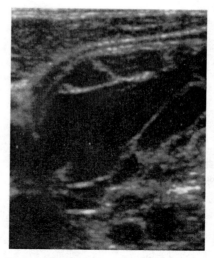

Peritesticular hematoma in patient with history of taking blood thinning drugs

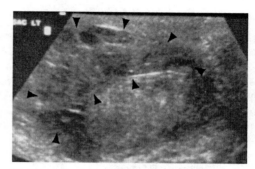

Fracture of testis: lower half of testis has no observable blood flow; moderately large peritesticular hematoma (between arrows)

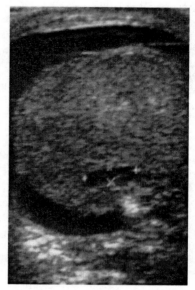

Small hematoma (between calipers)

ANOMALY	US APPEARANCE

TUMORS

EXTRATESTICULAR TUMORS
- may arise from spermatic cord or epididymis

1. ADENOMATOID TUMOR
- most common epididymal neoplasms
- arise from mesothelium
- slow growing and benign
- may range in size from a few millimeters to 5 cm

SS
- none

US
- well circumscribed of variable echogenicity

Diff. Dx.:
- sperm granuloma, leimyoma, fibroma, lypoma

GERM CELL TUMORS
- 90%–99% of malignancies

SS
- painful testicular mass
- metastatic disease to retroperitoneum, mediastinum, supraclavicular region

1. CHORIOCARCINOMA
- rare (< 1–3% of malignant primary tumors)
- small, highly malignant and can metastasize before being seen sonographically
- most common in 2nd and 3rd decades

SS
- gynecomastia secondary to high human chorionic gonadotropin levels

US
- mixed echogenic mass containing areas of hemorrhage, necrosis, and calcifications

2. EMBRYONAL CELL CARCINOMA
- 20%–30% of germ cell tumors
- 2nd most common germ cell tumor
- occur in younger age group than seminomas
- small size that seldom enlarge testis
- more aggressive than seminoma
- may invade tunica, distorting testicular contour
- infantile form: endodermal sinus or yolk sac tumor is most common germ cell tumor in infants

US
- more inhomogeneous and ill defined than seminomas, can contain cystic areas and echogenic foci with or without shadowing

3. SEMINOMAS
- 40%–50% of germ call tumors
- most common primary neoplasm
- peak incidence in 4th and 5th decades
- rare before puberty

SS
- elevated FSH levels
- most common tumor to arise with cryptorchidism

US
- focal hypoechoic mass, homogeneous texture with smooth or ill defined margins

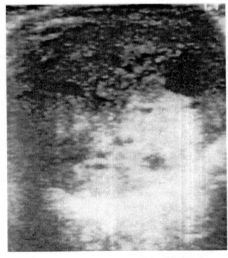

Transverse scan through testis containing malignant mixed germ cell carcinoma

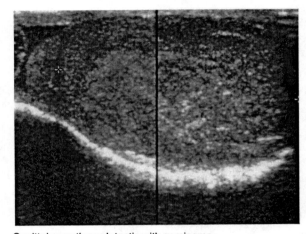

Sagittal scan through testis with seminoma

ANOMALY	US APPEARANCE

TUMORS (Continued)

4. TERATOMAS
- 5%–10% of primary testicular neoplasms
- 3 types; mature, immature, and teratoma with malignant transformation
- most common in infancy and early childhood and again in 3rd decade
- in adults is considered malignant, although can range from benign to malignant

US
- well defined inhomogeneous mass with cystic and solid areas, echogenic foci with shadowing

GONADAL STROMAL TUMORS
- tumors containing leydig, thecal, granulosa, or lutein cells in various combinations
- 3%–6% of testicular neoplasms and 20% occur in children

1. LEYDIG CELL TUMOR (HYPERPLASIA)
- unusual benign tumor (1%–3% of all testicular tumors)
- most common stromal tumor with incidence increased in 2nd to 5th decade
- difficult to differentiate from germ cell neoplasm
- can produce hormonal changes

SS
- painless mass, hynecomastia, impotenance, viralization secondary to hormone effects

US
- small, solid hypoechoic masses
- cystic change can occur when large

METASTASES
- testes are also sites for metastatic disease
- more common in elderly
- lymphoma/leukemia is most common
- lung and prostate are next in frequency
- can be multiple and bilateral

US
- focal mass or masses with variable echogenicity

Helpful Hint:
- all solid intratesticular masses should be considered malignant until proven otherwise, and a survey of the abdomen should be performed to rule out metastatic disease

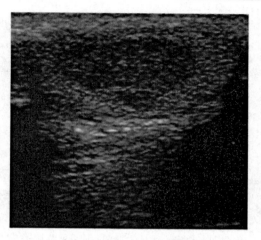

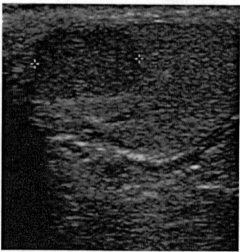

Seminoma in patient with history of undescended testicle that descended spontaneously as a youth

ANOMALY	US APPEARANCE

VARICOCELE

- dilated peritesticular veins that form as a result of incompetent valves
- occurs more frequently on left as the pressure on the left is higher (left spermatic vein drains into left renal vein, whereas the right internal spermatic vein drains directly into the lower pressure IVC)
- retroperitoneal masses should be considered when an isolated right-sided varicocele is present
- associated with male infertility

US

- numerous dilated, ectatic, and tortuous vessels in peritesticular region
- vein > 3 mm during Valsalva maneuver
- best visualized superior and lateral to testis
- when become large extend posterior and inferior to testis
- check renal veins for tumor/thrombus
- may enlarge when patient is scanned in upright position
- generally do not cause pain until they become quite large

Doppler:
- with normal respiration flow is often too slow to be detected
- with Valsalva maneuver or with patient standing the incompetent valves causes blood to flow rapidly and retrograde
- color Doppler is more sensitive than physical exam in detecting varicoceles

Helpful Hint:
1. scan patient standing OR
2. have patient perform Valsalva maneuver
- if veins are not obstructed from tumor or thrombus, there should be a change in their diameter

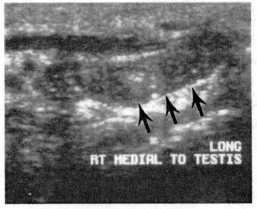

Thrombosed varicocele (arrows)

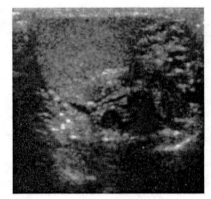

Multiple anechoic tubules adjacent to testicle: large varicocele

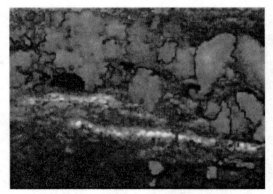

Color Doppler during Valsalva maneuver in varicocele

COMMON DIFFERENTIALS IN SCROTAL SONOGRAPHY

ACUTE SCROTAL PAIN	torsion of testicle or appendix testis epididymitis and epididymo-orchitis trauma strangulated hernias acute hydroceles abscess
PALPABLE MASS	epididymal cyst scrotal calculi seminoma
ENLARGED SCROTUM	hydrocele, hematocele epididymo-orchitis torsion neoplasm
ENLARGED TESTICLE	primary testicular tumors lymphoma orchitis acute or subacute torsion
ENLARGED EPIDIDYMIS	epididymitis tumor torsion
SMALL TESTES	chronic torsion undescended testicle postinfection atrophy
FLUID AROUND TESTIS	peritesticular abscess hydrocele hematocele pyocele
INHOMOGENOUS ECHOTEXTURE	tumor abscess hematoma pseudotumor (artifact that results from acoustic shadowing from transtesticular vessels: image testes in more than one plane to differentiate from true mass)

SCROTAL PATHOLOGY

EPIDIDYMIS	TESTIS	PAMPINIFORM PLEXUS	SCROTUM
acute epididymitis chronic epididymitis spermatocele	orchitis primary testicular tumors testicular torsion hemorrhage abscess lymphoma	varicocele	hydrocele pyocele inguinal hernia

F) TECHNICAL FACTORS

TRANSDUCER	• 5–7.5 MHz with short focus • stand-off pad required

TECHNIQUE	Scrotal examinations
	• patient lying supine on table
	  have the patient lift his penis onto his lower abdomen using a towel to cover and keep it in position
	  scrotum supported by a towel draped between the thighs
	  if the patient keeps his legs together, this will help keep the scrotum in a relatively stationary position on the towel
	  ample amount of gel to avoid undue pressure of scrotum
	  warm gel will reduce cremasteric responses that result in thickening of scrotal skin

DOPPLER	Optimize low flow detection by: decrease PRF/scale lower PRF lower wall filters increase Doppler gain or power high-frequency transducers (7 MHz) Tumor criteria • color Doppler findings are more dependent on the size of the lesion than on its histologic nature • lesions > 1.5 tend to be hypervascular and smaller lesions tend to be hypovascular
SCAN PLANES	• transverse and longitudinal scan planes including the epididymis
MINIMUM PROTOCOL	• longitudinal and transverse images of each testis including the lateral, medial, superior, and inferior aspects • longitudinal and transverse scans of head and tail of epididymis • document size • assess echogenicity (using split image to compare left and right) • evaluate extratesticular regions for presence of fluid, hernia, and other conditions • color and pulsed Doppler are used to evaluate vascular flow to the testicles
HELPFUL HINTS	1. for more accurate longitudinal measurement purposes only, it might be necessary to use the 5-MHz transducer, so that the whole length of the testis can be imaged at once 2. include a transverse scan of both testes at once, so that echogenicity can be more easily compared 3. if equipment has color Doppler, take a few seconds to examine the blood flow of each testis. This will aid in the times when you are required to judge if the perfusion of a testis is "normal."

CHAPTER 13 - SPLEEN AND LYMPHATIC SYSTEM
A) NORMAL ANATOMY AND SONOGRAPHIC APPEARANCE

SPLEEN		
DEFINITION		• largest mass of lymphatic tissue in body; therefore, the largest unit of the reticuloendothelial system • involved in systemic inflammations, metabolic disturbances, and hematopoietic disorders

STRUCTURE
1. CAPSULE
• dense connective tissue
2. PERITONEUM
• serous membrane that covers spleen
a) Lieno/splenorenal ligament
• attaches spleen to posterior abdominal wall
• 2 layers of peritoneum that contain the splenic vessels and pancreatic tail
• lies against splenic hilum
b) Gastrosplenic ligament
• 2 layers of peritoneum that contain short gastric vessels
• attaches spleen to greater curvature of stomach
3. HILUS
• vessels enter and leave at this point
• accessory spleens may be visualized in splenic hilum
a) Splenic artery and vein
4. VISCERAL SURFACE
• contoured to shape of organs adjacent to it
a) Gastric impression—stomach
b) Renal impression—left kidney
c) Colic impression—left flexure of colon
d) Pancreatic impression—tail of pancreas

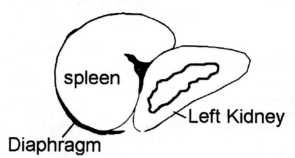

Longitudinal section through spleen and kidney

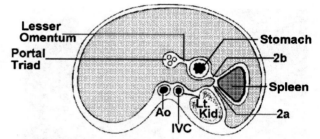

Cross section of abdomen focusing at level of spleen

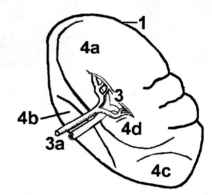

Splenic hilum

SIZE	**MASS** • normal spleen cannot be palpated and must be twice normal size to be felt • size varies with age, sex, and nutritional state Length = 12–14 cm Width = 7 cm Thickness (AP) = 3 cm	**WEIGHT FROM US MEASUREMENTS** Weight (g) = 0.43 × Length × Width × Thickness at Hilum Normal Range: Males = 180 g Females = 150 g
SHAPE	• wide range of normal configuration • crescent 1/2-moon shaped • varies according to shape of adjacent organs • smooth outer contour	
LOCATION	• left hypochondriac region • between fundus of stomach and diaphragm • left lateral margin of lesser sac • between 9th and 11th ribs • intraperitoneal except for its hilum • can be ectopic in location	

REGIONAL ANATOMY OF SPLEEN

SUPERIOR	smooth convex that conforms to adjacent concave surface of diaphragm
INFERIOR	splenic flexure of colon, left kidney
MEDIAL	gastric fundus, tail of pancreas
POSTEROLATERALLY	lower chest, upper abdominal wall
HILUS	tail of pancreas

US APPEARANCE

TEXTURE	ECHOGENICITY	PITFALL
• uniform, homogeneous, multiple low-amplitude echos • small vessels are seen within spleen as branching, anechoic round, or tubular structures	• more echogenic than normal renal cortex • medium-level echos • less echogenic or isoechoic to liver	• elongated left hepatic lobe can cross midline and appears between the spleen and diaphragm • less echogenic than spleen and therefore can mimic a perisplenic or subcapsular fluid collection

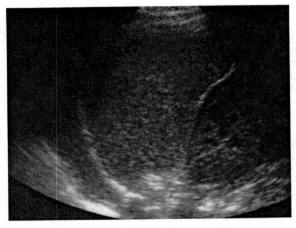

Sagittal spleen: left kidney interface

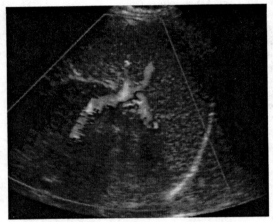

Coronal: color flow of splenic vein

LYMPHATIC SYSTEM

• all the structures in the body that are involved in the transport of lymph from tissues to the bloodstream

	LYMPH	LYMPH VESSELS	LYMPH NODES
DEFINITION	• watery transparent fluid • filtered by lymph nodes	• thin-walled vessels transporting lymph from the tissues	• discrete nodules of lymphoid tissue located along the lymphatic tract • also found in GI tract, lungs, bone marrow, spleen, and thymus
STRUCTURE	• contains lymphocytes, protein, and fat in the vessels draining bowel	• contains valves and 3 layers • resemble veins in structure	• encapsulated rounded body of lymphatic tissue • contain lymphocytes, B and T cells, plasma cells
SIZE	• fluid	• begin as tiny capillaries and merge to form larger vessels	• normally < 1 cm in size
LOCATION	• contained in the intercellular spaces of body	• drain along the major arteries, veins, and organs	• lie along lymph channels
COMMON SITES	• adjacent to vasculature (para-aortic, paracaval) • porta hepatis • retroperitoneum (peripancreatic, renal hilum) • pelvis side walls • mesenteric, perisplenic, perihepatic, retroperitoneal areas • CNS has no lymphatics		

US APPEARANCE	NORMAL	ABNORMAL	
	• normal lymph nodes are usually visualized sonographically	• enlarged lymph nodes are mostly seen if > 2 cm in size • with improving technical resolution and high-frequency transducers, some nodes smaller than 2 cm can be seen • appear as rounded, focal echo-poor lesions • can appear cystic to complex	

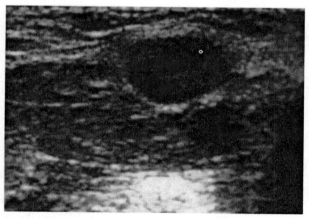

Lymph node

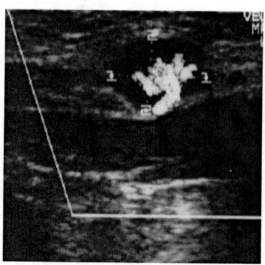

Arterial blood flow into lymph node

241

B) VASCULATURE

ARTERIAL SUPPLY → **SPLEEN** → VENOUS RETURN VIA PORTAL SYSTEM

Left Gastroepiploic Vein
↓
Celiac Axis → Splenic Artery → **SPLEEN** → (Splenic Vein + Superior Mesenteric Vein) = Portal Vein
↑ ↑
Short Gastric Veins Pancreatic Veins

C) PHYSIOLOGY

PURPOSE AND FUNCTION	
SPLEEN	• not essential to life, but is main component of reticuloendothelial system 1. Major secondary organ in immune system • reticular network traps antigen permitting it to come into contact wtih lymphocytes • production of B lymphocytes, which develop into antibody-producing plasma cells 2. Filter bloodstream of unwanted elements • phagocytizes bacteria and worn out and damaged RBCs and platelets 3. Storage and release of blood • in cases of demand such as hemorrhage • active role in blood formation during initial part of fetal life • storage of iron and other metabolites
PARENCHYMA	1. White pulp • lymphatic tissue, mostly lymphocytes arranged around splenic arteries (known as splenic nodules or malpighian corpuscles) • involved with immune system (antigen/antibody process) 2. Red pulp • venous component of spleen • lined by reticuloendothelial (macrophages) cells that phagocytose unwanted elements of the blood (e.g., abnormal RBCs, bacteria)
LYMPHATIC SYSTEM	1. formation of lymphocytes and monocytes 2. drainage of tissue fluid and protein back to the venous system 3. absorption and transport of fat from small bowel to bloodstream 4. main immune mechanism for the body 5. transportation of protein of the body into circulatory system

D) LAB AND OTHER TESTS

COMPLETE BLOOD COUNT (CBC)
- hematocrit (Hct)
- hemoglobin concentration (Hgb)
- erythrocyte indices
- white blood cell count (WBC)
- platelet quantification (Plt)
- peripheral blood smear (PBS)

	ELEVATED	DECREASED
HEMATOCRIT (HCT) • volume of packed RBCs in 100 mL of blood expressed as a percentage	• dehydration • polycythemia vera • diabetic acidosis	• acute blood loss • anemias • leukemias • Hodgkin's disease • multiple myeloma • anemias • cancers • kidney diseases • excessive IV fluids • Hodgkin's disease
HEMOGLOBIN (HB, HGB) • protein substance in RBCs composed of iron, which is an oxygen carrier	• dehydration • polycythemia • chronic obstructive lung disease	
ERYTHROCYTE (RBC) • suggest need for further investigation as they are not diagnostic	POLYCYTHEMIA • pulmonary disease • tumors • renal disease • endocrine disorders	PANCYTOPENIA • neoplasms • metabolic disorder • marrow infiltration • granulomas • infection
WHITE BLOOD COUNT (WBC) • function of relative rates of bone marrow and lymphoid leukocyte production, cell margination, and tissue consumption of leukocytes • measures number of WBCs in 1 μL of whole blood	• acute infection (e.g., pneumonia, meningitis, appendicitis) • leukemias • tissue necrosis (e.g., cirrhosis, burns) • stress (surgery, fever) • hematopoietic diseases (e.g., hypersplenism, aplastic anemia)	• viral infections • malaria

WHITE BLOOD CELL (WBC) DIFFERENTIAL

- evaluates morphology of 5 types of WBC (leukocytes)
- determines number and type of WBCs

	ELEVATED	DECREASED
1. BASOPHILS • increase during healing process	• inflammatory processes • leukemia • healing stage of infection or inflammation	• increase in steroids, i.e., stress, hypersensitivity reaction, pregnancy
2. EOSINOPHILS • increase during allergic and parasitic conditions	EOSINOPHILIA • allergic reaction • parasitic disease • collagen-vascular disease (phlebitis, thrombophlebitis) • cancer of bone, ovary, testicles, brain	• with an increase in steroid (produced by adrenal glands during stress or administered orally or by injection) i.e., stress (burns, shock), adrenocortical hyperfunction
3. LYMPHOCYTES • T cells attach to and destroy specific antigens • B cells attack invading microorganisms	LEUKOCYTOSIS • infection (chronic or viral) • lymphocytic leukemia • Hodgkin's disease • multiple myeloma • tissue necrosis	LEUKOPENIA • bone marrow depression • cancer, leukemia • influenza • measles, rubella • infectious hepatitis • mononucleosis
4. MONOCYTES • 2nd line of defense against bacterial infections and foreign substances • slower but larger than neutrophils; therefore can ingest larger particles of debris	MONOCYTOSIS • infections (e.g., TB, hepatitis, malaria) • monocytic lymphoma • lupus erythematosis • parasitic disease	
5. NEUTROPHILS (PMNS) • are the most numerous circulating WBC • respond more rapidly to inflammatory and tissue injury sites than other types of WBC	NEUTROPHILIA • infection, inflammation • drugs/toxins • endocrine disorders • hematologic abnormalities	NEUTROPENIA • infection, inflammation • chemicals and physical agents (e.g., chemo)
PLATELET COUNT (PLTS) • estimated as absent, reduced, adequate, or increased, or may be specifically quantitated	THROMBOCYTOSIS • reaction to surgery, malignancy, disease, drugs, inflammation • physiologic (exercise, stress) • myeloproliferative disorders (leukemia, multiple myeloma)	THROMBOCYTOPENIA • marrow injury • hereditary disorders • platelet destruction
NUCLEAR MEDICINE (SPLEEN) TSC-HEPATOSPLENIC SCAN	**INCREASED UPTAKE** • nonspecific • differential includes hepatocellular disease, underlying hematological abnormalities, recent infection	**COLD SPOT** • nonspecific • differential includes cyst, abscess, hematoma, neoplastic disease

E) ANOMALIES

ANOMALY	US APPEARANCE
CONGENITAL ANOMALIES <u>1. ACCESSORY SPLEEN (SPLENICULI)</u> • common, normal variant • 10% of population has ectopic spleens found near hilus of primary spleen • usually found in gastrosplenic ligament, tail of pancreas, bowel omentum or mesenteries • appear as small rounded homogeneous nodules isoechoic to spleen • usually 1–3 cm in size <u>Diff. Dx.:</u> • pancreatic tail pathology • left adrenal pathology • pathology of upper pole of left kidney <u>2. ASPLENIA</u> • rare, congenital absence of spleen • associated with congenital heart defects and situs inversus • hyposplenia is a more common finding <u>3. POLYSPLENIA</u> • rare, multiple retrogastric spleens • associated with biliary atresia and interruption of IVC with azygous vein continuation <u>4. WANDERING (FLOATING, ABERRANT) SPLEEN</u> • rare developmental anomaly due to a long mesentery • spleen moves around within abdominal cavity • may undergo torsion	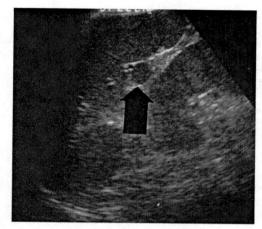 Accessory spleen in region of hilum of spleen (arrow) 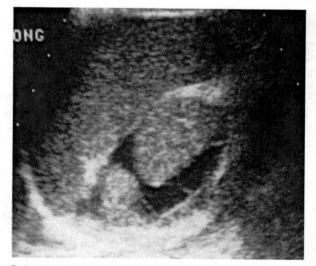 Polysplenia 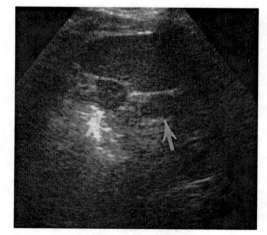 Two accessory spleens (arrows)

ANOMALY	US APPEARANCE

CYSTS
- uncommon

1. NONPARASITIC
i) True (Primary)
- Epidermoid
- epithelial-lined cysts are rare and are probably congenital
- occasional calcified wall
- commonly presents in young patients with LUQ pain
- large, solitary lesion
- Adult polycystic (kidney) disease
- congenital
  cystic lymphangiomas
  cavernous hemangiomas
  dermoid cysts

ii) False (Secondary)
- 80% of nonparasitic splenic cysts result from trauma
- represent hematomas that evolved into seromas
- lack a true epithelial wall
- more likely than epidermoid to have wall calcification

US
- hypoechoic or anechoic foci with well defined walls
- increased through transmission

2. PARASITIC (hydatid disease)
- echinococcus is only parasite that forms splenic cysts

US
- cystic lesions with internal septations and debris
- calcifications which are prominent within the wall

3. PANCREATIC PSEUDOCYSTS
- may occur within or adjacent to the spleen

Diff. Dx.:
Abscess—US appearance could simulate a cyst

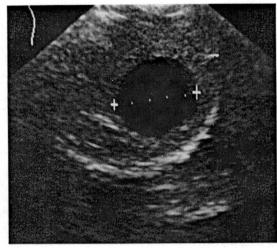

Moderate size splenic cyst (calipers)

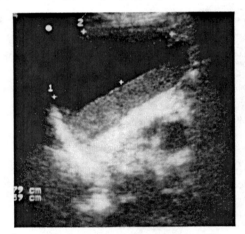

Large splenic cyst secondary to pancreatitis (pancreatic pseudocyst)

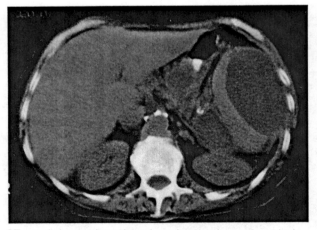

CT correlation to above (note hypodense subcapsular splenic cystic lesion)

ANOMALY	US APPEARANCE
GRANULOMATOUS DISEASE • may be secondary to acute or chronic inflammation that causes reactive hyperplasia **SS** • asymptomatic **US** • diffuse, multiple small echogenic calcifications in spleen (can have a single focus) representing calcified granulomas (e.g., old TB or histoplasmosis) • may or may not have acoustic shadowing	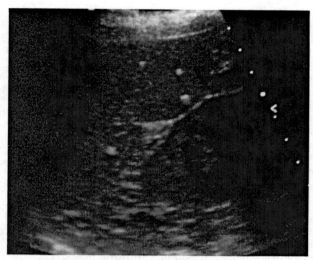 Focal small hyperechoic areas representing old granulomatous disease

ANOMALY	US APPEARANCE

INFARCT
• relatively common, may be large or small, multiple or single, and sometimes involve the entire organ
• occurs secondary to occlusion of splenic artery or any of its branches
• usually caused by cardiac emboli
• splenomegaly can predispose
• Etiology:
  subacute bacterial endocarditis (SBE)
  sickle cell anemia
  neoplastic or inflammatory/infectious involvement of splenic vessels
  hypotension
  pancreatitis
 	
SS
• LUQ pain
 	
US
• usually present as well defined wedge-shaped lesion with base toward subcapsular region (does not necessarily have to be wedge shaped)
• sonographic appearance varies according to time since onset
  early: hypoechoic mass
  later: hyperechoic due to fibrotic changes
	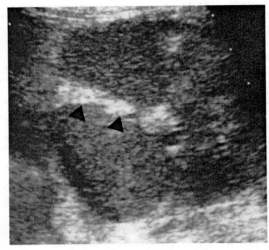
	Echogenic wedge-shaped area (arrows) representing an old splenic infarct

INFECTION/INFLAMMATORY PROCESS
1. ABSCESS
• uncommon
• high mortality
 	
SS
• pain, fever
• leukocystosis
 	
US
• ill-defined, irregular shape with thick and/or shaggy walls
• primarily hypoechoic but often containing echogenic foci (gas/debris)
• can occasionally have fluid–fluid level
• no increase through transmission
 	
2. AIDS
• splenomegaly and nonspecific lymphadenopathy may occur
• focal splenic lesions may be secondary to:
  pneumocystis
  atypical mycobacterium
  candida
  Kaposi's or lymphoma
 	
3. FUNGAL INFECTION
 	
4. TUBERCULOSIS
 	
Diff. Dx.:
• hematoma
• neoplasm
	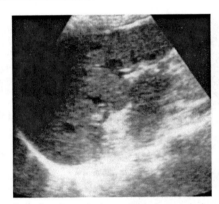
	Splenic tuberculosis: multiple hypoechoic lesions dispersed throughout spleen
	
	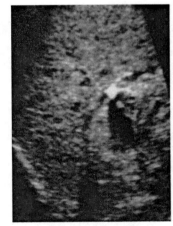
	Hypoechoic target lesions with central echogenic core in keeping with candida infection

ANOMALY	US APPEARANCE

LYMPHADENOPATHY
• can occur with infection/inflammation and malignancy

US

1. "sandwich sign"
• anterior and posterior node masses surround mesenteric vessels
• anterior displacement of aorta
2. "silhouette sign"
• organ compression or obscuration of outlines of paraortic structures

<u>General lymphadenopathy</u>
• solid, homogenous structures that generate low levels of internal echos usually hypoechoic
• large necrotic nodes can have inhomogeneous areas
• associated with acoustic enhancement

<u>Retroperitoneal lymphadenopathy</u>
• several nodes that have matted together can appear as lobular, smooth, or scalloped
• can obscure anterior margin of IVC and aorta
• testicular tumors commonly metastasize to retroperitoneal nodes

<u>Diff. Dx.:</u>
• retroperitoneal fibrosis
• abscess (especially psoas muscle)
• hematoma

<u>Mesenteric/omental nodes</u>
• multiple cystic or separated solid masses
• enlarged nodes can appear as a uniformly thick hypoechoic band-shaped structure when it occurs in the greater omentum

<u>Diff. Dx.:</u>
• abscess
• pancreatic pseudocyst
• fluid-filled loop of bowel
• hematoma

<u>SONOGRAPHIC DIFFERENTIAL FOR ADENOPATHY</u>
• lymphoma nodes—sonolucent
• metastatic disease nodes—complex
• posttherapy nodes—echogenic

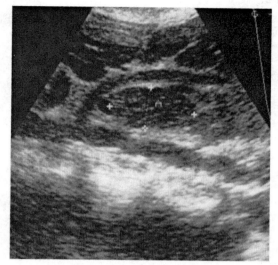

Lobulated hypoechoic solid nodule anterior to aorta

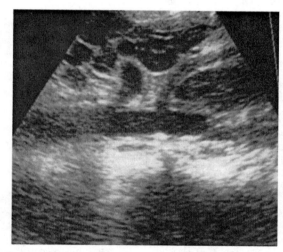

Lobulated solid nodules adjacent to aorta mainly around celiac axis

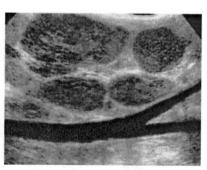

Coronal view of aorta with adjacent enlarged lymph nodes (Courtesy of Siemens SieScape)

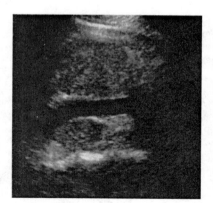

Longitudinal aorta with mass surrounding aorta in patient with primary testicular carcinoma

ANOMALY	US APPEARANCE

NEOPLASMS
- neoplastic involvement of spleen is rare except in lymphohematopoietic system tumors

BENIGN NEOPLASMS

1. CAVERNOUS HEMANGIOMA
- most common primary tumor of spleen
- some are better classified as hamartomas rather than as neoplasms

2. CYSTIC LYMPHANGIOMA
- second most common benign tumor

3. OTHER TYPES OF BENIGN SPLENIC TUMORS
- fibromas, osteomas, chondromas

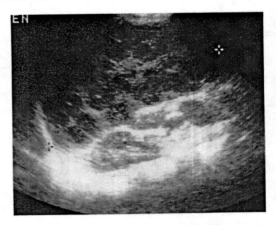

MALIGNANT NEOPLASMS

1. HEMANGIOSARCOMA
- primary malignancy that arises from the capsule
- rare
- usually metastasizes to liver

US
- inhomogeneous lesions

2. METASTASES
- uncommon to have spread to spleen
- most common primaries to spread to lymph and spleen are melanoma (most common), breast, lung, ovary, uterus, stomach, prostate

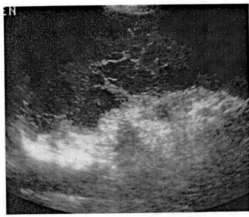

US
- focal hypoechoic (usually) or hyperechoic mass

LYMPHOMA
- primary malignancy that arises from lymphoid tissue
- most common splenic malignancy
- splenomegaly may occur
- solitary or multiple solid masses of varying size may occur within spleen

Lymphoma: enlarged spleen with multiple solid hypoechoic densities

1. BURKITT'S LYMPHOMA
- masses (pelvis, abdomen, and retroperitoneal locations) tend to be large and solitary
- increased incidence of ileocecal, mesenteric, or ovarian involvement
- well defined homogeneous masses that can appear hypo- or hyperechoic

2. HODGKIN'S (40%)
- generalized lymph node enlargement
- more common in males
- occurs between ages of 15–34 or after age 50
- 4% have mesenteric nodal involvement, 25% have para-aortic nodal involvement
- may involve spleen and not be detected by any imaging technique

3. NONHODGKIN'S (60%)
- majority of lymphomas
- occurs in all age groups with incidence increasing with age
- 50% have mesenteric disease and para-aortic nodal involvement

US
- Spleen
- spleen usually has a normal appearance although can be enlarged and can appear diffusely hypoechoic or show focal hypoechoic nodules (focal echogenic areas are rare)
- Renal lymphoma
  –appears as a diffusely enlarged kidney with an echo-poor cortex
- Hepatic lymphoma
  –multiple hypoechoic nodules
- Gastric lymphoma
  –thickened stomach wall

ANOMALY	US APPEARANCE

SPLENOMEGALY
• most common spleen abnormality
• enlarged if weight > 200 g, size > 14 cm in any dimension
• causes include:
  infections (e.g., CMV, hepatitis)
  congestive states (e.g., portal hypertension, heart failure)
  blood/lymphohematogenous disorders (e.g., Hodgkin's disease, lymphoma)
• immunologic and inflammatory (e.g., lupus)
• storage disease (e.g., Gaucher's disease)
• neoplasm (leukemia)
 	
SS
• palpable spleen
• discomfort after eating due to impingement on stomach
 	
US
• size > 14 cm in any dimension (see specific causes)
	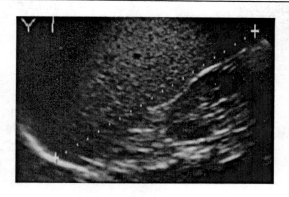

TRAUMA/RUPTURE OF SPLEEN
• most commonly involved organ in upper abdominal trauma
• different appearances and location depending on where trauma occurred
• spontaneous rupture can occur in certain disease states when spleen is enlarged and fragile
• three main types of lacerations:
  1. subcapsular
  2. intraparenchymal
  3. capsular
 	
SS
• LUQ pain, left shoulder pain, left flank pain, hypotension
• ↓ hematocrit
 	
US
• free intraperitoneal fluid (blood) secondary to capsular tear
• variable appearance depending on age of injury:
• Early
  inhomogenous and hypoechoic
• With clot formation
  more echogenic and isoechoic to splenic parenchyma
• Subcapsular hematomas:
  peripheral hypoechoic lens-shaped mass that displaces the splenic parenchyma inward and the capsule outward
	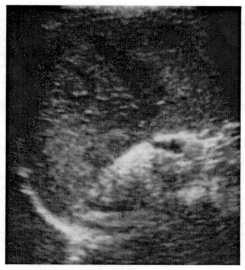
	Splenic injury: irregular area of mixed echogenicity representing splenic hematoma/contusion
	
	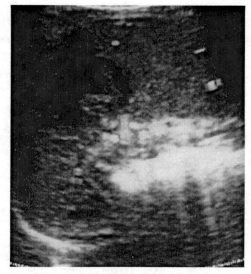
	Splenic injury: absence of flow within affected area

DIFFERENTIAL OF SONOGRAPHIC APPEARANCES OF SPLEEN

DIFFUSE	DECREASED ECHOGENICITY lymphoma granulomatous disease congestion (cirrhosis) malignancy disorders		CALCIFICATIONS TB, histoplasmosis splenic artery atherosclerosis post-traumatic cyst	
FOCAL	ANECHOIC-HYPOECHOIC lymphoma metastases infarct abscess splenic cysts		ECHOGENIC metastases hemangiosarcoma (mixed) hemangioma granulomatous disease	
ENLARGED	COMMON		UNCOMMON (many)	
	lymphoma portal hypertension mononucleosis leukemia		AIDS metastases Gaucher's disease multiple myeloma lupus	glycogen storage disease malaria hepatitis sickle cell disease TB

SPLENIC RELATIONSHIPS AND ASSOCIATED PATHOLOGY

ORGAN	RELATIONSHIP	CAN RESULT IN
PANCREAS	• splenorenal ligament attaches pancreatic tail to spleen's visceral layer	• exudation from pancreas can track along this ligament to produce perisplenic or intrasplenic fluid accumulation
LEFT KIDNEY	• upper pole of left kidney is adjacent to splenic hilum and medial surface of spleen • splenorenal ligament attaches left kidney perirenal space and visceral surface of spleen	• peripheral renal cyst may indent spleen
LEFT ADRENAL	• sits on top of left kidney; therefore, adjacent to spleen	• if enlarges can compress spleen, but hemorrhage of adrenal usually confined to perirenal space

F) TECHNICAL FACTORS

TRANSDUCER	3.5 or 5 MHz
PATIENT PREP	• none required • usually performed as part of abdominal US examination when patinet is NPO for 6–8 hours
TECHNIQUE	• start by having patient on the right side and gradually turn supine • spleen can also be imaged prone • transducer is placed near the left midaxillary line, either beneath or between the ribs • a high posterolateral approach is necessary to visualize spleen • deep inspiration is required Transverse: • scan far to the left posterior aspect as possible angling anteromedially Longitudinal: • pivot transducer 90 degrees to transverse scan plane
SCAN PLANES	• coronal plane with left lateral approach Longitudinal plane: • long axis of spleen with transducer perpendicular Transverse plane: • still in coronal scan plane rotate the transducer 90 degrees in to the transverse scan plane from the longitudinal plane
HELPFUL HINTS	• use patient's respiration to assist in visualization of spleen • if left kidney is easily visualized, check for an enlarged spleen that extends below kidney (normal spleen rarely extends that far)

CHAPTER 14 - URINARY BLADDER AND URETERS
A) NORMAL ANATOMY AND SONOGRAPHIC APPEARANCE

DEFINITION	BLADDER: • an extraperitoneal muscular, membranous distensible reservoir for urine excreted by kidneys and transported to bladder by the ureters • discharges urine through the urethra URETERS: • about 12-in. long narrow muscular tubes that transport urine from kidneys to bladder

STRUCTURE

BLADDER

1. APEX
• above neck
• most anterior, superior part
• medial umbilical ligament attaches

2. NECK
• lowers part, fixed behind symphysis pubis

3. BASE/FUNDUS OR POSTERIOR SURFACE (TRIGONE)
• triangular area between the insertion of the ureters and the urethra
• points anteriorly
• faces down and backward
• urethra (bladder neck) opens in apex of trigone
• ureters drain at superolateral angle at 2 points in base of trigone

4. URACHUS
• embryologic remnant that forms the middle umbilical ligament of the bladder
• if patent it creates an umbilical urinary fistula

5. URETHRA
• fibroelastic tube exiting trigone of bladder
• Male—conducts urine, spermatozoa, and various glandular secretions
  divided into three parts:
a) Prostatic
b) Membranous (through urogenital diaphragm)
c) Spongy (penile)
• Female—shorter in length (results in increased bladder infections in women)

6. URETER
• tube that carries urine from kidney to bladder
• 3 natural constrictions at levels of:
a) UPJ—hilum of kidney
b) Pelvic rim
c) Entrance (orifice) to posterior/lateral bladder wall

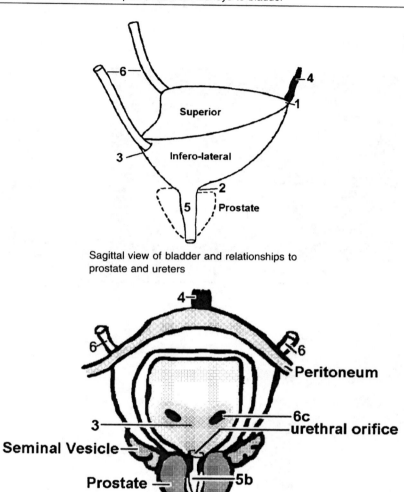

Sagittal view of bladder and relationships to prostate and ureters

Coronal view through bladder with relationships to prostate and ureters

BLADDER WALL

LAYERS

a) Mucosa
- innermost coat of epithelium containing rugae

b) Submucosa
- connective tissue adjoining the mucosa and muscular layers

c) Detrusor muscle
- 3 layers of muscle
- forms internal sphincter muscle around opening to urethra

d) Serosa
- outermost layer formed by peritoneum and covers only superior surface of bladder

DIMENSIONS

Distended = 3 mm
Nondistended = 6 mm

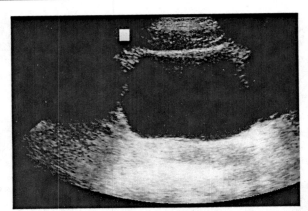

Distended bladder with normal wall size

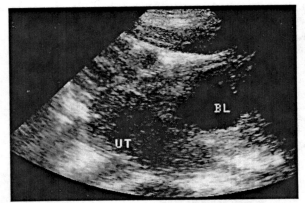

Nondistended bladder—cannot accurately measure wall

US APPEARANCE

BLADDER

- can only be examined sonographically when distended
- appears as an anechoic structure with smooth curved surface surrounded by a thin echogenic interface that represents the bladder wall
- anterior wall can be obscured owing to reverberation

Transverse plane: spherical, symmetrical appearance

Longitudinal plane: elliptical appearance

URETERS

- not normally visualized on US unless dilated

Ureteral jets:
- 1–3-second stream of urine visualized entering the bladder from the ureter
- when seen indicates ureteric flow is present

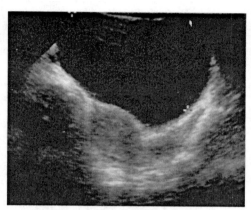

Longitudinal bladder with calipers placed for measuring bladder volume

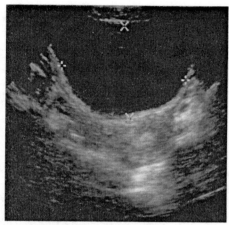

Transverse bladder: calipers measuring AP and TR dimensions

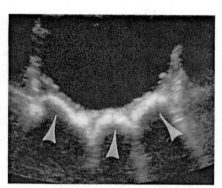

Transverse bladder: stool in colon can simulate pelvis mass (arrows)

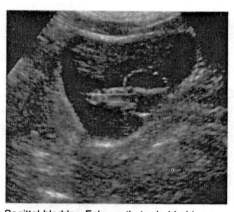

Sagittal bladder: Foley catheter in bladder

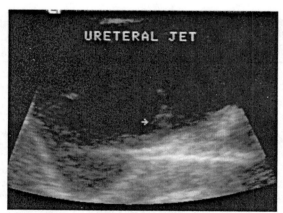

Urinary jets are seen as jets of low-intensity echos (arrow) enter bladder

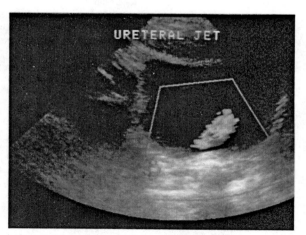

Left ureteral jet demonstrated with color Doppler

255

	BLADDER	URETERS
SIZE AND SHAPE	• both depend on urine volume Maximum Adult Volume: Volume = trans.×AP×L Postvoid residual of < 100 cc is not usually clinically significant	• 28–34 cm long • right usually shorter than left • diameter varies from 1–10 mm • > 8 mm is considered dilated
LOCATION	• pelvic cavity posterior to symphysis pubis • freely movable held in position by folds of peritoneum • extends upward and forward into abdominal cavity when distended	• originate in pelvis of kidney • enter pelvis and cross anterior to either the common iliac or external artery • terminate in base of bladder • retroperitoneal

REGIONAL ANATOMY OF BLADDER

	MALE	FEMALE
ANTERIOR	• pubis symphysis • abdominal wall • space of Retzius retropubic space filled with fat between the anteroinferior surface of bladder base and pubic bone	
POSTERIOR	• retrovesical pouch (peritoneal reflexion from the upper bladder to the rectum) • seminal vesicles • rectum	• uterus • cervix • vagina • rectum
SUPERIOR	• peritoneum • small intestine • sigmoid colon	• uterus • peritoneum • small intestine • sigmoid colon
INFERIOR	• levator ani muscle • urogenital diaphragm	• levator ani muscle • urogenital diaphragm

B) PHYSIOLOGY

	BLADDER	URETERS
FUNCTION	• reservoir for urine	• one-way conduits for urine from kidneys to bladder (retrograde can occur abnormally)
OPERATION	• an average of 1.2–1.5 L (40–50 oz) is voided per day • amount depends on quantity of fluid ingested and lost (kidney function, sweating, gastrointestinal factors, respiration) • retention controlled by sphincter muscles • due to its abdominal location in a child, the abdominal muscles play an important role in voiding in children	• muscles within ureters pass urine from kidney to the bladder by peristalsis

ANOMALIES OF BLADDER

ANOMALY	US APPEARANCE
CALCULI	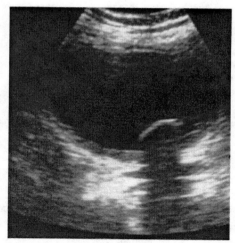
• develop from:	

CALCULI

• develop from:
  upper urinary tract and pass into bladder
  prolonged use of catheter (debris from catheter falls off and forms nidus for stone)
• any cause of bladder status such as outflow obstruction (e.g., enlarged prostate), neurogenic bladder, or tumor
• US may detect calculi that do not show on an IVP due to their density, because they are concealed by gas or feces, or they are mistaken as phleboliths

SS
• usually asymptomatic unless they obstruct bladder neck

US
• echodense structures producing acoustic shadow
• does not need to be calcified to be seen sonographically
• movement of calculi can be demonstrated by changing the patient's position

Diff. Dx.:
• blood clot (can occasionally see fluid–fluid level associated with this)

Bladder stone with shadow

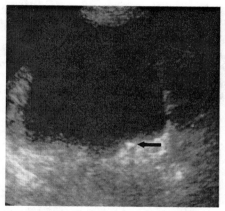

Transverse scan plane: UVJ stone with shadow (arrow)

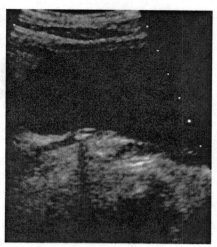

Longitudinal scan plane: UVJ stone at the UVJ (arrow)

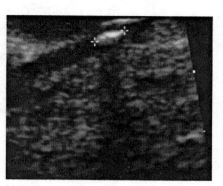

Magnified image of 5.5-mm stone within ureter

ANOMALY	US APPEARANCE

CYSTITIS

- infection or inflammation of the bladder
- secondary to diverticuli, obstruction fistulas, cystoceles, bladder neoplasms, kidney infections, neurogenic dysfunction
- more common in females where it is caused by ascent of bacteria in shortened urethra, pregnancy, coital trauma
- in males usually associated with prostatic disease

SS
- frequency, dysuria (burning during urination), lower abdominal pain over bladder region
- can experience nocturia, hematuria

US
- chronic cystitis may cause localized or general thickening of the bladder wall, pus–urine fluid level

Other types of cystitis include:

1. EMPHYSEMATOUS CYSTITIS
- seen in diabetics

US
- gas within bladder wall (usually secondary to *Escherichia coli* infection)

2. HEMORRHAGIC CYSTITIS
- secondary to chemotherapy

US
- bladder wall thickening with or without calcification
- echos seen within bladder secondary to blood

3. SCHISTOSOMIASIS INFECTION
- secondary to *Schistosoma haematobium* parasitic infection
- can lead to squamous cell carcinoma of the bladder

US
- bladder wall thickening with or without calcification

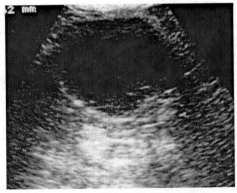

Transverse scan through bladder, showing nonspecific bladder wall thickening. Differential would include infection, inflammation, neoplasm.

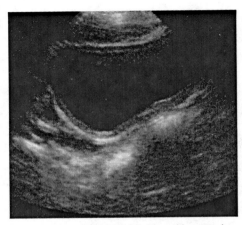

Transverse scan through bladder with posterior wall thickening: chronic cystitis

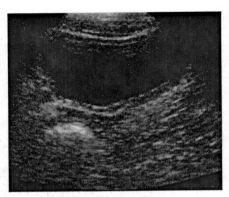

Longitudinal scan through bladder with chronic inflammation

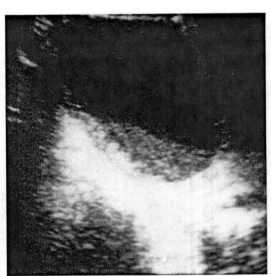

Bladder with fluid–fluid level in patient with hemorrhagic cystitis

ANOMALY	US APPEARANCE
DIVERTICULI • pouch-like evaginations of bladder wall • secondary to cystitis, bladder neck obstruction or can be congenital • region of urinary stasis and can become infected • can be as large as bladder; locate neck of bladder to identify SS • usually none specific to diverticuli • can be a site of urinary stasis that tends to become infected US • cystic buds with small necks that appear as pedunculated extensions to the bladder • enlarge as the bladder contracts, but disappear when bladder is empty • varying size and can be multiple • mostly seen in lateral bladder wall	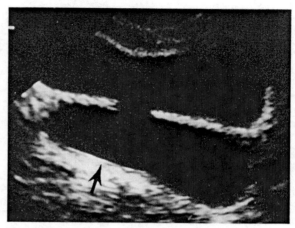 Sagittal bladder: large diverticulum (arrow) 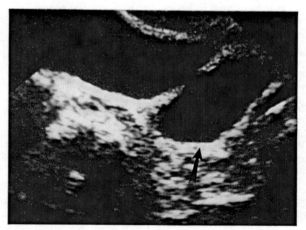 Transverse bladder: large diverticulum (arrow)

ANOMALY	US APPEARANCE

NEOPLASMS

1. PAPILLOMA
- rare benign tumor
- commonly occurs along lateral wall
- attached to wall by stalk and generally do not deform the bladder wall
- usually small (0.5–2 cm) in size

2. SQUAMOUS CELL
- 5% of malignant primary tumors
- occur primarily in men over the age of 50
- secondary to schistosomiasis infection, stones
- can be invasive, fungating tumors or infiltrative
- not papillary in nature but difficult to distinguish from TCC on US

3. TRANSITIONAL CELL CARCINOMA (TCC)
- 90%–95% of malignant primary tumors
- arises from transitional epithelium that lines the renal pelvis, ureter, and bladder
- occurs more frequently in men after the age of 50
- most common site is the bladder
- tend to be multiple

SS
- gross, painless hematuria with blood clots

4. METASTASES
- usually develop from:
  direct spread from kidneys, cervix, uterus, prostate, rectum
  lymphatic spread
  hematogenous spread

US
- focal thickening of bladder wall
- small to large, solid masses projecting from bladder wall
- are generally hypoechoic in nature but more echogenic than bladder wall
- malignant tumors may invade the wall, which obscures the echogenic outline of the bladder wall
- tumors on anterior wall are difficult to image due to focal zone and reverberation artifact

Diff. Dx.:
- focal thickening of wall (cystitis, trabeculae)
- blood clots
- BPH, prostatic carcinoma
- endometriosis

Helpful Hint:
- anomaly should be evident in 2 planes to avoid mistaking as artifact
- benign wall thickening usually does not project into bladder
- blood clots usually move with change in patient position, whereas neoplasms will stay fixed when patient changes position
- BPH is usually in a central inferior position

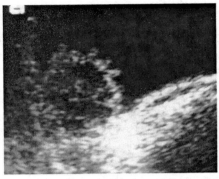

Magnified image of papillary tumor in bladder

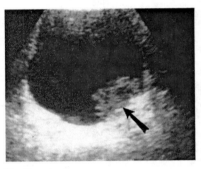

Papillary tumor

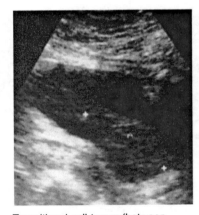

Transitional cell tumor (between calipers)

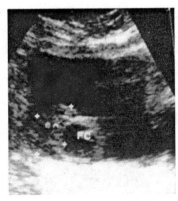

Clot (calipers) adjacent to Foley catheter (FC) should not be mistaken for neoplastic disease

ANOMALY	US APPEARANCE
OUTLET (BLADDER NECK) OBSTRUCTION • most commonly seen as secondary to: 1. BPH or Prostatic Carcinoma • wall thickening with trabeculation 2. Chronic Cystitis • chronic obstruction causes bladder wall thickening and trabeculation 3. Neurogenic (Atonic) Bladder • any dysfunction of the urinary bladder from CNS system disruption • subject to bladder calculi 4. Posterior Urethral Valves (PUV) • the most common cause of outlet obstruction in the male fetus and infant • congenital anomaly of a bladder outlet obstruction in male fetus • formation of rudimentary valves (membranous flaps) in region of posterior urethra • oligohydramnios in fetus 5. Ectopic Ureteroceles • medial and inferior to normal ureteral insertion site 6. Tumors • prostatic, TCC US • distended bladder • bilateral hydroureter and hydronephrosis • associated with diverticulum	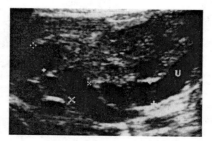 Fetal kidney shows a dilated ureter (U) and gross hydronephrosis (**) 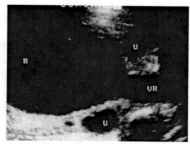 Coronal scan of a male fetus shows a dilated urinary bladder (B) with a thickened wall and a dilated posterior urethra (UR) giving a "key hole" appearance; both dilated ureters (U) are seen in cross section adjacent to the bladder (**)

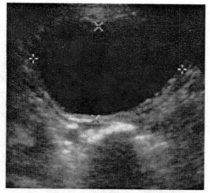

Significant postvoid residue in patient with BPH

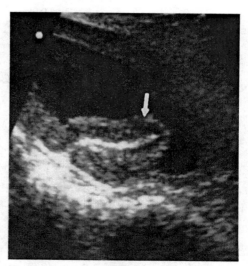

Neurogenic bladder with fold (arrow)

DIFFERENTIAL OF BLADDER ANOMALIES

THICKENED BLADDER WALL	• cystitis • neurogenic bladder • tumor (TCC) • adherent blood clot
ECHOGENIC FOCI	• catheters (echogenic circular [transverse scan plane] or linear [sagittal scan plane] artifact with balloon appearing as lucent mass) or other foreign bodies • blood clot • calculi • tumor • fungus ball

BLADDER VOLUME	DECREASED	INCREASED
	• large fixed pelvic masses • chronic infection • urinary and pelvic inflammatory disease • patients undergoing radiation therapy	• bladder neck obstructions (enlarged prostatic) • atonic bladder

LARGE POSTVOID RESIDUAL VOLUMES	• atonic bladders • bladder neck obstruction • long-standing cystitis • BPH • bladder tumor
TWO CYSTIC STRUCTURES IN PELVIS	• duplication very rare two separate bladders separated by peritoneum with each bladder receiving the ipsilateral ureter and each with its own separate urethra check uterus and GI tract • diverticulum • ovarian neoplasm • dilated ureter • ureterocele • pregnancy • uterine pathology • fluid collection (i.e., hematoma, seroma, ascites)
INTRALUMINAL MASS (FILLING DEFECTS)	• blood clot • benign polyp • calculi • malignant tumor (bladder or extension of prostate cancer)—fold/trabeculation • fungus ball • BPH

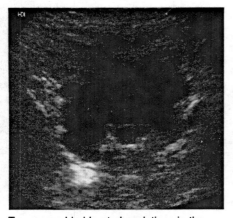

Transverse bladder: trabeculations in the bladder wall

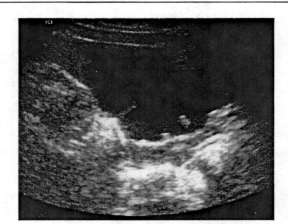

Sagittal bladder: trabeculations in the longitudinal scan plane

ANOMALIES OF URETERS

ANOMALY	US APPEARANCE

CONGENITAL ANOMALIES

1. BIFID/DUPLICATED URETERS
- associated with double collecting system
- embryologically 2 buds develop or one bud splits
- commonly joined within bladder producing a single ureteral orifice or joined midway to create a Y-shaped ureter

Upper pole ureter:
- ureters draining upper poles of kidney enter bladder medial and inferior to other ureter and obstructs (ectopic ureter)
- can be associated with ureteroceles
- in females (more common) can insert in trigone, urethra, perineum, uterus, vagina
- in males can insert in posterior urethra, seminal vesicle

Lower pole ureter:
- ureter draining the lower pole enters the bladder at the trigone region and can reflux

2. GARTNER'S DUCT—PARAOVARIAN CYSTS (females)
- results from incomplete obliteration of the atrophic mesonephric duct

SS
- none
- pain, swelling, dyspareunia

US
- cyst lying along anterolateral wall of vagina

3. SEMINAL VESICLE CYST (males)
- uncommon
- result from:
  incomplete absorption of mesonephric duct with ureter attached to side of seminal vesicle
- atresia of the ejaculatory duct creating a cyst
- usually presents in 20s or 30s

SS
- dysuria, pelvic pain, ejaculatory disturbances

US
- thin-walled cystic structure within seminal vesicle
- can be large

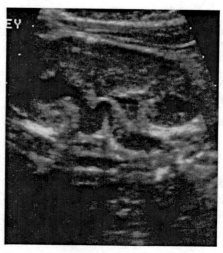

Hydronephrosis and hydroureter caused by obstruction of upper collecting system

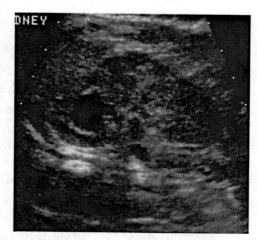

Hydronephrosis of upper pole in duplex system

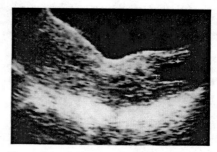

Transabdominal scan of uterus with a Gartner's duct cyst along the wall of the vagina (calipers)

ANOMALY	US APPEARANCE

HYDRO/MEGALOURETER

- large ureters
- associated with:
- congenital abnormalities such as
  - posterior urethral valves
  - urethral atresia, stricture
  - cloacal persistence
  - ureterocele
  - caudal regression anomaly
  - megacystis—internal hypoperistalsis syndrome
- obstruction of urine flow in ureter will have an enlarged ureter proximal to site of obstruction

US

- large anechoic tubular structure (with no vascular flow) descending from kidney to bladder
- usually is obscured in its midportion by bowel gas

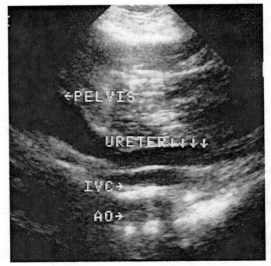

Right coronal longitudinal scan showing enlarged ureter (arrows)

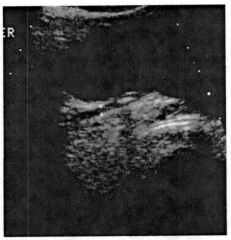

Longitudinal scan through lower ureter near UVJ junction: dilated ureter (between calipers) with stone

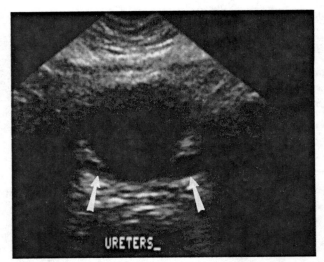

Transverse bladder through level of UVJ showing dilated ureters (arrows)

ANOMALY	US APPEARANCE
URETEROCELE • a cystic dilatation of the distal ureter into the bladder • can be associated with duplication of the renal collecting system • can be ectopic (ureter inserts into bladder in abnormal location) • chronic urinary stasis in dilated portion can lead to infection • may cause significant obstruction of ipsilateral ureter • a simple ureterocele is asymptotic and does not produce hydronephrosis US • thin-walled cyst is present at the site of entry of a (duplicated) ureter into the bladder • cystic lesion in bladder near UVJ • bladder wall may be thickened	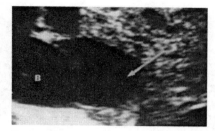 Sagittal scan of the urinary bladder shows an associated thin-walled cyst (arrow) that represents the site of entry of a dilated duplicated ureter 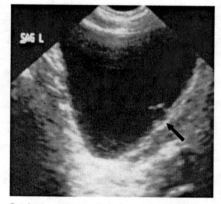 Sagittal scan: small ureterocele (arrow) 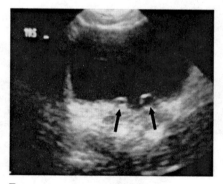 Transverse scan: small bilateral ureteroceles (arrows)

D) TECHNICAL FACTORS

TECHNIQUE	• patient in supine position with full bladder
	• in the suprapubic location angle scan:
	  Transverse scan plane: angle caudad and cephalad
	  Longitudinal scan plane: angle laterally out to iliac vessels

TRANSDUCER FREQUENCY	• prefer 5 MHz, or as high as possible
HELPFUL HINT	adjust TGC gains so that anterior surface of bladder is not lost in reverberation artifact

CHAPTER 15 - VASCULAR SYSTEM

A) NORMAL ANATOMY AND SONOGRAPHIC APPEARANCE

ANATOMY	
ARTERIES	**VEINS**

ARTERIES

- vessels that carry blood away from the heart to the tissues
- large are elastic, medium are muscular, small are arterioles

1. WALL
- 3 layers of tunica

a) Tunica interna (intima)
- inner layer composed of thin endothelium cells resting on connective tissue
- endothelial cells give the artery a smooth surface to aid blood flow

b) Tunica media
- thickest layer, but thickness varies depending on artery's function
- consists of elastic fibers (large arteries) with some smooth muscle (mainly medium-sized arteries) surrounded by fibrous tissue
- lumen size is regulated through smooth muscle cell contraction or relaxation

c) Tunica externa (adventitia)
- elastic and collagenous fibers enclosed by a fibrous tissue
- fibers run the length of the vessel
- adds great elasticity to the arteries

2. LUMEN

3. ARTERIOLES
- small arteries that deliver blood flow to capillaries
- as they get smaller in size their walls consist of little more than a layer of endothelium surrounded by a few smooth muscle cells

4. CAPILLARY
- microscopic vessels in tissues
- approximate size of RBC
- connect arterioles and venules and permit exchange of nutrients and wastes between blood and tissue through their walls
- composed of only one-cell thick endothelium tunica intima

VEINS

- convey blood from tissues back to heart
- contain less elastic tissue and smooth muscle in their walls compared to arteries
- many veins contain valves that prevent backflow of blood
- thin walled with lack of support and therefore can be easily compressed and invaded by neoplasms

1. WALL
- have same 3 layers as arteries but have much more fibrous tissue and much less smooth muscle and elastic tissue

a) Tunica interna (intima)
- inner endothelial lining with scant connective tissue
- poor internal elastic membrane

b) Tunica media
- consists of thin layer of smooth muscle surrounded by fibrous tissue

c) Tunica externa (adventitia)
- elastic and collagenous fibers enclosed by a fibrous tissue
- thin layer

5. VENULES
- groups of capillaries unite to form small veins
- collect blood from capillaries and drain it into veins
- important area in local inflammatory process

6. VALVES
- prevent reflux of blood back into dependent portions of the veins
- bicuspid in design
- number of valves increases toward the foot
- usually located immediately below the point of entry of a major tributary

a) Valve cusps

b) Valve sinus
- cephalad and surrounding the valve cusps
- dilatation allows extra space to aid in closure of the valve
- low blood flow at the base of the valve cusps in the sinuses often causes thrombus formation

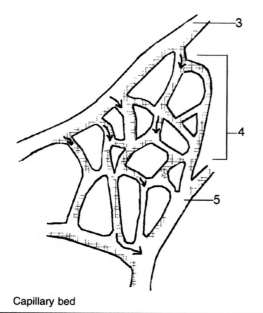

Capillary bed

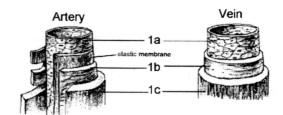

Artery and vein structure

VENOUS VALVE FUNCTION

- venous valves direct flow by keeping the blood moving back toward the heart in both the deep and the superficial veins
- in the perforating veins, the valves direct flow from the superficial to the deep veins
- valves, when functioning normally, prevent reflux of venous blood by trapping blood in their cusps or leaflets as they close
- venous valves open and close in conjunction with the action of the muscles

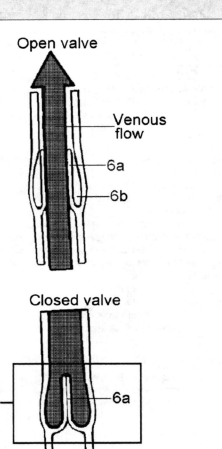

Open valve

Venous flow

6a

6b

Closed valve

6

6a

Valve (6), valve cusp (6a), and valve sinus (6b)

SONOGRAPHIC APPEARANCE

ARTERY	VEIN
• anechoic tubular vessel with medium echo reflections from the walls • occasionally echogenic blood may be seen to course through • noncompressible	• vein increased diameter with Valsalva • vein compressed in response to probe pressure • echo-free lumen with the exception of valve cusps • occasionally echogenic blood may be seen to course through • can be slightly larger in diameter than arterial counterpart

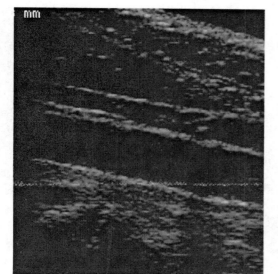

Longitudinal scan plane through carotid artery

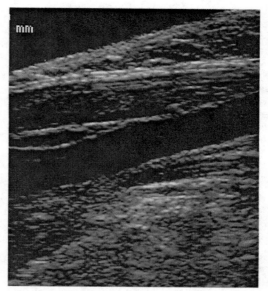

Longitudinal scan plane through jugular vein. Note that the walls are not as echogenic as in the carotid artery.

ANATOMY OF THE LOWER EXTREMITIES

ARTERIAL SYSTEM	VENOUS SYSTEM	
	# of valve	

ARTERIAL SYSTEM

1. COMMON ILIAC
- gives rise to 2 branches: internal and external iliac

2. INTERNAL ILIAC

3. EXTERNAL ILIAC
- continues distally to become common femoral artery
  a) inferior epigastric
  b) Deep iliac circumflex

4. COMMON FEMORAL
  a) Deep (profunda) femoral
- courses posterolaterally
- common collateral route when superficial femoral is obstructed
  b) Superficial femoral
- continues distally until it reaches Hunter's canal where it courses posteromedially behind the knee and becomes the popliteal

5. POPLITEAL
- bifurcates into the anterior tibial and the tibioperoneal trunk

6. CALF ARTERIES
  a) anterior tibial
- courses along anterior surface of interosseous membrane to become the dorsalis pedis artery in the foot
  b) posterior tibial
- direct continuation of popliteal artery
- created by bifurcation of tibioperoneal trunk
- takes an oblique-medial course to end behind the medial malleolus
- branches of this artery supply the foot
  c) peroneal (fibular)
- arises from posterior tibial artery, created by bifurcation of tibioperoneal trunk
- runs laterally ending at the fibula's posteromedial border

7. PLANTAR ARTERIES
Deep plantar branch: from the dorsalis pedis artery
Lateral plantar branch: from the posterior tibial artery
Metatarsal branches: supply the toes

VENOUS SYSTEM

# of valve	
0	**DEEP VEINS** • paired and accompanied by arteries that serve as sonographic landmarks **8. COMMON ILIAC** • empties into the IVC a) Internal iliac
0	b) External iliac
0–1	• joins internal iliac at sacroiliac joint to form common iliac vein
0–1	**9. COMMON FEMORAL** • ascends to groin to form external iliac at level of inguinal ligament
1–4	**10. SUPERFICIAL FEMORAL** • joins deep femoral vein to form common femoral vein
1–2	**11. DEEP FEMORAL (PROFUNDA)**
1–3	**12. POPLITEAL** • courses behind the knee adjacent to the popliteal artery • becomes superficial femoral at adductor canal
9	**13. CALF VEINS** a) anterior tibial • near ankle between shafts of tibia and fibula
9	b) posterior tibial • quite superficial at medial malleolus ankle level • usually paired, can have 3 or 4
7	c) peroneal • lie on lateral side of calf
	14. PLANTAR VEINS • unite to form deep plantar arch, which continues to form the posterior tibial veins
10–20	**SUPERFICIAL VEINS** • no arteries accompany these veins **15. GREATER (LONG) SAPHENOUS** • largest vein in body • often harvested as a graft for arterial reconstruction • originates near medial malleolus and empties into common femoral vein at the saphenofemoral junction; often duplicated • major collateral route
6–12	**16. LESSER (SHORT) SAPHENOUS** • originates posterior to lateral malleolus and empties into popliteal vein • posterior arch vein drains into it
	SINUSOIDS **SOLEAL SINUSOIDS** • drain muscle mass of calf into deep system **GASTROCNEMIAL SINUSOID** • drain gastrocnemius muscle into popliteal vein **COMMUNICATING (PERFORATING) SYSTEM** • connect deep and superficial venous systems • more common in calf • contain valves to direct blood flow to deep system

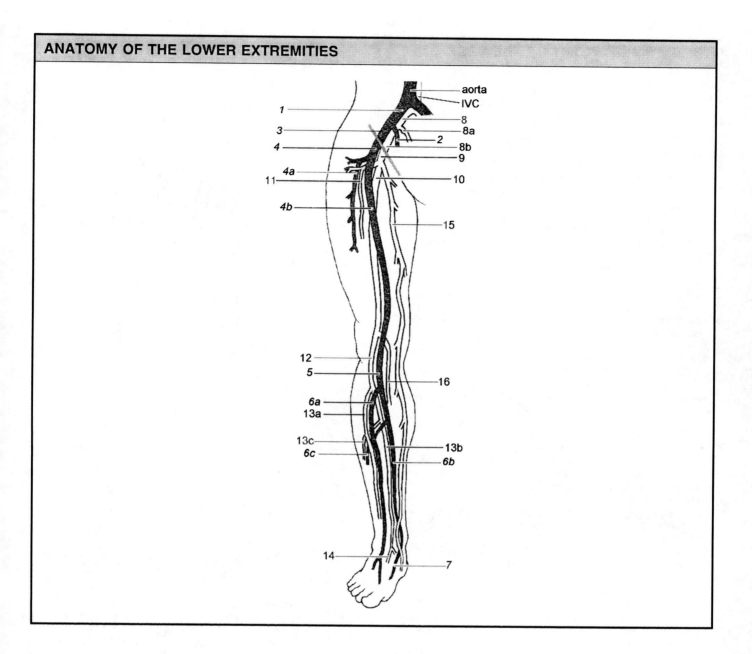

aorta
IVC
1
8
8a
3
2
4
8b
9
4a
10
11
4b
15
12
5
16
6a
13a
13c
6c
13b
6b
14
7

VASCULAR ANATOMY OF THE NECK

1. AORTA
a) Ascending
b) Arch
c) Descending

2. COMMON CAROTID ARTERY (CCA)
• both travel toward branch without branching until they reach level of thyroid
• located medial and deep to internal jugular vein
• bifurcates at 3–4 cervical vertebral body into internal and external branches
a) Right (RCCA)
• originates from brachiocephalic (innominate) artery
• widens into carotid bulb
b) Left (LCCA)
• second major branch off the aortic arch
• can arise from the base of the innominate artery
• arises directly from the transverse portion of the arch
c) Bulb
• expanded portion of CCA before it bifurcates into the ICA and ECA
• common site of plaque and intimal thickening

3. INTERNAL CAROTID ARTERY (ICA)
• supplies anterior circulation to brain
• no extracranial branches
• **larger** and more lateral branch of CCA in a transverse scan plane
• orientated posteriorly, toward the mastoid process

4. EXTERNAL CAROTID ARTERY (ECA)
• supplies neck, scalp and face with blood
• the **smaller** and more medial branch of CCA in a transverse scan plane
• oriented more anteriorly, toward face (medially) than the internal
• has several branches in neck:
  superior thyroid artery
  • identifying this branch soon after the bifurcation is an important means of differentiating the ECA from the ICA facial artery

5. VERTEBRAL ARTERIES
• originate from proximal subclavian arteries
• ascend superiorly and posteriorly and travel through transverse processes of cervical spine toward base of skull
• unite at base of brain to form basilar artery and the posterior circulation to brain
• collateral route for subclavian or innominate artery occlusion
• variable size, often very tortuous at its proximal end
• left is usually larger and may arise directly from arch in small population

6. SUPERIOR VENA CAVA

7. JUGULAR VEIN
a) Internal
• larger than and medial to external jugular
• anterior and lateral to CCA
b) External
• lies in more superficial position, lateral to internal jugular vein and carotid artery
• lies along posterior border of sternomastoid muscle
c) Anterior

8. THYROID ARTERIES
a) Inferior
b) Middle

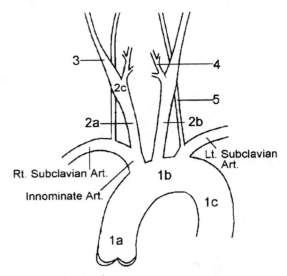

Arterial arch vessels

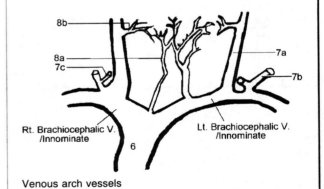

Venous arch vessels

ANATOMY OF UPPER EXTREMITIES

ARTERIES

1. BRACHIOCEPHALIC (INNOMINATE ARTERY)
• first great vessel off aortic arch
• branches into the subclavian artery and right common carotid artery

2. SUBCLAVIAN ARTERY
a) Left
• arises from transverse portion of arch
b) Right
• arises from innominate/brachiocephalic

3. AXILLARY ARTERY
• courses along the inner aspect of the arm
• bifurcates into brachial and deep brachial arteries

4. BRACHIAL ARTERY
• branches below the elbow into the radial, ulnar, and interosseous
a) Deep brachial
• largest branch of brachial

5. RADIAL (a) and ULNAR (b) ARTERIES
• supply hand

6. COMMON INTEROSSEOUS ARTERY

DEEP VEINS
• all deep veins travel with their respective arteries
7. BRACHIOCEPHALIC (INNOMINATE) VEIN
• formed by internal jugular and subclavian veins
• drain into the superior vena cava

8. SUBCLAVIAN VEIN
• is found above sternoclavicular joint and lateral aspect is below clavicle
• middle portion not visualized due to overlying clavicle
• patency can be checked through this area using augmentation
• lateral portion is imaged below the clavicle

9. AXILLARY VEIN
• becomes subclavian vein after takeoff of cephalic vein at outer border of 1st rib
• formed by brachial vein (deep) and basilic vein (superficial)
• requires arm raised and resting on table with palm face up exposing axilla

10. BRACHIAL VEIN
• ascends to form axillary vein at lower border of teres major muscle in upper arm
• may split into 2 separate trunks

11. RADIAL (a) and ULNAR (b) VEINS
• paired
• receive blood from deep and superficial arches of hand
• join to form brachial veins in proximal forearm

SUPERFICIAL VEINS
• not accompanied by arteries
12. CEPHALIC VEIN
• runs along lateral forearm and empties into axillary vein
• last vein to join the axillary vein before it becomes the subclavian vein at the level of the shoulder

13. BASILIC VEIN
• runs along medial arm and joins brachial vein to form axillary vein
a) Median basilic vein

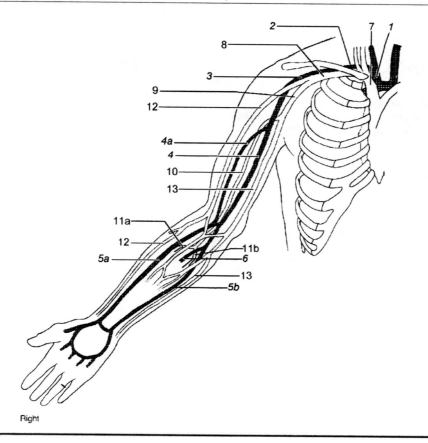

Right

PRINCIPAL RETROPERITONEAL VASCULATURE

ARTERIAL

1. AORTA
- anterior to spine and left of midline
- becomes more anterior as it descends into abdomen

2. CELIAC ARTERY (AXIS/TRUNK)
- 2–3 cm long
- first major branch of aorta
- arises at a perpendicular angle from the anterior aspect of aorta
- has 3 branches:

a) Common hepatic artery
- gastroduodenal artery branches off this artery and after that point becomes proper hepatic artery **(3)**
- landmark for the anterolateral aspect of the pancreatic head

b) Left gastric artery
- supplies stomach and esophagus

c) Splenic artery
- runs superior to pancreas on its course toward the spleen
- supplies spleen, pancreas, stomach

3. PROPER HEPATIC ARTERY
- enters porta hepatis with portal vein

a) Left, middle, and right hepatic arteries

4. GASTRODUODENAL ARTERY
- branch of common hepatic artery

5. SUPERIOR MESENTERIC ARTERY
- secondary major anterior branch of aorta
- lies posterior to pancreatic neck, then emerges and crosses anterior to the uncinate process
- supplies small bowel, portions of large bowel
- source of collateral circulation to lower extremities

6. RENAL ARTERIES
- arise off lateral aspect of aorta

a) Right renal artery
- only vessel that lies behind IVC

b) Left renal artery

7. INFERIOR MESENTERIC ARTERY (IMA)
- supplies transverse, descending and sigmoid colon and rectum
- arises anteriorly cranial to aortic bifurcation

8. COMMON ILIAC ARTERIES

a) External iliac artery
- supplies lower extremities
- gives off two dorsal branches: inferior epigastric and deep iliac circumflex arteries
- continues to become the common femoral artery

b) Internal iliac artery (hypogastric artery)
- bifurcates into anterior and posterior divisions
- supplies uterus, prostate, muscles of buttocks, urinary bladder

VENOUS

9. COMMON ILIAC VEINS (CIV)
- merge to right of midline to form IVC
- ascending lumbar veins arise from CIVs

a) External iliac vein

b) Internal iliac vein

10. INFERIOR VENA CAVA (IVC)
- courses cranially to right of midline along lumbar vertebral column through diaphragm to enter right atrium
- lies to right of aorta, posterior to pancreatic head
- returns blood from lower extremities and entire abdomen to heart

11. RENAL VEINS
- lie anterior to renal arteries

a) Right renal vein
- short course from right kidney to IVC

b) Left renal vein
- traverses between aorta and SMA to enter IVC

12. HEPATIC VEINS
- enter intrahepatic IVC just beneath diaphragm

a) Right, middle, and left hepatic veins

PORTAL SYSTEM
13. INFERIOR MESENTERIC VEIN

14. SUPERIOR MESENTERIC VEIN
- lies posterior to body and anterior to uncinate process of pancreas

15. PORTAL VEIN
- formed by confluence of superior mesenteric vein and splenic vein in the region of the neck of the pancreas

a) Right portal vein

b) Left portal vein

16. SPLENIC VEIN
- runs posterior to pancreatic body and tail on its course to the spleen
- anterior to the aorta and SMA
- caudad to celiac axis

Principle venous and arterial vasculature

Longitudinal line diagram through proximal aorta and surrounding relationships

Portal circulation line diagram

Relationships of principle vessels to organs

PHYSIOLOGY OF CIRCULATION

BLOOD FLOW REGULATION	Mechanisms that aid in flow 1. BLOOD PRESSURE • blood flows because of different pressures in various parts of the system • flows from high-pressure to low-pressure regions • average pressure in aorta is about 100 mm Hg • continually decreases through arterial and venous system to reach 0 mm Hg in right atrium 2. VEIN DIAMETER • venous vessels are larger in diameter, offering less resistance to flow 3. MUSCLE CONTRACTION • contraction of skeletal muscles around veins helps propel blood toward the heart
BLOOD PRESSURE	• defined as pressure exerted by blood on wall of any blood vessel Factors that affect arterial blood pressure: 1. CARDIAC OUTPUT • amount of blood ejected by left ventricle each minute = stroke volume $\times$ heart rate • blood pressure varies directly with cardiac output 2. BLOOD VOLUME • normal volume is about 5 L • blood pressure varies directly with blood volume 3. PERIPHERAL RESISTANCE • impedance to blood flow by the force of friction between blood and the walls of blood vessels • related to blood viscosity and blood vessel diameter • the smaller the vessel or the more viscous the blood, the higher the resistance then the higher the blood pressure
HEART RATE	• number of times heart contracts per minute • controlled by sympathetic and parasympathetic components of the autonomic nervous system • rate depends on frequency of sinoatrial node impulses

ARTERIAL VESSEL DOPPLER WAVEFORM CHARACTERISTICS

- normal wave form is triphasic with systolic forward flow followed by reverse flow in diastole
- influenced by following arterial properties:
  contractility—comes from smooth muscle
  vasoconstriction—decrease in size of lumen caused by sympathetic stimulation of smooth muscle, which contracts and narrows the vessel
- vasodilatation—increase in size of lumen when sympathetic stimulation is removed

HEAD AND NECK FLOW CHARACTERISTICS: ARTERIAL WAVEFORM (*Continued*)

COMMON CAROTID ARTERY

- high-velocity, laminar flow
- color persists during entire cardiac cycle due to low resistance of intracranial vascular bed, therefore Doppler signal does not go below the zero line

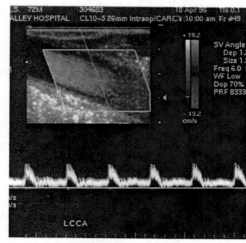

Common carotid artery

INTERNAL CAROTID

- low-resistance circuit to brain and therefore the flow continues during all of diastole

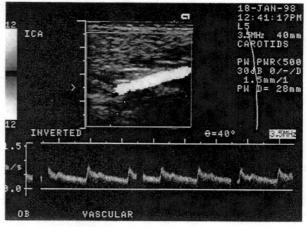

Internal carotid artery

EXTERNAL CAROTID

- pulsatile flow due to the high resistance of muscle beds provided by this vessel
- has a prominent dicrotic notch

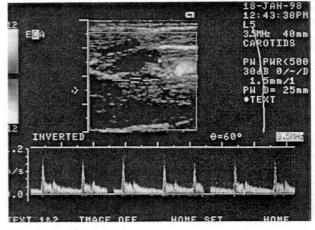

External carotid artery

VERTEBRAL ARTERY

- cephalad flow through the cardiac cycle with uniform flow pattern
- similar pattern as in ICA

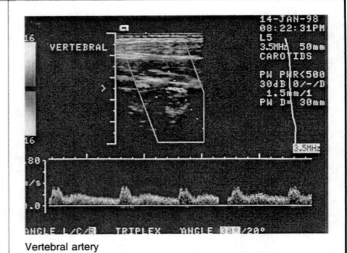

Vertebral artery

ABDOMINAL VASCULATURE FLOW CHARACTERISTICS

AORTA
- Suprarenal aorta
  low resistance signal
- Below renal arteries
  high-resistance signal with possible triphasic flow distally (since flow is influenced by peripheral circulation to legs)

CELIAC ARTERY
- low-resistance flow with forward flow in both systole and diastole
- more spectral broadening than aorta due to its small size

SUPERIOR MESENTERY ARTERY
- fasting: high resistance, nonfasting becomes low resistance
- turbulent flow not usually seen
- diastolic flow should double in postmeal state

HEPATIC ARTERIES
- same direction as portal vein, although is tortuous and flow may be toward or away from transducer especially in region of porta hepatis
- low-resistance signal

RENAL ARTERIES
- peak systole < 100 cm/sec
- low-resistance vascular bed
- high diastolic flow throughout cardiac cycle

ILIAC ARTERY
- triphasic flow pattern
- high impedance/resistance as it is a peripheral artery

EXTREMITIES
- triphasic due to the nature of the high-resistance vascular bed they flow to
- flow may be biphasic in elderly people

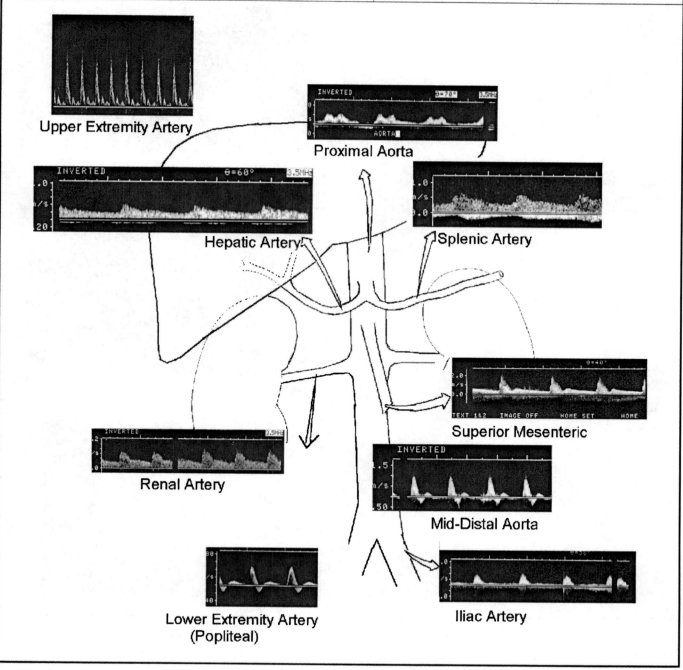

Upper Extremity Artery

Proximal Aorta

Hepatic Artery

Splenic Artery

Renal Artery

Superior Mesenteric

Mid-Distal Aorta

Lower Extremity Artery
(Popliteal)

Iliac Artery

NORMAL SONOGRAPHIC APPEARANCE OF VEINS

- spontaneous flow in patient at rest, which is influenced by
  respiration
  position of patient
  central venous pressure
  arterial inflow from muscular activity
  cardiac contraction

NECK AND EXTREMITY VENOUS FLOW CHARACTERISTICS

JUGULAR VEIN

- bidirectional flow that is more pulsatile than flow signals derived from the lower extremity (due to transmitted cardiac pulsations)
- distends during Valsalva maneuver

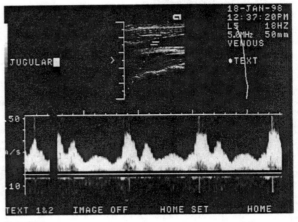

Jugular

UPPER EXTREMITY

- pulsatile bidirectional phasic flow pattern that varies with respiration
- more pulsatile than lower extremities

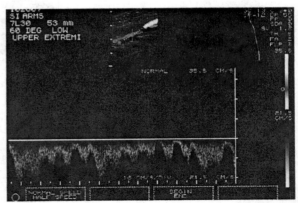

Upper extremity

LOWER EXTREMITY

- monophasic, unidirectional centripetal flow

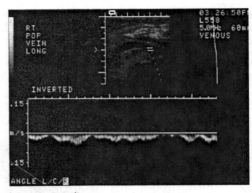

Lower extremity

ABDOMINAL VENOUS FLOW CHARACTERISTICS

IVC
- waveform is many components due to respiratory variations and proximity to the right atrium
- caliber is quite variable

HEPATIC VEINS
- pulsatile flow pattern dependent on cardiac cycle and pressure variation in right atrium
- same waveform as IVC
- should drain into IVC

PORTAL VEIN
- hepatopedal flow
- low-velocity continuous venous signal
- respiratory variation is present
- pulsation in flow is seen in tricuspid regurge

SPLENIC VEIN
- normal flow is toward midline

RENAL VEIN
- examined sonographically usually to rule out thrombosis
- low-velocity, continuous signal

ILIAC VEIN
- can have pulsations from adjacent artery
- continuous low-flow signal

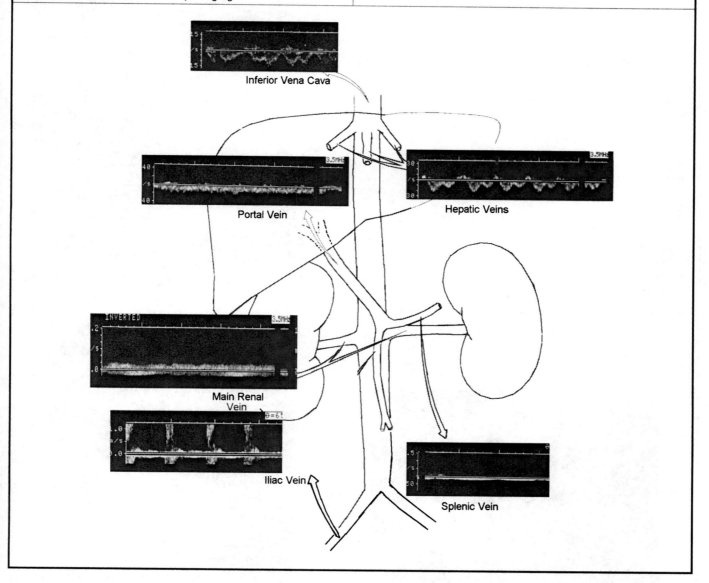

Inferior Vena Cava

Portal Vein

Hepatic Veins

Main Renal Vein

Iliac Vein

Splenic Vein

C) ANOMALIES

ANOMALY	US APPEARANCE
ANEURYSMS 1. ABDOMINAL AORTIC ANEURYSM (AAA) • mainly caused by atherosclerosis; less commonly due to mycotic or dissecting lesions • incidence increased in older population, especially men • majority occur below origin of renal arteries and involve mid or distal aorta • can involve proximal aorta, origin of renal arteries, SMA, and celiac artery • can extend into one or both common iliac arteries Thrombus: • thrombus is commonly eccentrically located within an aortic aneurysm and is usually anteriorly or anterolaterally located • high-amplitude linear echos may frequently be seen along the luminal surface of thrombus SS • none • pulsatile abdominal mass, back pain US • aorta diameter > 3 cm in maximum dimension (outer wall to outer wall) • determine extent of aneurysm as defined with respect to the bifurcation and/or renal arteries • findings can include aortic wall calcification and intraluminal thrombus (medium to low-level echos, more common along the anterior and lateral walls) Pitfall: • mild dilatation or tortuosity in a vessel can give the appearance of a true aneurysm when improperly measured Differential Diagnosis for Pulsatile Abdominal Mass: • retroperitoneal tumor/mass • fibroid uterus • paraortic lymph nodes	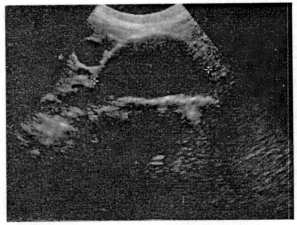 Longitudinal scan through saccular aortic aneurysm 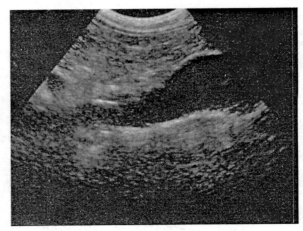 Longitudinal scan through fusiform aortic aneurysm

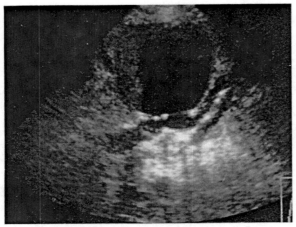

Aneurysm of left iliac artery: note thrombus within it

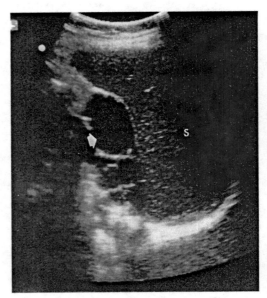

Splenic artery aneurysm (arrow), spleen (S)

ANOMALY	US APPEARANCE

2. AORTIC RUPTURE
• most commonly occurs in aneurysms > 5 cm in diameter

SS
• acute abdominal pain, shock (hypotension), expanding abdominal mass

US
• may rupture into several retroperitoneal compartments
• retroperitoneal mass or fluid collection along exterior edge of aorta
• may displace one or both kidneys
• can extend along psoas muscles

3. FALSE ANEURYSM/PSEUDOANEURYSM
• hematomas that have maintained some communication with the arterial lumen by means of a puncture site
• do not have layers of intima, media, and adventitia
• communicating channel is of variable size and length
• Postsurgical
  develop in association with surgical placement of bypass graft
  develop from penetrating trauma to native arterial wall (e.g., postarterial catheterization)
• Trauma
  penetrating trauma such as knife and bullet wounds

US
• flow through channel to and from aneurysm
• swirling luminal blood flow within the pseudoaneurysm
• variable amounts of mural thrombus
• synchronous pulsatility of arterial and pseudoaneurysm walls

Doppler:
• disorganized, pulsatile flow with low-velocity signals in a hypo or anechoic mass adjacent to an artery—if fully clotted, no flow will be present

Treatment:
US can aid in compression repair by:
identifying precisely where compression should be applied
• using the transducer to apply pressure on the neck of the aneurysm
• color and pulsed Doppler can determine successful obliteration of flow

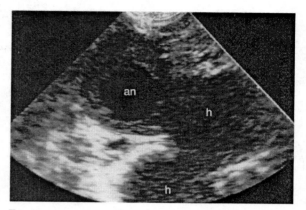

Transverse sonogram through a ruptured aneurysm (an) with adjacent hematoma formation (h)

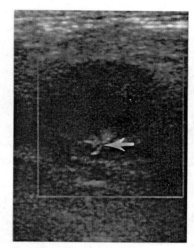

Pseudoaneurysm adjacent to femoral artery. Arrow indicates the color jet in neck.

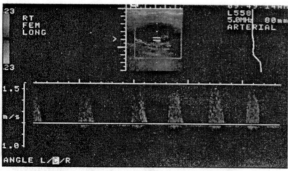

Spectral Doppler of flow in neck of pseudoaneurysm

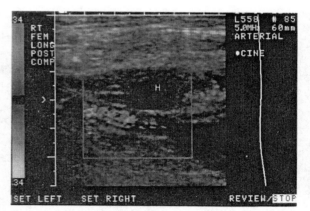

Postcompression of pseudoaneurysm shows flow in femoral artery with anechoic hematoma (H) and no flow between the two structures

SURVIVAL CRITERIA BASED ON SIZE OF ANEURYSM

< 5 cm	maximum survival rate with 1% rupture rate
5–6 cm	significant aneurysm with 75% 1-year survival rate
> 6 cm	50% survival of 1 year
> 7 cm	25% survival rate for 1-year and 75% risk of fatal rupture

CLASSIFICATIONS OF ANEURYSMS

CLASS	TYPE	DIAGRAM	DEFINITIONS
FALSE	DISSECTING	Type A — Ascending aorta; Type A Ascending & Descending; Type B Descending aorta	• inner wall (intima) pulls away from other 2 walls causing a tear in the tunica intima • results in hemorrhage between walls Type A: • involves any part of ascending aorta Type B: • involves only descending aorta
	PSEUDO-ANEURYSM (PA)		• pulsating hematoma connected to the lumen of the artery by a means of channel (neck) of variable size and length
TRUE	BERRY		• small spherical aneurysm • 1–1.5 cm • occurs usually within cerebral circulation • communicates with vessel by a small opening

CLASSIFICATIONS OF ANEURYSMS

CLASS	TYPE	DIAGRAM	DEFINITIONS
	FUSIFORM	 b	• all walls of vessel dilate almost equally • creates a tubular dilation • usually occurs below renal arteries to aortic bifurcation
	SACCULAR	 c	• less common • localized, spherical outpouching of vessel wall • does not involve entire circumference • usually due to trauma • usually larger than fusiform type MYCOTIC—aneurysm due to bacterial infection

OTHER MORE COMMON ANEURYSMS INCLUDE

CAROTID ARTERY	• focal dilatation anywhere along the carotid artery • may occur in combination with plaque, thrombus, calcification, or dissection
POPLITEAL ARTERY	• often bilateral • associated with AAAs • unlikely to reach point of rupture • mural thrombus can cause peripheral embolization and thrombosis of distal arteries, which causes limb ischemia and possible amputation • < 2 cm is considered small
RENAL ARTERY	• commonly develop as a complication of large-bore renal biopsy • can cause hypertension • hypoechoic fluid masses contiguous with the renal artery
SPLANCHNIC ARTERIES	• aneurysm of the digestive arterial system • may be congenital, atheroslerotic, traumatic, mycotic, or inflammatory in origin • can be fusiform or saccular

ANOMALY	US APPEARANCE

AORTIC DISSECTION

- can be referred to dissecting aneurysm
- intimal lining (inner wall) of aorta separates from the rest of the wall
- hemorrhage occurs between dissected intima and aortic wall, which creates a false lumen
- etiology is unclear but associated with hypertension, Marfan's syndrome, pregnancy, aortic valve disease, congenital cardiac anomalies, Cushing's syndrome, pheochromocytoma, catheter-induced needle wounds

SS

- severe chest pain that can mimic cardiac pathology
- abdominal, extremity, and/or back pain, hypotension, shock

US

- thin intraluminal flap that moves with aortic pulsations
- difficult to differentiate between true and false lumen

Doppler:
- demonstrates arterial blood flow in true and false lumen (on both sides of the thin membrane)

Pitfall:
- if the false lumen becomes thrombosed, it may be impossible to differentiate between dissection and intraluminal thrombus

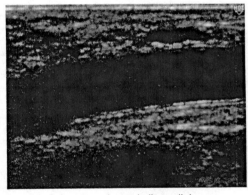

Longitudinal sonogram through the proximal portion of the abdominal aorta (a) in a patient with a dissection (carets, intimal flap)

	Type A	Type B
Involvement	any dissection involving ascending aorta	any dissection involving only descending aorta
Other	high mortality associated with Marfan's syndrome	lower mortality and better prognosis

AORTIC/ARTERIAL GRAFTS

- used when the aneurysm is either removed or are placed within the graft
- two attachment points of tube:
  proximal part is anastomosed to the proximal aorta
  distal portion has two sleeves that are anastomosed to either common iliac, external iliac, or femoral artery
- US beneficial in assessing complications such as false aneurysms, hemorrhage, infection or occlusion, degeneration of graft material
- some fluid surrounding graft site in the first 3 postoperative months can be expected

US

- tube with discrete echogenic borders
- end-to-end anastomosis appears as two tubes on top of each other (one is the native aorta, the other is the graft)

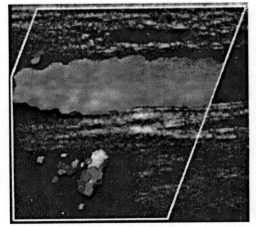

Arterial graft: note echogenic linear lining

Color flow within graft

ANOMALY	US APPEARANCE

ARTERIOSCLEROSIS/ATHEROSCLEROSIS
- term given to describe a number of pathologic conditions in which there are thickened and hardened arterial walls with loss of elasticity
- most common pathology of abdominal aorta seen sonographically

ATHEROMATOUS PLAQUE/ATHEROMA
- abnormal deposits of lipids that result in the degeneration of the endothelial lining of the arteries
- contains smooth muscle cells, macrophages, lymphocytes, collagen, elastic with central cholesterol crystals, calcium, and cellular debris
- thrombosis results from the interaction of platelets and clotting factors at the site of the lesion
- most commonly occurs at the bifurcation of arteries possibly due to the turbulence that normally arises there

US
- aorta often dilated and tortuous and may lie in midline or slightly to right of midline

Plaque Appearances:
- all plaque produces at least **minimal stenosis**
- appearance depends on severity as atheromas can undergo hemorrhage, necrosis, or calcification
- generally noted as echogenic material that encroaches on arterial lumen and produces a flow void in color Doppler image
- note echogenicity, extent, thickness, and how much it narrows the lumen (use transverse scan plane)

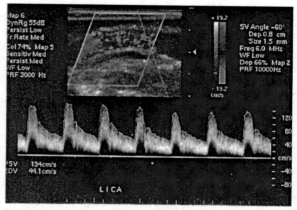

Moderate stenosis of internal carotid artery with peak systolic velocity of 1.34 m/sec

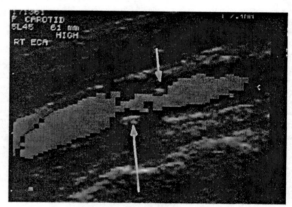

Plaque in carotid artery interrupting normal flow (arrows)

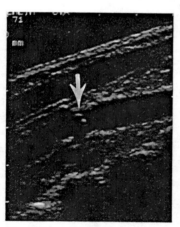

Plaque in carotid artery (arrow)

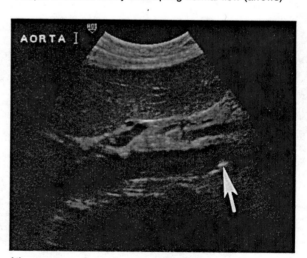

Atheromatous plaque in aorta (arrow)

GENERAL PLAQUE COMPOSITION AS RELATED TO SONOGRAPHIC ECHOGENICITY

fibrofatty	least echogenic, iso or hypoechoic to sternomastoid muscle
fibrous	hyperechoic to sternomastoid muscle, hypoechoic to arterial adventitia
dystrophic calcification	very hyperechoic, distal acoustic shadows

PERIPHERAL ARTERIAL DISEASE

- part of more generalized involvement of the arteries from atherosclerosis
- symptoms usually appear in people 50 years and older
- men more predisposed than women
- risk factors same as coronary and carotid artery disease
  smoking
  elevated cholesterol levels
  hypertension
  diabetes
- growth of atherosclerotic plaque that causes reduction in the diameter of the artery
- a 60% or greater stenosis can be considered hemodynamically significant
- can be progressive or abrupt
- slow growth sometimes allows time for collateral circulation to develop
- acute onset can cause ischemia, which leads to tissue changes and ultimately to loss of limb
- treatment includes bypass surgery, angioplasty, atherectomy, stent placement, thrombolytic medications

US Role:
- general arterial survey with assessment for narrowing, thrombosis, atherosclerotic plaque, calcification, aneurysmal dilatation
- postoperative monitoring of
1. bypass graft patency
2. bypass complications (pseudoaneurysms, hematoma)

DIAGNOSTIC DOPPLER CRITERIA FOR CAROTID ARTERY DISEASE

- velocity values are valid for all transducer frequencies using a Doppler angle of 60 degrees

% DIAMETER REDUCTION	ICA VELOCITY	WINDOW	SPECTRAL BROADENING	REPORT DESCRIPTION
0	peak < 1.25 m/sec	clear	none	normal
1–15	peak < 1.25 m/sec	clear	none—minimal in deceleration phase of systole	• wall irregularities • not hemodynamically significant
16–49	peak < 1.25 m/sec	none	throughout systole	• minor stenosis • not hemodynamically significant
50–79	peak > 1.25 m/sec	none	marked throughout	• moderate stenosis • hemodynamically significant • color flow aliasing possible
80–99	end > 1.4 m/sec	none	marked throughout	• severe stenosis • hemodynamically significant
OCCLUDED	no signal	—	—	• occlusion • CCA could have unilateral flow to zero or reversed

ANOMALY	US APPEARANCE

AV SHUNTS/ANASTOMOSES/FISTULAE

- an abnormal physical communication between artery and vein by which the capillary bed is bypassed
- shunts can also be used from the portal vein to IVC (portocaval shunt), mesenteric vein to IVC (mesocaval shunt), and splenic vein to renal vein (splenorenal shunt) in treating portal hypertension

1. CONGENITAL
- larger ones are source of obvious skin discoloration, etc.

2. ACQUIRED
- secondary to trauma, surgery, inflammation
- major cause of fistulas
- distention of recipient vein that contains high-velocity signals resembling those of an artery
- feeding artery has low-resistance flow (high diastolic)

3. CREATED VOLUNTARILY
i) Dialysis shunt
- AV shunt created for use during renal dialysis
ii) Surgical
- Doppler is used for determining shunt patency and hemodynamic results of the surgery
- Portocaval anastomosis
  - surgical creation of a connection between the portal vein and the vena cava
  - flow visualized through anastomosis
  - dilation of IVC
- Mesocaval anastomosis
  - connection between the mesenteric vein and the vena cava
  - difficult to visualize
  - reversed flow in IMV
- Splenorenal anastomosis
  Proximal—reversed flow in splenic vein
  Distal—anastomosis between splenic vein and left renal vein anterior to aorta
- Transjugular intrahepatic portosystemic shunts (TIPS)—see Chapter 7

US
Doppler:
AV fistulae: focal areas of both forward and reversed flow
arterial component = increased flow velocities and decreased RI
venous component = increased pulsatility

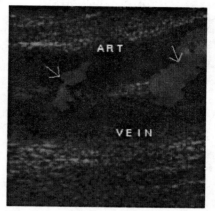

Fistula between artery and vein (arrows)

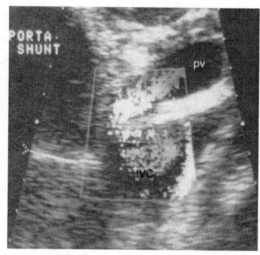

Portocaval shunt

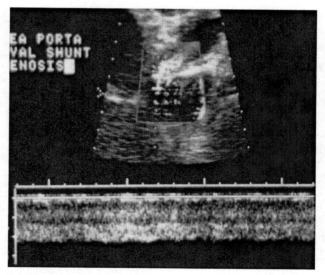

Portocaval shunt

ANOMALY	US APPEARANCE

BAKER'S CYST (POPLITEAL BURSITIS)

- not a vascular anomaly but included in this section as can be seen on sonographic evaluation of leg veins
- posterior herniation of knee joint synovium through capsule into the popliteal fossa
- can rupture, which can cause acute inflammation, pain, and swelling that can extend down into the posterior calf

SS
- felt as a swelling in popliteal space
- decreased mobility
- if ruptures, can cause pain and swelling

Diff Dx.:
- popliteal aneurysm
- if ruptures, can be confused with venous thrombophlebitis

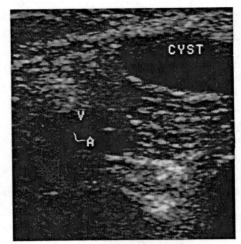

Transverse scan through popliteal fossa shows popliteal vessels (VA) and an adjacent popliteal cyst as an anechoic structure with through transmission

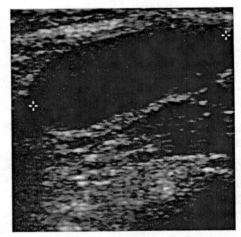

Longitudinal section through popliteal cyst measuring 5 cm in length

IVC FILTERS

- can be placed in IVC to prevent blood clot from traveling to heart and pulmonary arteries from the lower extremity
- used when anticoagulation therapy fails to prevent pulmonary emboli from venous thrombosis
- optimal location is between renal veins and IVC bifurcation

US
- bright hyperechoic foci in IVC

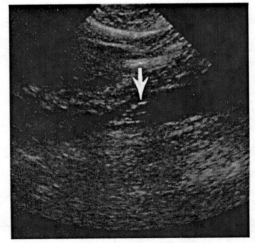

Longitudinal scan through IVC with filter (arrow)

ANOMALY	US APPEARANCE

IVC TUMORS

- several ways in which the IVC can be affected by tumor pathology:
  - peritoneal or retroperitoneal masses compress or deviate IVC
    adrenal, pancreatic head, liver tumors, retroperitoneal lymphadenopathy, AAA, hepatomegally, retroperitoneal fibrosis
  - direct invasion from adjacent tumor
    uncommon: but seen with retroperitoneal sarcomas, renal cell carcinoma, and hepatocellular carcinoma
  - venous extension of tumor from a vein draining into IVC
    seen with hepatomas and renal cell carcinomas
  - primary tumor of the IVC
    primary malignant tumor such as leiomyosarcoma may arise in wall of IVC, but this is rare

US
- intraluminal echogenic nodules

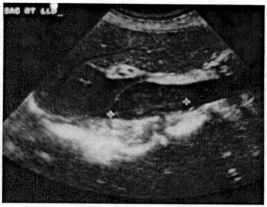

Spread of renal cell carcinoma within IVC (calipers)

ANOMALY	US APPEARANCE

RENAL VASCULAR DISEASE

1. RENAL ARTERY STENOSIS (RAS)

- occurs in:
  children rarely—secondary to dehydration, catheterization
  adults—secondary to severe atherosclerosis, trauma, arteritis,
  aneurysm,
  fibromuscular hyperplasia
- infarction in an avascular region in the kidney caused by arterial occlusion
- bilateral renal artery occlusion can be a cause of renal failure

GRAY SCALE US

- US examination is very time consuming and requires a high level of sonographic skill
- focal infarction gives rise to echogenic or hypoechoic areas that may have a mass effect
- eventually infarct atrophies causing parenchymal thinning

Diff. Dx:

- angiomyolipoma
- cavernous renal hemangioma
- renal cell carcinoma
- oncocytoma
- metastases

Doppler:

- entire length of artery must be visualized (can take from 30–60 minutes per kidney to examine completely) with Doppler signals obtained from the origin to the renal hilum
- suggestive of RAS are:
  renal-to-aortic peak systolic ratio > 3.5
  velocities > 180 cm/sec with poststenotic turbulence

Pitfalls:

- visualization of renal arteries may be impossible due to bowel gas, obesity, etc

2. RENAL VEIN THROMBOSIS

- impedance to renal venous flow caused by intrinsic or extrinsic compression of renal vein
- most commonly occurs in:
  neonates–secondary to dehydration, sepsis
  adults—secondary to nephrotic syndrome, glomerulonephritis, tumor, trauma, pregnancy (maternal diabetes), transient hypertension
- slow clot formation allows venous collaterals to form

SS

- hematuria, flank pain, hypertension, renal failure

US

- increased renal size with decreased echogenicity
- thrombus presents as echogenic intraluminal focus

Late stage:

- cortex becomes echogenic with preservation of CMJ differentiation
- thrombus may be visible within renal vein
- with bland thrombus the vein does not dilate, contrary to tumor thrombus, which can dilate the vein

Doppler:

- increase in intrarenal arterial impedance (absent or reversed diastolic flow)
- absence of venous flow

Hint:

- do not mistake reversed diastolic arterial flow for pulsatile venous flow
- due to recanalization of renal vein, presence of renal venous flow does not always exclude diagnosis

---

Renal artery-to-aortic ratio (RAR)

- take midstream Doppler waveforms from aorta at level of SMA recording highest peak systolic velocity
- take spectral waveforms of origin, proximal, mid, and distal segments of renal artery and record peak systolic velocity

$$RAR = \frac{Renal\ peak\ systolic\ velocity}{Aortic\ peak\ systolic\ velocity}$$

- normal RAR > 3.5

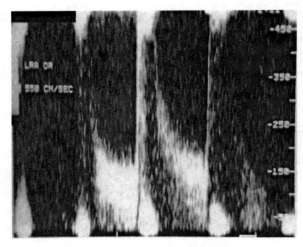

Doppler spectral tracing of proximal left renal artery stenosis demonstrating increased velocities of 550 cm/sec. The RAR was > 3.5.

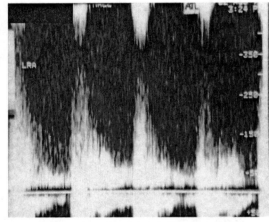

Doppler spectral tracing distal to the stenosis demonstrating poststenotic turbulence

ANOMALY	US APPEARANCE

VEIN THROMBOSIS

- risk factors:
- venous stasis
  prolonged immobilization, pregnancy, post-trauma, surgery
- hypercoagulability
  oral contraceptives, malignant state
- injury to venous intimal surface
  indwelling catheter, trauma
- prior history of DVT, pulmonary emboli
- 40% will resolve spontaneously, 20% will progress
- as clot ages it adheres to vein walls and causes partial or complete occlusion
- clot may retract and the vein may reopen
- collateral vessels may persist following recanalization
- overdiagnosis runs the risk of complications of therapy

SS
- swelling of limb
- pain and tenderness
- if clot embolizes to lung, symptoms can include dyspnea, tachypnea, tachycardia, chest pain

US
- see chart below

Pitfalls:
- inability to visualize segments of deep venous system due to bowel gas, large/obese or muscular patients
- poor technique when compressing
- recanalized vessels may have thick walls, which inhibit compressibility

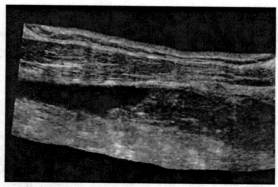

Jugular vein thrombus (Courtesy of Siemans SieScape)

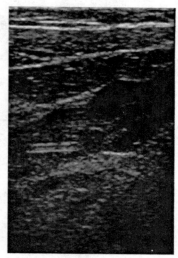

Axillary vein containing clot surrounding subclavian line (parallel echogenic lines)

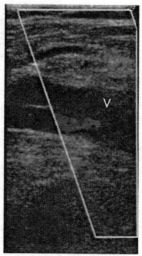

Occluded popliteal vein (V) adjacent to patent popliteal artery

Same as above with vein marked by calipers

(continued)

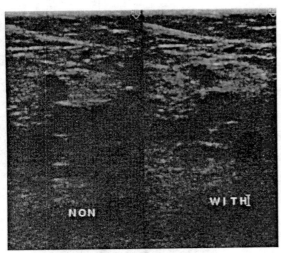

Noncompression of popliteal vein (non, no compression: with, with compression of transducer on vein)

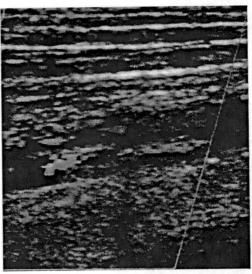

Nonoccluding thrombus of femoral vein. Note trace of color flow through clotted area in vein.

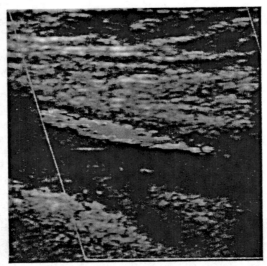

Echogenic clot in femoral vein near bifurcation

DEEP VENOUS THROMBOSIS SONOGRAPHIC FINDINGS

MAJOR DIAGNOSTIC CRITERIA OF CLOT	MINOR DIAGNOSTIC CRITERIA OF CLOT
• noncompressibility of veins • visualization of intraluminal clot • absent Doppler shift signal	• no alteration in flow by Valsalva or augmentation • no venous pulsation • absence of visible flow • absence of valve motion
FRESH/ACUTE THROMBUS	**CHRONIC/ORGANIZED THROMBUS**
• anechoic or hypoechoic • homogeneous • usually will fill entire vein • usually distends vein beyond normal size • vein walls will not compress adequately • soft thrombus can compress slightly with probe pressure • no collaterals visible	• moderately echogenic and can be difficult to visualize • calcified thrombi will have acoustic shadowing • well attached to vein wall • irregular surface if recanalization is occurring • chronic thrombosed veins will be smaller than artery • collateral veins are usually present

Chronic echogenic thrombus in
femoral vein (arrow)

Acute hypoechoic thrombus in femoral vein

295

ANOMALY	US APPEARANCE

VERTEBRAL ARTERY ABNORMALITY

- vertebral artery is best seen between the cervical spine's transverse processes
  - Nonvisualization/absent flow
    - occluded
  - Small size
    - size is normally variable
    - < 2 mm is abnormal and check for stenosis at origin
  - Increased velocity
    - > 40 cm/sec peak systole + flow disturbance suggests stenosis
  - Decreased velocity/blood volume
    - severe stenosis at origin
    - obstruction or distal obstruction of vertebral or basilar arteries or their tributaries in the brain
  - Abnormal flow direction
    - reversed flow secondary to <u>SUBCLAVIAN STEAL PHENOMENON</u>
    - this occurs when there is a stenosis of the proximal subclavian artery (after the innominate and before the vertebral artery takeoff)
    - blood bypasses the stenosis by going through the head and down the vertebral artery in a retrograde fashion

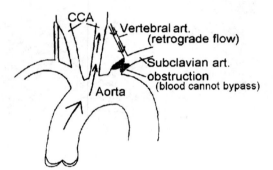

Subclavian steal

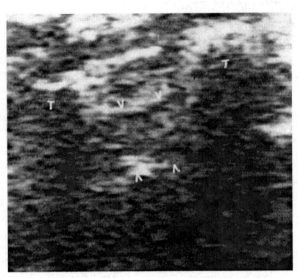

The vertebral artery (arrows) is vaguely seen between the transverse process (T), but flow is not evident on this Doppler image.

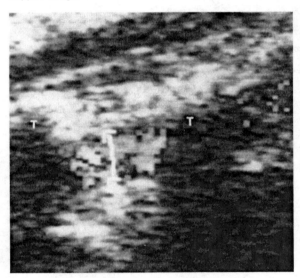

Flow is evident in the enlarged (5 mm) contralateral vertebral artery (cursor)

GRAY-SCALE (2-DIMENSIONAL) IMAGING

FUNCTION	• used as a road map for identification for the placement of Doppler US, identify areas of plaque and thrombus formation and also plaque characterization
PLAQUE MORPHOLOGY	• still under investigation and not widely used for patient management • Homogeneous plaque 　tends to be stable over time • Inhomogeneous with hypoechoic defects 　correlated with presence of intraplaque hemorrhage 　tend to break down and produce emboli • Echogenic plaque 　calcification is echogenic with acoustic shadowing
TECHNIQUE	• longitudinal and transverse scans vessel • highest possible frequency transducer
MEASURING VESSELS	DIAMETER • at point of maximum stenosis 　1. measure artery true lumen 　2. measure diameter of residual lumen $$\% \text{ of diameter stenosis} = \frac{\text{residual lumen diameter (2)}}{\text{vessel diameter (1)}} \times 100$$ AREA • using area method 　1. trace outside circumference of artery (sq mm) 　2. trace inner circumference of residual lumen (sq mm) $$\% \text{ of diameter stenosis} = 1 - \frac{\text{residual lumen area (2)}}{\text{vessel area (1)}} \times 100$$
COMPRESSION	• should be performed routinely on venous examinations • highly sensitive and specific for identification of venous thrombosis • with mild external pressure from US transducer, the veins should collapse (the lumen disappear) throughout their course • best performed in transverse plane to ensure that the transducer does not roll off the vein • poor technique is a main cause of vein noncompressibility

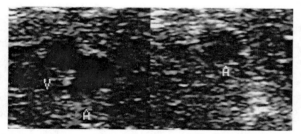

Split image of transverse scan plane through popliteal fossa. On the right shows both the artery (A) and vein (V) with no compression. On the left the transducer has compressed the popliteal vein, leaving only the artery visible.

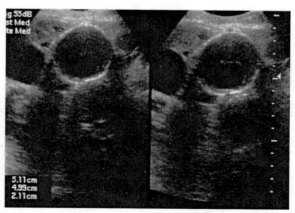

Transverse through aortic aneurysm measuring diameter of patent lumen and of vessel

297

DOPPLER ULTRASOUND

DEFINITION
- using the Doppler effect, movement of scatters (blood cells) are detected by analyzing a change in frequency of a US beam after it is reflected off of them
- measured in Hertz (Hz) = cycles per second (units of frequency)
- in clinical US, typically range from -10 kHz to $+10$ kHz
  Positive shift: occurs when source and receiver are approaching each other
  Negative shift: occurs when source and receiver are moving away from each other

BENEFIT
- can give information about blood flow velocity (magnitude and direction)
- adds physiologic information to the anatomic, morphologic information obtained from gray-scale imaging

DOPPLER SHIFT
- the difference between the frequencies of transmitted and received waves
- is a frequency shift as a result of motion between the sound source (sound waves) and the receiver (RBCs)
- proportional to the velocity of relative motion between the transducer and the moving blood depends on direction (cosine of the angle) between the sound beam and reflector direction of motion

$$\text{Doppler shift } (\Delta f) = \frac{2fV \cos \theta}{c} \qquad\qquad \text{Velocity of blood flow} = \frac{c \, \Delta f}{2f \cos \theta}$$

Where:

Δf = Doppler shift frequency between the transmitted wave and echo received from a moving target

f = transmitted (insonant) frequency*

V = blood flow velocity (reflector/particle speed)

C = speed of sound in body (propagation speed) 1540 m/sec

θ = Doppler angle (angle between direction of blood and direction of sound)*
  optimum angle of incidence is from 45°–60°

*operator controlled factors

If Reflector is:
- stationary THEN → returning frequency = transmitted frequency → **NO SHIFT**
- moving away from transducer THEN → returning frequency < transmitted frequency → **NEGATIVE SHIFT**
- moving toward transducer THEN → returning frequency > transmitted frequency → **POSITIVE SHIFT**

TECHNIQUE
- center stream angle of insonation < 60° and an appropriate sample volume size for the vessel width are used to document velocity spectral patterns
- use appropriate Doppler wall filter (50–100 Hz) so that low-amplitude, low-velocity signals associated with minimal or preclusive disease may be recognized
- freezing the 2-dimensional image will improve a Doppler spectrum that is weak or noisy
- often low-frequency transducer may be needed to elicit a Doppler signal due to weaker amplitude of echos from RBCs

COMPARISON OF	CONTINUOUS WAVE DOPPLER	PULSED DOPPLER
DEFINITION	• defects Doppler-shifted signals by continuous and simultaneous transmission of sound and reception of echos	• detects Doppler-shifted signals by collecting samples from separate ultrasonic pulses in the same location
CRYSTALS	2 crystals • one crystal is constantly sending out US energy and one is continuously listening	1 crystal • alternates between sending and receiving
RESOLUTION	no range resolution echos can come from anywhere along length of beam	range resolution echos can come only from area being investigated (sample volume)
VELOCITY CONSIDERATIONS	able to measure very high velocities	limited maximum velocity high velocities appear as negative (aliasing) this occurs at the Nyquist limit
	always producing pulse Duty Factor = 1	producing pulse Duty Factor = 0.001-0.01 receiving sound sample volume

TYPES OF DOPPLER

PULSED DOPPLER	• also known as range-gated Doppler • depth of Doppler detection is determined by the gate (sample volume) • pulsed mode of sound transmission investigates the Doppler shift in a specific region known as the sample volume • calculates the blood velocity • cursor must be placed parallel with blood flow to provide an accurate velocity reading • can refer to color and spectral Doppler
SPECTRAL DOPPLER	• combination of either continuous wave or pulsed Doppler with a spectral display • frequencies are graphed as they appear in time It can evaluate: 1. TIMING: when the signal occurs in relation to the cardiac cycle 2. DURATION: how long the signal lasts 3. DIRECTION: where the signal is going—away or toward the transducer 4. VELOCITIES: the amplitude gives us the maximum and mean velocities of the spectrum 5. FREQUENCY RANGE: spectral broadening shows the range of frequencies present
DUPLEX ULTRASOUND	• US machine that can combine anatomic and flow information simultaneously or sequentially = pulsed Doppler + spectral display + real-time imaging system • advantage is that the real-time image allows placement of a US Doppler beam in the correct anatomic location • can refer to both color and spectral Doppler

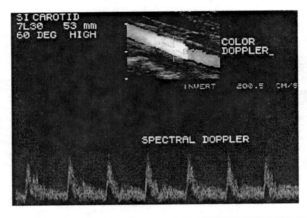

EVALUATING ARTERIES WITH DOPPLER

TURBULENCE	• disorganized, chaotic blood flow travels at a greater range of velocities and in a variety of nonaxial directions within the vessel • occurs with stenosis
SPECTRAL BROADENING	Spectral Broadening: • represents range of frequencies at any given time • appears as the width of Doppler spectrum • increases in proportion to stenosis severity • larger spectral broadening in small vessels • difficult to quantify Spectral Window: • clear space between arterial signal and baseline • large number of frequencies causes the spectral window to fill in Pitfalls: • spectral broadening is also caused by high Doppler gain, high-power settings, and large sample volumes
ALIASING ARTIFACT	• spectral display has spectrum wrapping around or folding over the baseline • occurs when blood is moving too fast in combination with a too low pulse repetition frequency Doppler settings (i.e., when the Doppler shift attains the Nyquist limit = 1/2 the pulse repetition rate) • increasing the pulse repetition frequency will solve this problem • often associated with pathology (significant stenosis)

FLOW PATTERN	High-Resistance Waveform
	• little, no, and possible reversed flow in diastole (tracing will approach, touch, or cross the baseline)
	• feed muscular beds
	  e.g., distal aorta, external carotid arteries, fasting SMA
		Low-Resistance Waveform
		• forward flow in diastole that is well above baseline
		• feed major life-supporting organs
		  e.g., renal, hepatic, internal carotid arteries

FLOW DIRECTION	• documented with spectral Doppler tracing and color flow imaging

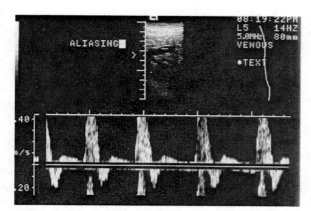

Aliasing: wrapping of the signal around baseline indicating too rapid a blood flow for the Doppler settings

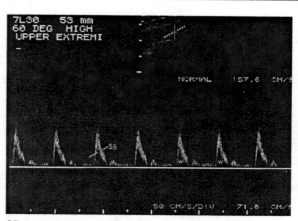

SB, spectral broadening between the white lines; W, spectral window

EVALUATING VEINS WITH DOPPLER

NONPULSATILITY	• most veins do not pulsate and therefore are considered nonpulsatile (exceptions include hepatic and IVC) • pulsatility is **not** an indication of obstruction or thrombosis Differential for pulsatile venous waveforms include: fluid overload (CHF, dialysis, IV fluid replacement) venous valvular incompetence tricuspid regurgitation
PATENCY	Augmentation • patient's extremity is manually compressed distal to examination site (augmentation in lower extremity can be done by having the patient plantar flex the foot) • this creates an audible increase in flow • confirms patency of the vein between the site of interrogation and the site of compression • can be observed with partial venous occlusion and appears as a real response • documented by pulsed Doppler rather than color Doppler to avoid misinterpretation of color information due to wrong settings or motion artifact
COMPETENCE	Valsalva Maneuver • competent venous valves cause venous flow to be interrupted during a Valsalva maneuver or proximal limb compression • patient takes in a breath and holding it bears down • used to help evaluate competence of valves and patency of deep venous system in abdomen and pelvis • documented by pulsed Doppler
SPONTANEITY OF FLOW/PHASICITY	• documented with spectral Doppler tracing and color flow imaging • venous sounds are in phase with the respiratory cycle • loss of the phasicity in the spontaneous venous signal indicates an obstruction in the venous system between the area being examined and the diaphragm

302

SONOGRAPHIC APPEARANCE OF DOPPLER OF VEINS

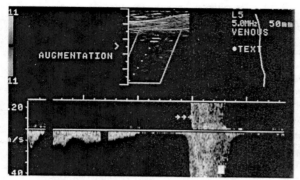

Augmentation: squeezing the area inferior to the site causes the exaggerated flow (arrows)

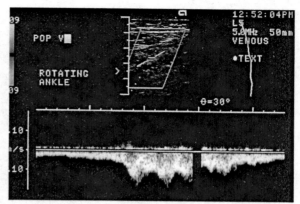

Augmenting the vein can also be achieved by having the patient move a part more distal to the vein. In this scan plane, augmented flow is achieved in the popliteal vein with the patient rotating the ankle.

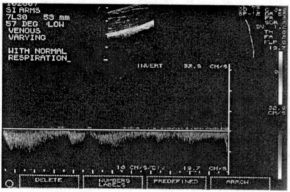

Venous flow varying with normal respiration

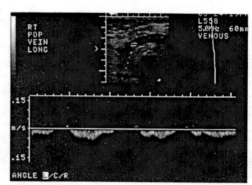

Pulsatility of popliteal vein in 89-year-old patient could be caused by CHF and is not a sign of obstruction.

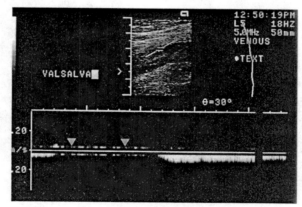

Valsalva maneuver caused a cessation of flow (arrows). Normal flow resumed when patient began to breath normally again.

MEASURING ARTERIAL BLOOD FLOW

ARTERIAL VELOCITY	• velocity is proportional to the Doppler frequency shift and to the increase of cos θ • image vessel so that the Doppler angle is < **60°**
PEAK SYSTOLIC VELOCITY	• most reliable Doppler parameter for gauging severity of stenosis • measured at site of stenosis • the longer the stenosis the lower the velocity • peak velocity not routinely used to diagnose disease in the abdomen with the exception of the renal arteries • area of maximum velocity is at a point just beyond maximum stenosis • the greater the stenosis the higher the velocity • for extreme stenosis the velocity will approach zero as stenosis approaches 100%
PEAK END-DIASTOLIC VELOCITY	• remains normal with arterial stenosis of < 50% diameter reduction • > 50% stenosis, increases in proportion to severity of narrowing
RESISTIVE INDEX (RI) = $$\frac{\text{S (peak systole)} - \text{D (end diastole)}}{\text{S (peak systole)}}$$	• also known as Pourcelot index • approaches 1 when diastolic velocity approaches zero • increases when resistance to flow goes up • important to measure at end of diastole (point right before the next systolic upstroke) and not where diastolic flow ends • parenchymal organs usually have RI < 0.7
PULSITIVITY INDEX (PI) = $$\frac{\text{S (peak systole)} - \text{D (end diastole)}}{\text{V (mean velocity)}}$$	• also known as the impedance • mean is the mean flow velocity throughout the cardiac cycle, which is usually calculated automatically by the US machine • truer indication of vascular resistance than the resistive index • value of PI increases with increasing resistance • used to evaluate blood flow to tumors or masses
SYSTOLIC/DIASTOLIC RATIO = $$\frac{\text{S}}{\text{D}}$$	• simple older index • value declines as resistance declines • will become infinity when diastolic velocities reach zero • can be used in the abdomen to compare the systolic velocity of the main renal artery to that of the aorta to assess whether renal artery stenosis is present
VELOCITY RATIO $$\frac{\text{A \{peak systolic v at site of stenosis\}}}{\text{B \{peak systolic v 2–4 cm prox/N\}}}$$	• used to compare two different velocities • can also be used to compare main renal artery to that of aorta to assess for renal artery stenosis

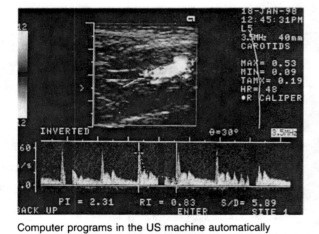

Computer programs in the US machine automatically calculate the RI, PI, and S/D ratio when one waveform has been traced out.

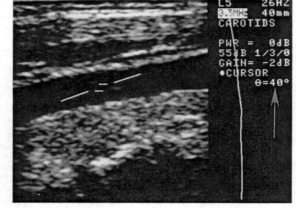

Cursor should be placed mid vessel and sample volume adjusted to correct width. The angle must be set < 60°. This angle is at 40° (arrow).

COLOR DOPPLER/POWER DOPPLER

COMPARISON	COLOR (FLOW) DOPPLER	POWER (ANGIO) DOPPLER
DEFINITION	• superimposes color on all or part of the gray-scale image • displayed colors normally range from red to blue • direction of blood flow is relative to the selected angle of Doppler detection • velocity, frequency, and energy can be depicted by the variation in color hue and brightness	• colors correspond to power or intensity of the Doppler signal rather than to its frequency or velocity • extension of auto correlation process of conventional (mean-frequency) color Doppler
ADVANTAGES	• decreases examination time by providing flow information from a large area faster with less operator dependence than spectral Doppler • demonstrates physiologic and pathologic blood flow changes (e.g., can evaluate clot as being totally or partially obstructive) • evaluates blood flow in vessels that are not accessible to compression, i.e., subclavian	• increased flow sensitivity, which allows for rapid evaluation of flow • angle independence • evaluation of organ perfusion (good for spleen, testicles, kidneys) • detection of low flow (infarction, ischemia)
PITFALLS AND DISADVANTAGES	• lack of color can be due to: no blood flow in that particular area flow that is perpendicular to the US beam shadow from structure (plaque) that prevents color from being detected beneath it VELOCITY SCALE • acts as a filter by emphasizing vessels with higher velocities and will not display slower ones next to the vessel wall • if set too high, vessel will not fill with color and can appear as a clot-filled vessel • if set too low, color aliasing can occur	• does not provide flow direction information
CRITICAL FACTORS	• tortuous arteries can create problems as certain angles will show a lack of color • minimize color sample box can improve color sensitivity and frame rates • motion artifact can distort image (i.e., respiration, movement of bowel gas)	
GAIN	• increase color gain until background fills with color speckles, then decrease until they disappear • color will not overwrite gray scale, therefore too high a gray-scale gain will have to be lowered for good color fill-in	

TECHNIQUE

AORTA TECHNIQUE

- scan usually with patient in supine position
- coronal scans are helpful in patients with overlying bowel gas or that are obese

MEASURING CORRECTLY

- accurately measure maximum cross-sectional diameter from outer wall to outer wall
- a transverse scan plane and/or a tilted probe can create a widened vessel due to obliquity
- the best way to overcome these artifacts is to demonstrate the aorta in a longitudinal scan plane, using the maximum AP diameter as the point where you measure

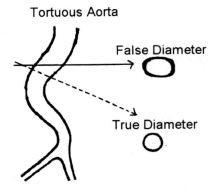

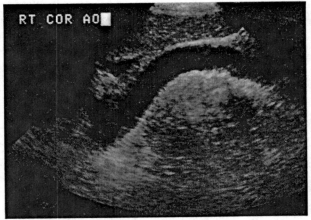

Right coronal view of aorta: tortuous aorta such as this one can cause problems when trying to measure accurately

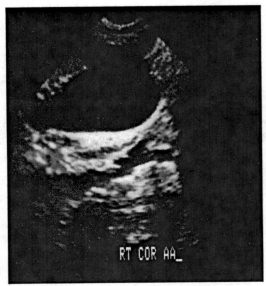

Right coronal approach can sometimes give a better demonstration of bifurcation into iliacs

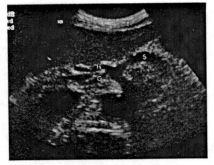

Transverse scan plane through aorta at level of celiac axis showing trifurcation into common hepatic (H), splenic (S) and left gastric (G) arteries

IVC TECHNIQUE
- marked change in caliber with respiration (inspiration should cause it to partially collapse due to decreased pressure within thoracic cavity)
- many tributaries but most cannot be seen due to their small size
- renal and hepatic veins are most consistently seen

US APPEARANCE
- appears as anechoic structure to the right of midline
- more oval in shape than aorta

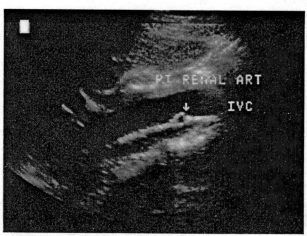

Longitudinal scan through IVC

ABNORMAL CALIBER AND POSITION

1. TOO LARGE
- caused because of proximal obstruction due to:
  right-sided heart failure (CHF)
  chronic pulmonary disease
  pulmonary hypertension
  pericardial effusion with tamponade
  constrictive pericarditis
  right atrial tumor
  tricuspid valve disease
  hepatomegaly

US
- loss of normal respiratory variation of caliber
- slow blood flow

2. TOO SMALL
- can be compressed and displaced anteriorly by right renal artery aneurysm, enlarged retroperitoneal lymph nodes

3. DISPLACEMENT
- mass in posterior, caudate or right hepatic lobe of liver
- right renal artery aneurysm
- lymphadenopathy
- tortuous aorta
- right kidney or adrenal mass
- retroperitoneal tumors (e.g., leiomyosarcoma)

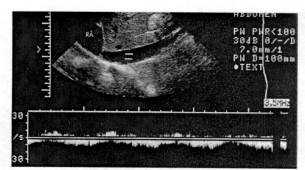

Longitudinal proximal IVC: as it courses near the heart, it turns anteriorly before it terminates in the right atrium (RA)

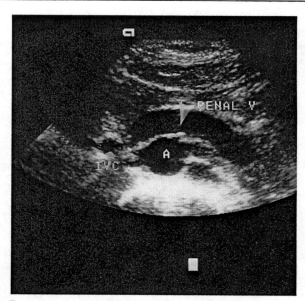

Transverse level through mid IVC and aorta. Left renal vein transverse across aorta (arrowhead)

EXTREMITIES TECHNIQUE

UPPER	LOWER
• patient supine with head tilted away from affected side • affected arm is abducted to allow for evaluation of the axilla • starting in axilla move distally in transverse plane	• patient examined 10°–15° head up tilt position • knees slightly flexed and hips externally rotated • apply gel along whole course, which allows for continuous uninterrupted examination of vessels • scan beginning at groin and extending downward along medial aspect of thigh to the adductor canal • patient turned prone or decubitus to visualize popliteal vessels Transverse Scan Plane: • used for compression Longitudinal Scan Plane: • optimizes color and pulsed Doppler examinations
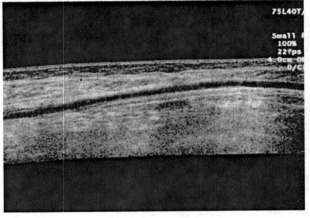 Longitudinal scan along saphenous vein in leg (Courtesy of Siemans SieScape)	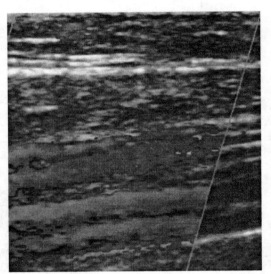 Flow in calf veins

CAROTID TECHNIQUE

TRANSVERSE SCAN PLANE
• begin at clavicle and move cephalad
Identify:
  CCA, carotid bulb, ECA, ICA
  areas of plaque or obstruction
Measure:
  residual lumen size and percent diameter reduction
Identify:
  CCA, carotid bulb, ECA, ICA, vertebral artery
		LONGITUDINAL SCAN PLANE
		• begin at clavicle and move cephalad
		  plaque—extent and characteristics
		  other areas of obstruction
		  confirm cephalad flow
		  velocity waveform configuration
		Measure:
		  cardinal Doppler parameters
		luminal narrowing from color Doppler image

ICA OR ECA?	ICA	ECA
WAVEFORM	• low-resistance flow with diastolic flow well above baseline • lower intensity color present throughout diastole	• higher resistance flow similar to an extremity flow peaks then drops to near the baseline
DIAMETER	larger	smaller
LOCATION	posterior/lateral	anterior/medial
BRANCH	none	has a branch near origin
TAP OF SUPERFICIAL TEMPORAL ARTERY	• no pulsations	• superficial temporal artery is a branch of ECA, therefore pulsations produced by tapping immediately anterior to the tragus of the ear are transmitted to ECA and appear on waveform

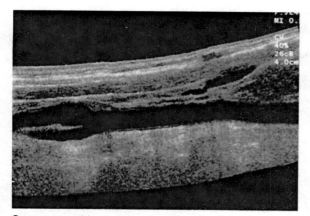

Common carotid artery showing bifurcation into external and internal carotid arteries (Courtesy of Siemens)

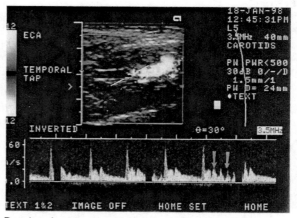

Doppler of external carotid artery. Small transmitted pulses (arrows) from tapping ensure that the signal is coming from the ECA.

BIBLIOGRAPHY

1. Anderhub B. *General Sonography: A Clinical Guide.* St. Louis: Mosby, 1995.
2. Bisset R. and Khan A. *Differential Diagnosis in Abdominal Ultrasound.* London: Bailliere Tindall, 1990.
3. Goldberg B. and Kurtz A. *Atlas of Ultrasound Measurements.* Chicago: Year Book Medical Publishers, 1990.
4. Kawamura D. *Diagnostic Medical Sonography: Abdomen and Superficial Structures,* 2nd ed. Philadelphia: Lippincott-Raven Publishers, 1997.
5. Kapid W. and Elson L. *The Anatomy Coloring Book.* New York: Harper & Row, 1993.
6. Kee, J.L. *Handbook of Laboratory and Diagnostic Tests with Nursing Implications,* 2nd ed. Norwalk, CT: Appleton & Lange, 1994.
7. Kurtz A.B. and Middleton W.D. *Ultrasound: The Requisites.* St. Louis: Mosby, 1996.
8. Netter F.H. *Atlas of Human Anatomy.* Summit, NJ: CIBA-GEIGY Corp., 1989.
9. Odwin C., Dububsky T. and Fleisher A. *Appleton & Lange's Review for the Ultrasonography Examination.* Norwalk, CT: Appleton & Lange, 1993.
10. Robbins S. *Pathologic Basis of Disease,* 5th ed. Philadelphia: WB Saunders, 1994.
11. Rumack C., Wilson S. and Charboneau W. *Diagnostic Ultrasound.* St. Louis: Mosby, 1992.
12. Sacher R. and McPherson R. *Widmann's Clinical Interpretation of Laboratory Tests,* 10th ed. Philadelphia: FA Davis Co, 1991.
13. Sadler T.W. *Langman's Medical Embryology,* 5th ed. Baltimore: Williams & Wilkins, 1985.
14. Sauerbrei E., Nguyen K. and Nolan R. *Abdominal Sonography.* Philadelphia: J. B. Lippincott, 1993.
15. Taylor K., Burns P. and Wells P. *Clinical Applications of Doppler Ultrasound.* New York: Raven Press, 1995.
16. Thomas C. *Taber's Cyclopedic Medical Dictionary,* 17th ed. Philadelphia: FA Davis, 1989.
17. Thompson J.S. *Core Textbook of Anatomy.* Philadelphia: J. B. Lippincott, 1977.
18. Tortora G. *Principles of Anatomy and Physiology,* 6th ed. New York: Harper & Row, 1990.
19. Williamson M.R. and Williamson S.L. *Gamuts in Ultrasound.* Philadelphia: WB Saunders, 1992.
20. Zollo A.J. *Medical Secrets.* Philadelphia: Hanley & Belfus, Inc. 1991.

Index

A

Abdomen
  arterial flow characteristics in, 279
  cross section of, 189
  muscles of, 193
  ultrasound of, 74
  venous flow characteristics in, 281
Abdominal wall
  anatomy of, 193
  anomalies of, 194–195
  technical factors and, 206
  US appearance of, 193
Abscess(es)
  amebic, 136
  appendiceal, 63
  breast, 29
  diverticular, 64
  hepatic, 136
  pericholecystic, 46
  peritoneal cavity, 196
  prostatic, 216
  pyogenic, 136
  renal, 100, 101
  scrotal, 230
  seminal vesicle, 217
  splenic, 248
  submandibular
    US appearance of, 154
Acid phosphatase (ACP/SAP) test
  prostate gland and, 213
Acinar cells
  pancreatic, 175
Acoustic shadowing
  in gallbladder sonography, 55
ACP/SAP test. See Acid phosphatase (ACP/
  SAP) test
ACTH test. See Adrenocorticotropic hormone
  (ACTH) test
Acute lobar nephronia (acute focal bacterial
  nephritis), 94
Acute tubular necrosis
  in kidney transplant failure, 106
  renal failure in, 102
Adenocarcinoma
  pancreatic, 178
  prostatic, 215, 217
Adenolymphoma (Warthin's tumor), 153
Adenoma
  adrenal gland, 5
  gallbladder, 52
  liver, 142
  parathyroid, 161
  pleomorphic
    salivary gland, 153, 154
  thyroid, 162
Adenomatoid tumor
  extratesticular, 234
Adenomyomatosis (hyperplastic
  cholecystosis)
  of gallbladder, 52, 53

Adenopathy
  sonographic differential for, 249
Adhesions, 71
Adrenal glands
  adult, 1, 2
  anatomy of
    normal, 1
  anomalies of
    adenoma, 5, 8
    adrenogenital syndromes, 6
    carcinoma, 5, 9
    cysts, 5
    hemorrhage, 5, 8
    hyeraldosteronism, 6
    hypercortisolism, 6
    hyperfunction of cortex, 6
    insufficiency, 6
    tumors, 7, 8, 9
  approaches to, 10
  arterial supply to, 3
  fetal, 2
  infant, 1
  lab tests and, 4
  masses in
    displacement of regional anatomy by, 4
    origin of, 4
  neonatal, 2
  physiology of, 3
  structure of, 1
  technical factors and, 10
  US appearance of, 2
  vasculature of, 3
Adrenal insufficiency (hypoadrenalism)
  primary and secondary, 6
Adrenocorticotropic hormone (ACTH) test, 4
Adult polycystic kidney disease (APKD), 85
Adventitia
  of large bowel, 58
AIDS cholangitis, 18
Alanine aminotransferase (ALT) values, 128
Albumin values, 128
Aldosterone test, 4
Aliasing artifact
  in Doppler ultrasound, 301
Alkaline phosphatase (Alk Phos, ALP)
    values, 128
  gallbladder and, 41
  pancreas and, 177
  parathyroid glands and, 160
  prostate gland and, 213
Ampulla of Vater (sphincter of Oddi), 169
Amylase, 175
  blood study, 177
  pancreas and, 177
  urine study, 177
Anal canal, 57
Anastomoses, 289
Aneurysm(s)
  abdominal aortic, 282
  carotid artery, 285

  classification of, 284–285
  false, 283, 284
    dissecting, 284
    pseudoaneurysm, 284
  popliteal artery, 285
  renal artery, 285
  splanchnic artery, 285
  survival criteria for, 284
  true
    berry, 284
    fusiform, 285
    saccular, 285
Angiomyolipoma
  renal, 83
Angiosarcoma (hemangiosarcoma)
  hepatic, 143
Aorta
  anatomy of, 272
  blood flow characteristics of, 279
  disssection of, 286
  grafts of, 286
  retroperitoneal, 274
  rupture of, 283
  ultrasound technique in, 306
APKD. See Adult polycystic kidney disease
  (APKD)
Appendicitis, 63
Appendix
  with fecolith, 63
  inflammation/infection of, 63
  size and location of, 58
  structure of, 57
  ultrasound technique for, 74
Areola, 23, 24
Arterioles
  anatomy of, 267
  renal, 81
Arteriosclerosis, 287
Arteriovenous (AV) fistulas
  renal arterial, 106
Arteriovenous shunt, 289
Artery(ies)
  adrenal gland, 3
  anatomy of
    normal, 267
  breast, 26
  Doppler ultrasound evaluation of, 301
  grafts of, 286
  of head and neck, 272
  hepatic, 123, 125
  of lower extremities, 270–271
  mammary, 26
  mesentery, 172, 274, 279
  pancreatic, 175
  peripheral, 288
  popliteal, 270, 271
  portal, 126
  renal, 79, 80, 81
    calcification of, 107
  retroperitoneal, 274

Artery(ies) (*continued*)
   of salivary glands, 152
   splanchnic, 285
   subclavian, 272, 273
   thoracic, 26
   of upper extremities, 273
   US appearance of, 269
Ascariasis
   biliary, 15
Ascending colon, 57
Ascites
   exudative and transudative, 197
Asplenia, 245
Artery(ies)
   thoracic, 26
Atheroma, 287
Atheromatous plaque, 287
Atherosclerosis, 287
Atresia
   biliary, 15
Axillary artery, 26, 273
Axillary vein, 273

B

Baker's cyst (popliteal bursitis), 290
Bartholin duct, sublingual, 151
Basilic vein, 273
Basophils, 244
Benign prostate hyperplasia (BPH), 214
Bifid ureters, 263
Bile
   function of, 41
Bile ducts, 11–22
   anatomy of, 11–13, 36
   anomalies of
      ascariasis, 15
      atresia, 15
      Caroli's disease, 17
      cholangiosarcoma, 16
      cholangitis, 18
      choledochal cyst, 19
      choledocholithiasis, 20
      cystadenocarcinoma, 16
      cystadenoma, 16
      cystic, 11
      differential pathology of, 21
      metastasis to, 16
      neoplasms, 16
      pneumobilia, 21
      wall thickening, 21
   common, 11, 12, 14
   compression of, 21
   dilated, 21
   hepatic, 11
   hepatic artery and, 13
   intrahepatic, 11
   physiology of, 14
   structure of, 11
   technical factors and, 22
   US appearance of, 13–14
Biliary tree
   abnormal in relation to gallbladder, 22
   normal and dilated, 13
Bilirubin measurement
   gallbladder and, 41
   pancreas and, 177
   urine and, 129

Bilomas
   peritoneal cavity, 198
Biopsy
   breast, 34
   transrectal ultrasound scanning with, 218
Bladder
   anatomy of
      normal, 256
      regional, 256
   anomalies of
      calculi, 257
      cystitis, 258
      differential of, 262
      diverticula, 259
      metastases to, 260
      neoplastic, 260
   in hydronephrosis, 93
   physiology of, 256
   urinary
      structure of, 253
   US appearance of, 255
   wall of, 254
Bladder neck
   outlet obstruction of
      causes of, 261
Blood flow
   arterial
      on Doppler ultrasound, 301
      pulsativity index of, 304
      resistive index of, 304
      ultrasound measurement of, 304
      velocity of, 304
      velocity ratio of, 304
   regulation of, 276
   venous
      on Doppler ultrasound, 302
Blood glucose
   conditions affecting, 176
Blood pressure, 276
Blood urea nitrogen (BUN) determination, 82
Bowel
   large. *See* Large bowel
   small. *See* Small bowel
   thickening of, 73
BPH. *See* Benign prostate hyperplasia (BPH)
Brachial artery, 273
Brachial vein, 273
Brachiocephalic (innominate) artery, 272, 273
Brachiocephalic (innominate) vein, 272, 273
Breast (mammary glands), 23–25
   anatomy of, 23
   anomalies of
      carcinoma, 28–29
      cysts and cystic structures, 29–30
   arteries and veins in, 26
   augmentation/prosthesis of
      rupture of, 27
   development of, 26
   lymphatics in, 26
   physiology of, 26
   sonography of
      in biopsy of, 34
      in cyst aspiration, 34
      documentation of, 33
      indications for, 32
      patient position for, 32
      scan planes in, 32

      in stereotactic biopsy, 34
      technical factors in, 32–35
      transducer in, 32
   structure of, 23
   ultrasound lesions in
      interpretation of, 35
   US appearance of
      age-related changes in, 24
      normal, 24–25
   vasculature of, 26
Budd-Chiari syndrome, 146
Burkitt's lymphoma, 250

C

Calcification
   renal, 107
Calcinosis
   renal
      cortical, 84
      medullary, 84
Calcium levels
   parathyroid glands and, 160
Calf arteries, 270, 271
Calf veins, 270, 271
Calyceal diverticula calcification, 107
Candida lesions
   hepatic, 136
Capillary
   anatomy of, 267
Carboxypolypeptidase, 175
Carcinoma
   adrenal gland, 5, 9
   breast, 28
      infiltrating lobular, 28
      invasive ductal, 28
      ultrasound for, 29
   colorectal, 69
   gastric, 69
   gastrointestinal, 69
      sonographic appearance of, 70
   hepatocellular, 143
   liver function tests in, 129
   parathyroid gland, 161
   renal
      transitional cell, 97
   renal cell, 96
   thyroid gland
      anaplastic, 163
      follicular, 163
      medullary, 163
      papillary, 163
Carcinomatosis
   peritoneal, 201
Cardia
   structure of, 56
Caroli's disease, 17, 22
Carotid artery disease
   Doppler criteria for, 288
Carotid artery(ies)
   aneurysm of, 285
   common, 272
   external, 272
   flow characteristics of: arterial waveform, 277–278
   internal, 272
   ultrasound technique and, 309
Catecholamines, 4

Cavernoma
 in portal hypertension, 148
Cavernous hemangioma
 splenic, 250
Cecum, 57
Celiac artery
 axis/trunk, 274
 blood flow characteristics of, 279
Cephalic vein, 273
Cholangiosarcoma
 biliary, 16
 hepatic. *See* Angiosarcoma
  (hemangiosarcoma)
Cholangitis
 AIDS-related, 18
 of bile ducts, 18
 recurrent pyogenic, 18
 sclerosing, 18
Cholecystitis
 acute
  acalculous and calculous, 44, 45
 chronic, 45
 complications of, 46–47
 emphysematous, 46
 gangrenous, 46
 pericholecystic abscess in, 46
 xanthogranulomatous, 47
Choledochal cysts, 22
Choledocholithiasis
 of bile ducts, 20
Cholelithiasis, 48
 sonographic appearance of, 49
Cholesterolosis
 of gallbladder, 52, 53
Choriocarcinoma, 165
 testicular, 234
Chymotrypsin, 175
Circulation
 physiology of, 276
Cirrhosis
 of liver, 130
 liver function tests in, 129
CIVs. *See* Common iliac veins (CIVs)
Colitis
 neutropenic, 72
 ulcerative, 67
Collecting duct
 renal, 81
Collecting system
 calcification of, 107
 renal
  anatomy of, 76
  duplication of, 111
  structure of, 75
Colon. *See also* Large bowel; Mesocolon
 ascending, 57
 descending, 57
 metastases to, 70
 transverse, 57
Color (flow) Doppler, 305
Column of Bertin, 110
Common bile duct (CBD), 11
 enlarged, 14
 pancreas and, 172
 size of, 12
Common carotid artery, 155
Common iliac veins (CIVs), 274
Common interosseous artery, 273

Competence
 of veins
  on Doppler ultrasound, 302
Complete blood count (CBC)
 spleen and, 243
Conn's syndrome (hyperaldosteronism), 6
Cooper's ligaments, 23, 24
Core biopsy
 of breast
  sonography in, 34
Coronary ligaments, 119
 hepatic, 187, 188, 189
Corpora amylacea
 echogenicity of, 210
Cortex
 adrenal, 1, 2
 hyperfunction of, 6
 masses in, 4
 physiology of, 3
 renal
  anatomy of, 76
  calcification of, 107
  calcinosis of, 84
  cysts of, 89
  disease of, 107
  structure of, 75
Cortisol test, 4
Courvoisier's gallbladder, 50
Courvoisier's sign, 22
Cretinism, 165
Crohn's disease (ileitis/regional enteritis/
  granulomatous enterocolitis), 67
 comparison with ulcerative colitis, 68
Crura
 of diaphragm, 191
  US appearance of, 192
Cryptorchidism (undescended testis), 226
Cushing's syndrome (hypercortisolism), 6
Cystadenocarcinoma, 22
 biliary, 16
Cystadenoma, 22
 biliary, 16
Cystic disease
 renal, 85–88
Cystic duct
 of gallbladder, 36
  sonogram of, 38
Cystic tumors
 pancreatic
  mucinous and serous, 179
Cyst(s). *See also* Pseudocyst(s)
 adrenal, 5
 breast
  hemorrhagic, 29, 30
  simple, 30
 choledochal, 18
 duplication, 65
 echinococcal, 137
 epidermoid, 228
 epididymal, 227
 hepatic, 137, 138
  nonparasitic, 137, 138
  parasitic, 137, 138
 intratesticular, 228
 mesenteric/omental, 198
 pancreatic, 180
 paraovarian, 263
 parapelvic, 98

 pararenal, 98
 prostatic, 216
 renal, 89
  dialysis-associated, 89
  hemorrhagic/infected, 89
  parapelvic/pararenal, 89
  simple cortical, 89
 salivary gland, 153
 seminal vesicle, 217, 263
 splenic, 246
 testicular, 228
 thyroglossal duct, 162
 thyroid, 162
 tunica albuginea, 227
 urachal, 205

D
Descending colon, 57
Desmoid tumors
 of abdominal wall, 201
Dexamethasone suppression test (DST), 4
Diaphragm
 movement of
  measurement of, 191
 structure of, 191
 technical factors and, 206
 US appearance of, 192
Diverticula, 64
Diverticulitis, 64
Diverticulosis, 64
Doppler flow studies
 of kidney transplant, 104, 105
Doppler ultrasound
 of arteries, 277, 301
 color (flow), 305
 continuous wave, 299
 duplex, 300
 of kidney, 115
 power (angio), 305
 pulsed, 299, 300
 spectral, 300
 of vasculature, 298
  comparison of continuous wave and
   pulsed, 299
 of veins, 301
Doppler wave forms
 of head and neck arteries, 277–278
Double arc sign, 40
Duct of Santorini. *See* Pancreatic duct (duct
  of Santorini)
Duct(s)
 ejaculatory, 207
 lactiferous, 23
 mammary, 23
 parotid, 151
 sublingual, 151
 thyroglossal, 162
Ductus (vas) deferens/seminal duct
 anatomy of
  normal, 219–220
 structure of, 219
Duodenum, 169
 structure of, 56

E
Effusion
 pleural, 203, 206

Effusion (*continued*)
  into scrotum, 233
Ejaculatory ducts, 207
Electrolyte levels, 82
Embryonal cell carcinoma, 234
Empyema
  in acute cholecystitis, 46
Endocrine regulation
  kidney in, 81
Endoscopic ultrasound, 74
Enteritis
  regional, 67
Enterocolitis
  granulomatous, 67
Eosinophilia, 244
Eosinophils, 244
Epidermoid cyst
  testicular, 228
Epididymis
  anatomy of
    normal, 219–220, 221
  anomalies of
    cysts, 227
    enlarged, 237
  Doppler US appearance of, 221
  pathology of, 237
  physiology of, 224
  structure of, 219
  vasculature of, 223
Epididymitis, 230
Epididymo-orchitis, 230
Epinephrine (adrenaline), 3
Erythrocyte (RBC) count
  spleen and, 243
Esophagus, 155
  structure of, 56
Extremities
  vascular system of
    lower, 270–271
    ultrasound technique and, 308
    upper, 273

F
Falciform ligament, 119, 187, 188, 189
Fat liver, 131–132
Fecal blood test, 61
Fecaliths, 59
Feces
  examination of, 61
Femoral veins, 270, 271
Fetoprotein (AFP) values, 128
Fibroadenoma
  of breast, 31
Fibrocystic change
  of breast, 31
Fibrolipomatosis. *See* Renal sinus
    lipomatosis (fibrolipomatosis)
Fibrosis
  retroperitoneal, 204
Fine needle aspiration (FNA)
  of parathyroid glands, 168
  of thyroid gland, 168
Fine needle aspiration biopsy (FNAB)
  sonography in, 34
Fistula(s)
  renal, arteriovenous, 106

urachal, 205
vascular, 289
Fluid collection
  extraperitoneal *versus* intraperitoneal,
    206
  peritoneal, 198–199
  pleural *versus* subdiaphragmatic, 206
  retroperitoneal *versus* intraperitoneal,
    206
  subcapsular *versus* intraperitoneal, 206
Fluid regulation
  kidney in, 81
FNA. *See* Fine needle aspiration (FNA)
Focal nodular hyperplasia (FNP)
  hepatic, 133
Foramen of Winslow (epiploid/omental
    foramen), 186, 187, 189
Fungus balls
  renal, 94

G
Galactoceles, 29, 30
Gallbladder, 36–56
  anatomy of, 36–37
  anomalies of
    adenoma, 52, 53
    adenomyomatosis, 52
    carcinoma
    cholecystitis, 44
    cholelithiasis, 48–49
    cholesterolosis cholesterol polyp, 52,
      53
    congenital, 49
    contracted, 39–40
    Courvoisier's gallbladder, 50
    enlarged, 50
    hydropic, 50
    metastasis to, 42–43
    sludge in, 51
  appearance differential of, 54
  and bile function, 42
  biliary tree abnormalities and, 22
  differential for masses of, 54
  fossa shadowing of, 54
  lab tests and, 41
  nonvisualization of, 54
  normal, 37–38
  physiology of, 41
  structure of, 36
  structures mimicking, 54
  technical factors in, 55
  US appearance of
    "wes" triad/"double arc" sign, 40
    visualization error and, 40
  wall thickness of, 52, 53, 54
Ganglioneuroma
  of adrenal medulla, 7, 9
Gartner's duct, 263
Gastrin test, 61
Gastroduodenal artery, 274
  pancreas and, 172
Gastrointestinal tract, 56–74
  anatomy of, 56–58
    sonographic, 59
  anomalies of
    appendiceal mucocele, 62

appendicitis, 63
carcinoma, 69
diverticular disease, 64
duplication cysts, 65
hypertrophic pyloric stenosis, 66
inflammatory bowel disease, 67
lymphoma, 69
malignancies, 69
metastases to, 70
obstruction, 71
  causes of, 71
pseudomyxoma peritonei, 62
typhlitis, 72
lab tests and, 61
operation of
  chemical, 60
  mechanical, 60
  physiology of, 60
size and location of, 58
structure of, 56–58
ultrasound of
  abdominal, 74
  endoscopic, 74
Germ cell tumors
  testicular, 234–235
Globulin values, 128
Glomerulonephritis, 94
Glomerulus, 81
Glucagon, 175
Glucocorticoids, 3
Glucose testing
  pancreas and, 177
Glutaminic pyruvic transaminase (SGPT)
    values, 128
Glycogen storage disease: type 1 von
    Gierke's, 133
Goiters
  simple and multinodular, 164
Gonadal stromal tumors, 235
Gonadocorticoids, 3
Graft(s)
  aortic/arterial, 286
Graves' disease, 165
Gray-scale imaging
  of vasculature, 297

H
Hartman's pouch
  sonogram of, 38
Hashimoto's disease, 166
Haustra, 57
HB. *See* HBG; Hemoglobin (HB)
HBG. *See* HBG; Hemoglobin (HB)
HCC. *See* Hepatocellular carcinoma (HCC)
HCT. *See* Hematocrit (HCT)
Head
  arterial flow characteristics of, 278
Heart rate, 276
Hemangioma
  cavernous, 140
Hemangiosarcoma (angiosarcoma). *See*
    Angiosarcoma (hemangiosarcoma)
  splenic, 250
Hematocele, 229
Hematocrit (HCT)
  spleen and, 243

Hematologic disease
  liver function tests in, 129
Hematoma(s)
  abdominal wall, 194, 195
  breast, 29
  hepatic, 141
  intratesticular, 233
  parenchymal, 90
  periphrenic, 90
  peritoneal cavity, 198
  renal, 90, 100
  subcapsular, 90
Hematuria, 82
Hemoglobin (HB, HBG)
  spleen and, 243
Hemorrhage
  adrenal, 5, 8
  peritoneal cavity, 198
  renal, 100
Hemorrhagic cysts
  of breast, 29, 30
Hepatic arteries, 274
  blood flow characteristics of, 279
  location of, 13
Hepatic duct, 36
Hepatic veins, 274
  flow characteristics in, 281
Hepatitis
  acute and chronic, 143
  liver function tests in, 129
Hepatitis panel, 128
Hepatoblastoma, 144
Hepatocellular carcinoma (HCC), 143
Hepatoduodenal ligament, 119
Hepatogastric ligament, 119
Hernias, 71
  abdominal wall, 194, 195
Hodgkin's lymphoma, 250
Hookwire localization
  presurgical
    sonography in, 34
Horseshoe kidney, 113
HPS. *See* Hypertrophic pyloric stenosis
  (HPS)
Human chorionic gonadotropin test, 224
Hydatid cyst
  hepatic, 137–138
Hydatidiform mole, 165
Hydrocele, 229
Hydronephrosis
  fetal and maternal, 92
  types and causes of, 93
  unilateral mild, 91
  US appearance of, 92
Hydroureter, 264
Hyoid bone, 155
Hyperadrenalism, 6
Hypercortisolism. *See* Cushing's syndrome
  (hypercortisolism)
Hyperglycemia, 176
Hyperplasia
  parathyroid, primary, 161
Hyperthyroidism
  causes of, 161, 165
Hypertrophic pyloric stenosis (HPS), 66
Hypoadrenalism. *See* Adrenal insufficiency
  (hypoadrenalism)

Hypoglycemia, 176
Hypothyroidism
  causes of, 161, 165

I

IJV. *See* Internal jugular vein (IJV)
Ileitis, 67
Ileocecal sphincter, 57
Ileocecal syndrome, 72
Ileum
  structure of, 56
Iliac arteries, 270, 271
  blood flow characteristics of, 279
  common, 274
Iliac vein(s)
  common, 270, 271, 274
  external, 270, 271
  flow characteristics in, 281
  internal, 270, 271
Infantile polycystic kidney disease (IPKD),
  86
Infarct
  splenic, 248
  testicular, 233
Inferior vena cava (IVC), 274
Inflammatory bowel disease, 67
Innominate artery. *See* Brachiocephalic
  (innominate) artery
Insulin, 175
Intercostal arteries, 26
Internal jugular vein (IJV), 155
Intestinal malrotation, 71
  US appearance of, 71
Intravenous catheter
  filters in, 290
  tumors of, 291
  ultrasound technique and, 307
  venous flow characteristics and, 281
Intussusception, 71
IPKD (infantile polycystic kidney disease),
  86
Islet cell tumor, 181
Islets of Langerhans, pancreatic, 175, 176
IVC. *See* Inferior vena cava (IVC)

J

Jaundice
  obstructive
    liver function tests in, 129
Jejunum
  structure of, 56
Jugular vein, 272
  flow characteristics in, 280
  internal, 155

K

Kidneys, 75–108. *See also* Renal; Renal
  failure
  anatomy of, 76
    regional, 77
    vascular, 76, 79
  anomalies of
    acute lobar nephronia, 94
    agenesis, 109

    benign tumors, 83
    bilateral small, 108
    calcification, 84, 107, 108
    column of Bertin/renal column
      hypertrophy, 110
    congenital, 109
    cystic disease, 85–86
    cystic mass, 108
    cysts, 89
    ectopic, 112
    enlarged, 108
    extrarenal pelvis, 112
    hematoma, 90
    horseshoe, 113
    hydronephrosis, 91
    hypoplasia, 109
    inflammatory disease, 94–95
    junctional parenchymal defect, 114
    malignancy, 96–97
    multicystic dysplastic, 88
    multiple cystic structures in, 108
    parapelvic/pararenal cysts, 98
    pediatric neoplasms, 99
    perinephric collections, 100, 101
    pyonephrosis, 91, 92
    splenic hump, 114
    variants of normal, 109
  arteries of, 79
  blood flow pattern of, 79
    anatomy of, 79
    Doppler, 79
  collecting system in
    duplication of, 111
  collecting system of, 75
  cortex of, 75
  cystic area at hilum, 108
  echogenicity of, 78
  function of, 81
  lab tests and, 82
  medical disease of, 107
  medullary, 75
    cystic, 87
  operation of, 81
  physiology of, 81
  pseudokidney, 114
  renal vessels of, 79–80
    relationship between, 80
  sonography of
    differentials in, 108
    Doppler, 115
    positions in, 115
    technical factors in, 115
    technique in, 115
    transducer in, 115
  splenic relationship to, 252
  structure of, 75
  transplantation of
    Doppler flow studies in, 104, 105
    failure of, 106
    US roles in, 104
  transplanted
    abnormal Doppler findings in, 106
    graft rupture and, 106
  US appearance of, 101
  vascularity of, 79–80
  veins of, 79
Klatskin tumor, 22

L

Lactic acid dehydrogenase (LDH) values, 129
Lactiferous sinuses, 23
Large bowel, 58
  anatomy of
    sonographic, 59
  appendix of, 58
  intestinal wall of, 58
  structure of, 57
  ultrasound technique for, 74
LCA. *See* Liver cell adenoma (LCA)
Lesser sac (lesser omental bursa), 186, 187, 189
Leukemia
  testicular neoplasms from, 231
Leukocytes
  evaluation of, 244
  gallbladder and, 41
Leukocytosis, 244
Leukopenia, 244
Leydig cell tumor (hyperplasia)
  testicular, 235
Ligamentum teres (round ligament), 119, 122
Ligamentum venosum, 119
Lipase, 175
  pancreas and, 177
Lipomatosis
  renal sinus, 103, 107
Liver, 116–148
  anatomy of
    gross, 116
    ligaments of, 119
    lobar, 116–117
    normal, 120
    segmental, 118
  anomalies of
    glycogen storage disease
      type 1 von Gierke's, 133
    hematoma, 141
  anterior and posterior views of, 189
  bare area of, 119
  caudate lobe, 116, 118
  coronary ligaments of, 188
  diaphragm interface with, 192
  diffuse anomalies of, 130–134
    cirrhosis, 130
    differentials with sonographic findings in, 135
    fatty change in, 131–132
  echogenicity of, 121–122
    fissures and, 121
    parenchyma and, 121
  focal anomalies of, 136–144
    abscess/inflammatory lesions, 136
    adenoma, 142
    cavernous hemangioma, 140
    differentials with sonographic findings, 145
    focal nodular hyperplasia of, 139
    malignancy of, 143–144
    metastases to, 144
  hepatic, 187, 188, 189
  hepatitis and, 134
  lab tests and, 128–129
  left lobe of, 116, 117, 118
  physiology of, 127
  right lobe of, 116, 117, 118
  structure of, 116

vascular anomalies of
  Budd-Chiari syndrome, 146
  portal hypertension/obstruction, 147–148
vasculature of
  blood supply and drainage in, 124
  comparison of hepatic, 123
  hepatic vessels and origins in, 125
  portal systemic venous collaterals and, 126
Liver cell adenoma (LCA), 142
Liver function tests, 129
Lobes
  breast, 23, 24
Longus colli muscle, 155
Lower extremities
  arterial flow characteristics in, 279
  vascular system of, 270–271
    arterial, 270, 271
    venous, 270, 271
  venous flow characteristics in, 280
Lung
  diaphragm interface with, 192
Lymphadenopathy
  AIDS-related, 248
  mesenteric/omental, 249
  retroperitoneal, 249
Lymphangioma
  cystic
    splenic, 250
Lymphatics
  of breast, 26
  of thyroid and parathyroid glands, 158
Lymphatic system
  anatomy of, 241
  physiology of, 242
  technical factors and, 252
  US appearance of, 241
Lymph nodes
  breast, 23, 24, 25
Lymphocele
  renal, 100, 101
Lymphoceles
  retroperitoneal and peritoneal, 198, 199
Lymphocytes, 244
Lymphoma
  mesenteric, 201
  renal, 96
  submandibular
    US appearance of, 154
  testicular neoplasms from, 231

M

Mammary glands. *See* Breast (mammary glands)
Mastitis, 30
MCDK. *See* Multicystic dysplastic kidney (MCDK)/cystic renal dysplasia
Medulla
  adrenal, 1
    masses in, 4
    physiology of, 3
    sonographic appearance of, 2
  renal
    calcinosis of, 84
    cystic, 87
    disease of, 107
    structure of, 75

Medullary carcinoma
  of breast, 28
Megaloureter, 264
Menopause
  breast in, 26
Mesenteric artery(ies)
  inferior and superior, 274
Mesenteries
  anatomy of, 187, 188–189
  anomalies of
    mesenteritis, 200
  lymphadenopathy of, 249
  technical factors and, 206
Mesenteritis, 200
Mesentery artery(ies)
  blood flow characteristics of, 279
Mesoappendix, 57
Mesoblastic nephroma (fetal renal hamartoma), 99
Mesocolon, 57. *See also* Colon
  sigmoid, 187, 188, 189
  transverse, 187, 188, 189
Mesothelioma, 201, 202
Metastases
  from adrenal masses, 4
  to adrenal medulla, 7, 8
  to biliary system, 16
  to gastrointestinal tract, 70
  to kidney, 96
  to liver, 144
  to testes, 235
  to thyroid gland, 165
Mineralocorticoids, 3
Mirrizzi syndrome, 20, 22
Monocytes, 244
Monocytosis, 244
Mucinous carcinoma
  of breast, 28
Mucocele
  appendiceal, 62
Mucosa
  of gastrointestinal tract, 58
Mucous membrane
  of gastrointestinal tract, 58
Multicystic dysplastic kidney (MCDK)/cystic renal dysplasia, 88
Muscle(s)
  abdominal, 193
  head and neck, 151
  muscularis propria, 58
  pectoralis, 23, 24, 193
Myxedema, 165

N

Neck
  arterial flow characteristics and, 278
  vascular system of, 272
  venous flow characteristics in, 280
Neoplasm(s)
  abdominal wall, 194
  salivary gland, 153
  seminal vesicle, 217
Nephritis
  acute focal bacterial. *See* Acute lobar nephronia (acute focal bacterial nephritis)
Nephroblastoma (Wilms' tumor), 97, 99

Nephrocalcinosis
    renal medullary, 107
Nephrolithiasis (renal stones/calculi), 84, 107
Nephron, 81
Nephrotoxicity
    chronic
        renal failure in, 102
Neuroblastoma
    of adrenal medulla, 7, 9
Neurogenic tumors
    retroperitoneal, 201
Neurovascular bundles
    of thyroid and parathyroid glands, 156
Neutropenia, 244
Neutrophilia, 244
Neutrophils (PMNS), 244
Non-Hodgkin lymphoma, 250
Norepinephrine (noradrenaline), 3
Nuclear medicine
    spleen, 244

O
Occlusion
    renal arterial
        Doppler findings in, 106
Omental bursae
    lesser. See Lesser sac (lesser omental
        bursa)
Omentum
    greater and lesser, 187, 188, 189
    lesser, 119
Omohyoid muscle, 155
Oncocytoma
    renal, 83
Orchitis, 230–231
    acute and chronic, 230
    granulomatous, 230
Oriental cholangitis (recurrent pyogenic), 18
Outlet obstruction
    bladder neck, 261

P
Pampiniform plexus, 237
Pancreas, 169–184
    anatomy of
        normal, 169, 171
        regional, 170–171
        sonographic, 172
    anomalies of, 178–183
        adenocarcinoma, 178
        annular pancreas, 171
        cystic tumors of, 179
        cysts, 180
        islet cell tumor, 181
        pancreas divisum, 171
        pancreatitis, 182–183
    differential diagnosis in region of, 184
    ductal system of, 169
    echogenicity of, 174
        with aging, 174
    lab tests and, 177
        blood studies, 177
        urine studies, 177
    physiology of, 175
    splenic relationship to, 252
    technical factors and, 184

US appearance of, 173
vasculature of, 172, 175
Pancreatic duct (duct of Santorini), 169
Pancreatitis
    acute, 182
    chronic, 182–183
    moderate (edematous), 182
    severe (acute hemorrhagic/necrotizing),
        182
Pancytopenia, 243
Papilla
    duodenal, 169
Papillary carcinoma
    of breast, 28
Papillary necrosis
    renal, 107
Papilloma
    of bladder, 260
    of breast, 31
Paracolic gutters, 186, 187, 189
Pararenal space, 190, 191
Parathormone, 159
Parathyroid glands
    anatomy of
        normal, 156
        regional, 155
    echogenicity of, 156
    fine needle aspiration of, 168
    lab tests and, 160
    percutaneous biopsy of, 168
    physiology of, 159
    technical factors and, 168
    US appearance of, 156, 157
    vasculature of, 158
Parathyroid hormone
    parathyroid glands and, 160
Parenchyma
    hepatic, 121, 127
    physiology of, 242
Parotid gland
    sonographic appearance of, 152
    structure of, 151
Parotid (Stensen's) duct, 151
Patency
    of veins on Doppler ultrasound, 302
Pectoralis muscles, 23, 24, 193
Pelvic cul-de-sacs, 186, 187, 189
Percutaneous biopsy
    of parathyroid glands, 168
    of thyroid gland, 168
Perforation
    of gallbladder
        in acute cholecystitis, 46
Peripheral arterial disease, 288
Perirenal space, 190, 191
Peritoneal cavity
    anatomy of, 185, 186, 187, 189
        normal, 185
    anomalies of
        abscess, 196
        ascites, 197
        cystic collections and cysts, 198–199
        pleural effusion, 203
    technical factors and, 206
Peritoneum. See also Retroperitoneum
    anatomy of
        normal, 185
    anomalies of

neoplastic, 201–202
    pleural effusion, 203
    technical factors and, 206
    visceral, 58
Periurethral glands, 207
pH
    of urine, 82
Pheochromocytoma
    of adrenal medulla, 7, 9
Phosphorus determination, 82
Phrenic artery, 3
Phrygian cap, 37, 38
Plantar arteries, 270, 271
Plantar veins, 270, 271
Plaque
    atheromatous, 287
    composition and echogenicity of, 288
    gray-scale imaging of, 297
Platelet count (PLTS), 244
Platysma muscle, 155
Pleural effusion, 203, 206
Pneumobilia, 21
Polycystic disease
    hepatic, 137, 138
    renal failure in, 102
Polycythemia, 243
Polyp
    cholesterol, 52, 53
Polysplenia, 245
Popliteal artery, 270, 271
    aneurysm of, 285
Popliteal bursitis. See Baker's cyst (popliteal
        bursitis)
Porcelain gallbladder, 46
Portal circulation, 275
Portal hypertension, 147
    types of, 148
Portal system
    mesenteric veins, 274
Portal veins, 123, 124, 125, 274
    flow characteristics in, 281
    obstruction pf, 147
Power (angio) Doppler, 305
Pregnancy
    breast in, 26
Prostate gland. See also Seminal vesicles
    anatomy of
        normal, 209
        regional, 209
        zonal, 207
    anomalies of
        abscess, 216
        adenocarcinoma, 215
        benign prostate hyperplasia, 214
        cyst, 215
        prostatitis, 216
    coronal view of, 207, 208
    echogenicity of, 210–211
    in hydronephrosis, 93
    lab tests and, 213
    physiology of, 212
    structure of, 207
    technical factors and, 218
    US appearance of, 210–211
        transabdominal, 211
Prostate specific antigen (PSA) test, 213
    normal values for, 213
Prostatitis, 216

Prostatodynia, 215
Proteinuria, 82
Prothrombin (PT/PTT) values, 129
Pseudoaneurysm, 283
Pseudocyst(s). *See also* Cyst(s)
    pancreatic, 100, 180, 198, 199
    splenic, 246
Pseudokidney, 114
Pseudomyxoma peritonei, 201, 202
    gastrointestinal, 62
Puberty
    breast in, 26
Pyelonephritis
    acute, 94, 95
    chronic, 95
        with urolithiasis, 95
    renal failure in, 102
    xanthogranulomatous pyelonephritis, 95
Pylorus
    structure of, 56
    ultrasound technique for, 74
Pyocele, 229
Pyonephrosis, 91, 92

R

Radial artery, 273
Radial vein, 273
Radioactive iodine uptake (RAIU) I-131
    uptake
    thyroid gland and, 160
RAS. *See* Renal artery stenosis (RAS)
Rectum, 57
Rejection
    acute
        of kidney transplant, 106
Renal. *See also* Kidneys
Renal arteries, 3, 274
    acute occlusion of
        in kidney transplant failure, 106
    aneurysm of, 285
    blood flow characteristics of, 279
Renal artery stenosis (RAS), 292
Renal failure
    acute, 102
    causes of, 102
    chronic, 103
Renal insufficiency, 103
Renal pelvis
    in hydronephrosis, 93
Renal sinus lipomatosis (fibrolipomatosis),
    103
Renal veins, 274
    flow characteristics in, 281
    thrombosis of, 292
Rete testis, dilated, 228
Retroperitoneum. *See also* Peritoneum
    anatomy of
        normal, 190
        regional, 191
    anomalies of
        fibrosis, 204
        fluid collections in, 206
        lymphadenopathy, 249
        neoplastic, 201–202
    structure of, 190–191
    technical factors and, 206
    vasculature of, 274–275
Rivinus duct, sublingual, 151

S

Salivary glands
    anatomy of
        normal, 151
    anomalies of
        cysts, 153
        enlargement, 153
        inflammation/infection, 153
        tumors, 153
    physiology of, 152
    technical factors for, 154
    US appearance of, 152
    vasculature of, 152
Saphenous veins, 270, 271
Sarcoma
    retroperitoneal, 201
Scalenus muscle, 155
Scrotum
    anatomy of
        normal, 219–220
    anomalies of
        calcification, 225
        effusion into, 233
        epidido-orchitis, 230
        epididymitis, 230
        hematocele, 229
        hernia into, 228
        hydrocele, 229
        infection/inflammation of, 230–231
        pyocele, 229
    differentials in sonography of, 237
    Doppler US appearance of, 221
    pathology of, 237
    physiology of, 224
    structure of, 219
    technical factors and, 238
    vasculature of, 223
Seminal vesicles, 207. *See also* Prostate
        gland
    anatomy of, 212
    anomalies of, 217
        congenital absence of, 217
        cysts of, 263
        dilation of, 217
    physiology of, 212
    technical factors and, 218
    US appearance of, 212
Seminomas
    testicular, 234
Serosa
    of large bowel, 58
Serum amylase determination, 61
Serum glutamic oxaloacetic transaminase
        (SGOT) values, 128, 129
Serum glutamic pyruvic transaminase
        (SGPT), 128
Sex hormones, 3
SGOT. *See* Serum glutamic oxaloacetic
        transaminase (SGOT)
SGPT. *See* Glutaminic pyruvic transaminase
        (SGPT) values; Serum glutamic
        pyruvic transaminase (SGPT)
Sialadenitis, 153
Sialolithiasis, with sialadenitis/infection, 153
Sialosis, 153
Sigmoid colon, 57
Sludge
    in gallbladder
        types of, 51

Small bowel, 188
    anatomy of
        sonographic, 59
    cross section of, 58
    size and location of, 58
    structure of, 56
    ultrasound technique for, 74
SMA syndrome, 71
Somatostatin, 175
Spermatic cord
    anatomy of
        normal, 219–220
    structure of, 219
    torsion of, 232
Spermatocele, 227
Sphincter of Oddi. *See* Ampulla of Vater
        (sphincter of Oddi)
Splanchnic arteries
    aneurysm of, 285
Spleen, 239–252
    anatomic relationships and associated
        pathology, 252
    anatomy of, 239
        regional, 240
    anomalies of
        abscess, 248
        AIDS-related, 248
        congenital, 245
        cysts, 246
        granulomatous disease, 247
        infarct, 248
        infection/inflammatory process, 248
        neoplasms, 250
        pseudocysts, 246
        rupture, 251
        splenomegaly, 251
    differential sonographic appearances of,
        252
    echogenicity of, 240
    lab tests and, 243–244
    metastases to, 250
    physiology of, 242
    structure of, 239
    technical factors and, 252
    trauma to, 251
    US appearance of, 240
    vasculature of, 242
    wandering, 245
Splenic flexure, 57
Splenic hump (dromedary hump), 114
Splenic vein, 274
    flow characteristics in, 281
    pancreas and, 172
Splenomegaly, 251
    AIDS-related, 248
Squamous cell carcinoma
    of bladder, 260
    of breast
        invasive ductal, 28
Stensen's duct. *See* Parotid (Stensen's) duct
Stereotactic biopsy
    of breast
        sonography in, 34
Sternocleidomastoid muscle, 151, 155
Stomach
    anatomy of
        sonographic, 59
    antrum of, 172
    metastases to, 70

size and location of, 58
structure of, 56
ultrasound technique for, 74
Strap muscles, 155
Subclavian artery, 272, 273
Subclavian steal phenomenon
in vertebral artery abnormality, 296
Subclavian vein, 273
Subhepatic space, 186, 187, 189
Sublingual ducts, 151
Sublingual glands, 151
Submandibular gland, 151
Submandibular (Wharton's) duct, 151
Subphrenic space, 186, 187, 189, 191
Superior mesenteric artery
pancreas and, 172
Superior mesenteric vein
pancreas and, 172
Superior vena cava, 272
Suprarenal vein, 3
Suspensory ligaments, 23

T

TCC. See Transitional cell carcinoma
(TCC)
Teratoma(s)
retroperitoneal, 201
testicular, 235
Testes/testicles
anatomy of
normal, 219–220, 221
anomalies of
calcification, 225
cryptorchidism, 225
cysts, 227–228
fracture, 233
germ cell tumors, 234–235
gonadal stromal tumors, 235
hematoma, 233
metastases to, 235
neoplasms, 231
orchitis, 230–231
torsion, 232
varicocele, 236
Doppler US appearance of, 221–222
lab tests and, 224
lymphatic drainage of, 223
metastasis to, 235
pathology of, 237
physiology of, 224
structure of, 219
technical factors and, 238
vasculature of, 223
Testosterone test, 224
Thoracic arteries, 26
Thrombocytopenia, 244
Thrombocytosis, 244
Thrombosis
deep venous
sonographic findings, 295
renal vein, 292
venous, 293, 294
Thrombus
fresh/acute, 295
Thyroglossal duct
cyst on, 162
Thyroglossal duct cyst, 162
Thyroid arteries, 272

Thyroid gland
anatomy of
normal, 156
regional, 155
anomalies of
adenocarcinoma, 163
adenomas, 162
carcinoma, 163
cysts, 162
goiters, 164
thyroiditis, 166
echogenicity of, 156
hormones of, 159
lab tests and, 160
nodules on
benign and malignant, 167
cold and hot, 167
percutaneous biopsy of, 168
physiology of, 159
radionuclide scans of, 167
structure of, 155
technical factors and, 168
US appearance of, 156, 157
vasculature of, 158
Thyroiditis, 165, 166
subacute and acute, 165, 166
Thyroid stimulating hormone (TSH) level, 160
Thyroxine (T_4), 160
Trachea, 155
Transitional cell carcinoma (TCC)
of bladder, 260
Transrectal ultrasound scanning (TRUS)
biopsy with, 218
indications for, 218
patient preparation for, 218
technical factors for, 218
Transverse colon, 57
Triangular ligaments, 187, 188, 189
Triiodothyronine (T_3), 160
TRUS. See Transrectal ultrasound scanning
(TRUS)
Trypsin, 175
TSC-hepatosplenic scan, 244
Tubular carcinoma
of breast, 28
Tubules
renal, 81
Tunica albuginea cysts, 227
Turbulence
of arterial blood
on Doppler ultrasound, 301
Typhlitis (neutropenic colitis/ileocecal
syndrome), 72

U

Ulcerative colitis, 67
comparison with Crohn's disease, 68
Ulnar artery, 273
Ulnar vein, 273
Uncinate process, of pancreas, 170
Upper extremities
vascular system of, 273
venous flow characteristics in, 280
Urachal cysts, 205
Urachal sinus
cysts and fistulas of, 205
Urachus
anatomy of, 253

Ureter
in hydronephrosis, 93
Ureterocele, 265
Ureters
anatomy of, 253
normal, 256
anomalies of
congenital, 263
hydroureter, 264
megaloureter, 264
ureterocele, 265
physiology of, 256
size and shape of, 256
technical factors and, 265
US appearance of, 255
Urethra
anatomy of, 253
in hydronephrosis, 93
prostatic, 207
Urine urea nitrogen, 82
Urine volume, 82
Urinoma, 100, 101
in perinephric space, 198

V

Valves
anatomy of, 267
Varicocele
peritesticular, 228
Vascular system. See also Artery(ies);
Vein(s)
anatomy of
normal, 267–268
anomalies of, 282–296. See also
Aneurysm(s)
anastomoses, 289
aneurysms, 282–285
aortic dissection, 286
aortic grafts, 286
arterial grafts, 286
arteriosclerosis, 287
arteriovenous shunts, 289
atheroma, 287
atheromatous plaque, 287
atherosclerosis, 287
Baker's cyst, 290
carotid artery disease, 288
fistulae, 289
intravenous catheter filters, 290
intravenous catheter tumors, 291
peripheral arterial disease, 288
renal vascular disease, 292
vein thrombosis, 293–295
vertebral artery abnormality, 296
arterial blood flow
measurement of, 304
Doppler ultrasound of, 298–303, 305. See
also Doppler ultrasound
gray-scale imaging of, 297
of head and neck, 272
of lower extremities, 270–271
of neck, 272
of parathyroid glands, 158
physiology of
arterial vessel Doppler waveforms in,
277
circulation in, 276

Vascular system, physiology of (*continued*)
   head and neck flow characteristics of,
     277–278
  physiology of circulation in
    abdominal flow characteristics of, 279
    blood flow regulation and, 276
    blood pressure and, 276
    heart rate and, 276
  of retroperitoneum, 274–275
  of salivary glands, 152
  of thyroid gland, 158
  of upper extremities, 273
  US appearance of, 269
  US techniques for
    abnormal caliber and position, 307
    aorta, 306
    carotid, 309
    extremities, 308
    intravenous catheter, 307
  venous valves in
    anatomy of, 268
Veins(s)
  abdominal
    flow characteristics in, 280

adrenal gland, 3
anatomy of
  normal, 267
breast, 26
Doppler ultrasound evaluation of, 302
of head and neck, 272
hepatic, 123, 125, 127
of lower extremities, 270–271
  deep, 270, 271
  superficial, 270, 271
mammary, 26
pancreatic, 175
portal, 126
renal, 79, 80
retroperitoneal, 274
of salivary glands, 152
of upper extremities, 273
  deep, 273
  superficial, 273
US appearance of, 269, 280
  Doppler, 303
Venous thrombosis, 106, 293, 294
Venous valve
  function of, 268

Venules
  anatomy of, 267
Vertebral arteries, 272
  abnormality of, 296
  flow characteristics of: arterial waveform,
    278

W
Warthin's tumor (adenolymphoma), 153
Wes triad, 40
Wharton's duct. *See* Submandibular
    (Wharton's) duct
White blood cells
  in urine, 82
White blood cell (WBC) count
  gallbladder and, 41
White blood cell (WBC) differential, 244
White blood count (WBC)
  spleen and, 243
Wilms' tumor. *See* Nephroblastoma (Wilms'
    tumor)

CPSIA information can be obtained at www.ICGtesting.com
Printed in the USA
LVOW11s0511180714

394812LV00052BA/6/P